Designing and Using
Assistive Technology

This book is printed on recycled paper. ♲

Designing and Using Assistive Technology

The Human Perspective

edited by

David B. Gray, Ph.D.
Washington University School of Medicine
St. Louis, Missouri

Louis A. Quatrano, Ph.D.
National Center for Medical Rehabilitation Research
National Institute of Child Health and Human Development
National Institutes of Health
Bethesda, Maryland

and

Morton L. Lieberman, Ph.D.
Sandia National Laboratories
Albuquerque, New Mexico

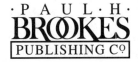

·P·A·U·L·H·
BROOKES
PUBLISHING CO.

Baltimore • London • Toronto • Sydney

Paul H. Brookes Publishing Co.
Post Office Box 10624
Baltimore, Maryland 21285-0624

Typeset by Brushwood Graphics, Inc., Baltimore, Maryland.
Manufactured in the United States of America by
The Maple Press Company, York, Pennsylvania.

This work may be reproduced in whole or in part for the official use of the
U.S. government or any authorized agency thereof.

The conference on which this book is based was sponsored by the National
Institute of Child Health and Human Development of the U.S. Public Health
Service.

The case study appearing on page 240 represents an actual person and actual
circumstances and is published with the individual's written permission. The
other case studies described in this book are composites based on the authors'
experiences; these case studies do not represent the lives or experiences of
specific individuals, and no implications should be inferred.

Library of Congress Cataloging-in-Publication Data

Designing and using assistive technology: The human perspective /
  edited by David B. Gray, Louis A. Quatrano, and Morton L. Lieberman.
    p.   cm.
    ISBN 1-55766-314-9
    1. Self-help devices for the disabled.   I. Gray, David B.   II. Quatrano,
Louis A.   III. Lieberman, M.L. (Morton L.)
RM698.D47   1998
617'.03—DC21   97-17087
                                                                     CIP

British Cataloguing in Publication data are available from the British Library.

Contents

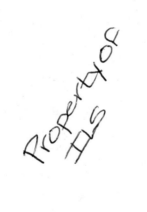

About the Editors

David B. Gray, Ph.D., Professor and Associate Director of Research, Program in Occupational Therapy, Washington University School of Medicine, 4444 Forest Park, St. Louis, Missouri 63108-2292. Dr. Gray is on the boards of Paraquad, an independent living center located in St. Louis; the World Institute on Disability in Oakland, California; and the National Advisory Board for the Functional Electrical Stimulation Center in Cleveland, Ohio. He is a member of the North American Collaborating Center for the revision of the *International Classification of Impairments, Disabilities, and Handicaps* (ICIDH). With the support of the Centers for Disease Control and Prevention (CDC) and the National Center for Health Statistics, he is conducting studies of the influence of environmental access on the social participation of individuals with disabilities. He serves on a National Institutes of Health (NIH) special emphasis peer review panel for Small Business Innovative Research grant applications and on the peer review board of the Paralyzed Veterans of America's Spinal Cord Injury Research Foundation.

Louis A. Quatrano, Ph.D., Director, Behavioral Sciences and Rehabilitation Engineering Program, National Center for Medical Rehabilitation Research, National Institute of Child Health and Human Development, National Institutes of Health, Executive Building, Room 2A03, 6100 Executive Boulevard MSC 7510, Bethesda, Maryland 20892-7510. Dr. Quatrano has worked at NIH since 1978. He has participated in research review and program development at NIH. He was involved in reviewing and assigning Small Business Innovative Research grant applications at NIH in the area of assistive technology. He is currently the National Center for Medical Rehabilitation Research (NCMRR) contact person for the Small Business Innovative Research program. The Applied Rehabilitation Medicine Research Branch of the NCMRR was instrumental in organizing the conference on behavioral adaptation to assistive technology and continues to support research in this important area.

Morton L. Lieberman, Ph.D., Distinguished Member of Technical Staff, Sandia National Laboratories, MS0309, Post Office Box 5800, Albuquerque, New Mexico 87185-0309. Dr. Lieberman is a chemist by training and has spent much of his career conducting materials research in fields including high-temperature chemistry, thin films, carbon composites, chemical vapor deposition, and energetic materials. He has performed project management and program development roles in defense areas including heatshield development, energetic material devices, and vehicular countermine systems, as well as in nondefense areas including coal liquefaction and assistive technology for people with disabilities. His most recent efforts have been in the development of an international project on lower-limb prosthetics.

About the Contributors

Adam Abdelhamied, Ph.D., ITT Corporation, 100 Kingsland Road, Clifton, New Jersey 07014-1993. Dr. Abdelhamied was a research associate fellow at the Center for Assistive Technology, State University of New York at Buffalo, at the time Chapter 14 was written.

Peter W. Axelson, M.S.M.E., Director of Research and Development, Beneficial Designs, Inc., 5858 Empire Grade, Santa Cruz, California 95060. Mr. Axelson is a rehabilitation engineer who sustained a spinal cord injury in a 1975 climbing accident while in the U.S. Air Force Academy. He continued his education at Stanford University, where he began applying engineering and design principles to overcome daily living hurdles faced by people with disabilities. In 1981, he founded Beneficial Designs, Inc., an engineering design firm dedicated to designing, developing, and testing assistive technologies. His accomplishments include developing the first chairlift-compatible mono-ski with a shock absorber, working to establish wheelchair-testing standards, developing seating systems for wheelchairs, and creating a system to assess outdoor hiking trails that will improve access to these trails for people of all levels of ability.

Carolyn M. Baum, Ph.D., OTR/C, FAOTA, Elias Michael Director, Program in Occupational Therapy, Assistant Professor, Occupational Therapy and Neurology, Washington University School of Medicine, 4444 Forest Park, St. Louis, Missouri 63108-2292. Dr. Baum studies the relationship of impairment in people with chronic neurological diseases and their performance in their daily lives and in the lives of their families, with the goal of designing and testing educational interventions and developing community-based care. She has held major policy positions as the President of the American Occupational Therapy Association; as President of the American Occupational Therapy Certification Board; and as a member of the Advisory Committee for the National Center for Medical Rehabilitation Research at the National Institutes of Health, the Rehabilitation and Engineering Committee at the Institute of Medicine, and the Cognitive Rehabilitation Committee of the McDonnell Foundation.

Nancy A. Brooks, M.A., Associate Professor, Department of Sociology, Wichita State University, 1845 North Fairmount Avenue, Wichita, Kansas 67260-0025. Ms. Brooks is an associate professor of sociology at Wichita State University in Kansas, where she specializes in the sociology of medicine and the sociology of technology. She has written numerous professional articles, is co-editor of the book *Women and Disability: The Double Handicap* (Transaction Press, 1985), and is co-author of the monograph *Framing the Artist: A Social Portrait of Mid-American Artists* (University Press of America, 1982). For many years, she has been actively involved in research on consumers' responses to assistive technology (AT). Ms. Brooks has had multiple sclerosis since 1967.

Rory A. Cooper, Ph.D., Chairman and Associate Professor, Departments of Rehabilitation Science and Technology, Bioengineering, and Mechanical Engineering, University of Pittsburgh, 7180 Highland Drive, Pittsburgh, Pennsylvania 15206. Dr. Cooper received bachelor's and master's degrees in electrical engineering from California Polytechnic State University, San Luis Obispo, in 1985 and 1986, respectively. He received a doctoral degree in electrical and computer engineering with a concentration in biomedical engineering from the University of California at Santa Barbara in 1989. He is an associate professor in the Departments of Rehabilitation Science and Technology, Bioengineering, and Mechanical Engineering at the University of Pittsburgh. He is also an associate professor in the Division of Physical Medicine and Rehabilitation within the Department of Orthopaedic Surgery at the University of Pittsburgh Medical Center. Dr. Cooper is also Director of the University of Pittsburgh/Veterans Affairs Medical Center (VAMC) Human Engineering Research Laboratories, which is a joint effort between the Highland Drive VAMC, the University of Pittsburgh, and the University of Pittsburgh Medical Center. Dr. Cooper was a bronze medalist in the Paralympic Games, Seoul, Republic of Korea, and was on the steering committee for the 1996 Paralympic Scientific Congress in Atlanta, Georgia.

George A. Covington, J.D., Advocate, Post Office Box 376, Alpine, Texas 79831. Mr. Covington is the former Special Assistant for Disability Policy (1989–1993) to the Vice President of the United States. He was the first person to serve full time as a White House aide on disability issues. Prior to joining the Vice President's staff, he worked on disability projects on the staff of Jim Wright, former Speaker of the U.S. House of Representatives. He is an attorney and former journalism professor whose career has spanned the fields of law, journalism, education, government, and disability civil rights. Since 1981, Mr. Covington has worked to change the mass media's portrayal of people with disabilities.

Jean Crosetto Deitz, Ph.D., OTR, Professor and Graduate Program Coordinator, Department of Rehabilitation Medicine, University of Washington, 1959 Pacific Street, N.E., Seattle, Washington 98195. Dr. Deitz is a fellow of the American Occupational Therapy Association, a member of the American Occupational Therapy Foundation Academy of Research, and a member of the National Advisory Board for Medical Rehabilitation Research. She has published extensively in the occupational therapy literature, with a focus on pediatrics, measurement issues, and evaluation of AT.

Patrick Fougeyrollas, Ph.D., Scientific Director, Québec City Rehabilitation Institute, Associate Professor, Department of Rehabilitation, Faculty of Medicine, Laval University, President, Québec Committee on the ICIDH, Canadian Society for the ICIDH, 525 Wilfried Hamel Boulevard East, Québec City, Québec G1M 2S8, CANADA. Dr. Fougeyrollas is Associate Professor in the Department of Occupational Therapy and Director of Professional and Scientific

Services at the University Institute of Rehabilitation and Social Integration Centre, Laval University. He has been President of the Canadian Society on the Classification of Impairments, Disabilities, and Handicaps since 1989 and is an active member of committees on classification of disablement for the World Health Organization, the United Nations, and the Council of Europe. Dr. Fougeyrollas is a founding member of the Research Network of Social Participation. His research focuses on the analysis of the interactive process between the individual and the environment in the realm of social participation of people with disabilities.

Laura N. Gitlin, Ph.D., Professor, Department of Occupational Therapy, Director, Community and Homecare Research Division, College of Health Professions, Thomas Jefferson University, 130 South 9th Street, Suite 2200, Philadelphia, Pennsylvania 19107. Dr. Gitlin is a sociologist and professor in the Department of Occupational Therapy at Thomas Jefferson University. She is also the Director of Research in the Center for Collaborative Research and directs a new initiative, the Community and Homecare Research Division. Dr. Gitlin is a funded researcher in the area of AT device use by older adults and the development and testing of environmental modification interventions to improve the daily functioning and quality of life of older adults and family caregivers.

Kenton R. Kaufman, Ph.D., P.E., Co-director, Biomechanics Laboratory, Associate Professor of Bioengineering, Mayo Clinic, Guggenheim Building 128, 200 First Street, S.W., Rochester, Minnesota 55905. Dr. Kaufman is a senior associate consultant in the Department of Orthopedics and Co-director of the Biomechanics Laboratory at the Mayo Clinic. His research focuses on the biomechanics of human movement. He is engaged in projects aimed at improving the mobility of individuals with disabilities. He also conducts research to decrease overuse injuries in military recruits. In addition, Dr. Kaufman has served the biomechanics community in several ways. He has served on National Institutes of Health Special Review Committees, was on the Working Group on Injury Prevention of the Armed Forces Epidemiological Board, and served as Chairman of the Ad-Hoc Committee for Accreditation and Standardization of the North American Society for Gait and Clinical Movement Analysis.

Rosanne Kermoian, Ph.D., Assistant Director, Institute of Human Development, University of California, Berkeley, 1203 Tolman Hall, Berkeley, California 94720. Dr. Kermoian is a developmental psychologist who has spent her career investigating the role of motor activity on psychological functioning. She is Assistant Director of the Institute of Human Development at the University of California, Berkeley, and is affiliated with the Rehabilitation Engineering Center at the Children's Hospital at Stanford University. Her research program focuses on the effects of locomotor experience on infant development and the effects of mobility devices on the development of children with physical disabilities.

P. Hunter Peckham, Ph.D., Professor of Biomedical Engineering, Case Western Reserve University, Department of Veterans Affairs, MetroHealth Medical Center, 2500 MetroHealth Drive, Cleveland, Ohio 44109. The focus of Dr. Peckham's professional career has been on the development of neural prostheses to aid people with disabilities. His initial research was on studying the fundamental physiological aspects of motor control by electrical stimulation, which resulted in the development of muscle-conditioning procedures and neural excitation techniques that are widely employed. His present focus is on clinical applications to restore functional movement and control to the upper extremities in individuals with spinal cord injuries. He has pioneered the development of neural prosthetic systems for control of the hand and arm, including implantable stimulators and sensors, and has successfully introduced this system into clinical usage. Dr. Peckham also has developed procedures that analyze movement restored through hand surgery and has provided techniques for measuring muscle properties intraoperatively that are incorporated into hand surgery education. He presently leads a multi-institutional study with five North American centers to evaluate the efficacy of the hand neuroprosthesis.

Marcia J. Scherer, Ph.D., M.P.H., Senior Research Associate, Director of Consumer Evaluations, Rehabilitation Engineering Research, Center on Technology Evaluation and Transfer, Senior Research Associate, Center for Assistive Technology, State University of New York at Buffalo, 515 Kimball Tower, Buffalo, New York 14214. Prior to her current appointment, Dr. Scherer was on the faculty of the National Technical Institute for the Deaf, Rochester Institute of Technology, for 10 years. Dr. Scherer has authored books and research articles on technology use, quality of life, and psychosocial influences on rehabilitation outcome. She is active in many professional organizations, including serving on the Board of Directors of the Rehabilitation Engineering and Assistive Technology Society of North America.

Jean Cole Spencer, Ph.D., OTR, Professor and Doctoral Program Coordinator, School of Occupational Therapy, Texas Woman's University, 1130 M.D. Anderson Boulevard, Houston, Texas 77030-2897. Dr. Spencer is Professor and Doctoral Program Coordinator in the School of Occupational Therapy at Texas Woman's University, Houston Center. Her doctorate in cultural anthropology is from Rice University, and her master's degree in occupational therapy is from Texas Woman's University. Dr. Spencer's research interests and publications deal with community participation of older adults and people with disabilities, cultural differences in adaptation to disability, and use of qualitative methods in clinical practice and research.

Stephen Sprigle, Ph.D., Research Director, Research Center for Rehabilitation Technology, Helen Hayes Hospital, Route 9W, West Haverstraw, New York 10993. Dr. Sprigle has worked as both a researcher and a service provider in rehabilitation engineering and AT. His research interests include wheelchair seating, posture, and pressure ulcer prevention. Clinical efforts have focused on addressing the seating, mobility, and AT needs of wheelchair users. In addition, Dr. Sprigle has designed and evaluated both commercial and customized assistive devices.

Steven A. Stiens, M.D., Spinal Cord Injury Staff Physician, Spinal Cord Injury Unit, Veterans Administration Puget Sound Health Care System, Assistant Professor, Department of Rehabilitation Medicine, University of Washington School of Medicine, BB 919 Health Sciences Building, 1660 South Columbian Way, Seattle, Washington 98108-1597. Dr. Stiens is an assistant professor of rehabilitation medicine at the University of Washington School of Medicine, where he practices spinal cord medicine within the Veterans Administration Puget Sound Health Care System. Prior to this appointment, Dr. Stiens was a member of the rehabilitation faculty of The Johns Hopkins University, Baltimore, Maryland, and acted as Director of the Rehabilitation Consultation Service at The Johns Hopkins Hospital in Baltimore. His interest in the interaction between the person and architecture led to a collaboration with his interior designer brother Doug on the project of redesigning a rowhome for a family with a paraplegic father; work on the development of Future Home, an adaptively designed living environment for people with disabilities; and educational work with Abilities Occupational Therapy Services, a firm that provides occupational therapy, medical, and architectural services to adaptively redesign environments for people with disabilities.

Margaret G. Stineman, M.D., Associate Professor, Department of Rehabilitation Medicine, University of Pennsylvania Medical Center, 101 Ralston-Penn Center, 3615 Chestnut Street, Philadelphia, Pennsylvania 19104-2676. Dr. Stineman, a former Robert Wood Johnson Foundation Clinical Scholar as well as a former Hartford Foundation Scholar in geriatric research, is Associate Professor of Rehabilitation Medicine, a Senior Fellow with the Leonard Davis Institute of Health Economics, a Fellow of the Institute on Aging, and an Associate Scholar in the Clinical Epidemiology Unit of the Center for Clinical Epidemiology and Biostatistics at the University of Pennsylvania. Dr. Stineman is interested in discovering ways in which technology can be applied to enhance the physical and social freedom of people with disabilities. This goal dictates the need to measure how adaptive technology affects how people perceive quality of life and function. She is the Principal Investigator on a project developing a prognostic staging system designed to establish the likelihood that people with disabilities can recover to specific levels of function. A major objective of the project is to reconcile the independent living and medical models of disability. She was also the Principal Investigator on the project that developed the Functional Independence Measure–Function Related Group (FIM–FRG) patient classification systems, which are being considered by the Health Care Financing Administration for possible incorporation into a new Medicare prospective payment system for medical rehabilitation.

Christine Wright-Ott, MPA, OTR, Occupational Therapist, Rehabilitation Engineering Center, Lucille Packard Children's Hospital, 725 Welch Road, Palo Alto, California 95014. Ms. Wright-Ott is an occupational therapist who has training in neurodevelopmental and infant treatment techniques. She is a member of a rehabilitation engineering team that specializes in providing AT assessments and intervention for children with physical disabilities as well as research and product development. She has authored several publications on assisted mobility for children with disabilities and is coauthor of the book *From Toys to Computers: Access for the Physically Challenged Child* (Wright & Nomura, 1991). She has established an early intervention mobility camp program for children with disabilities and has provided numerous presentations on mobility devices and techniques throughout the United States.

Foreword

As the assistive technology (AT) field has matured, it has been possible to move beyond the design of devices to the integration of these devices into total AT systems. The concept of an AT system includes the user (sometimes called the *consumer*), a task or activity to be done, and a context or environment in which the system functions. This is a much broader perspective, and it takes into consideration the use of assistive technologies and what makes that use practical and efficient as well as the process of matching the AT device or system to the needs of the user. In the latter case, emphasis has shifted from merely matching a device to a user's skills and needs to considering the entire system and how it can be matched with the user. This broadened perspective leads to consideration of previously understudied aspects such as cultural and age differences and how those affect AT systems. As the concern for effective use has developed, so has the recognition that it is not adequate to merely match technical specifications to the user's needs and skills. Therefore, strategies and training must be developed to achieve optimal performance in the use of the AT device. These must be developed in the community as well as in the clinic.

In this book, the editors have drawn together a set of chapters that follow these trends in AT development and delivery. There are common themes throughout the chapters. The most fundamental of these themes is that there must be a match established among users' needs and skills, the assistive technologies of choice, and the contexts in which the devices will be used. This book contains many examples of this holistic approach to AT applications. Within this common theme, the book features a wide variety of perspectives, approaches, models, and frameworks. This combination of a common theme and a variety of approaches to its implementation will be of value to researchers, AT practitioners, AT suppliers, and consumers of assistive technologies.

The book also features a variety of professional disciplinary perspectives. These include medical, engineering, rehabilitation, and educational perspectives as well as a consumer focus. This diversity of perspectives is evident in discussions relating to the book's common theme, and it adds to the richness of the text. The reader can easily discern the basic differences among these professional approaches by reading different chapters. These approaches include the classical medical model of professionally directed intervention and the more current consumer-focused model of equal participation by the consumer in decision making regarding assistive technologies. The strengths and weaknesses of each approach can be appreciated by studying this book.

From theoretical models and frameworks to evaluation of outcomes of AT use, this book offers a wealth of information to the reader. The many discussions of example projects, research studies, assessment strategies, descriptions of engineering development of assistive technologies, and consumer use and evaluation studies add an important level of detail that will help readers to apply the information to their own work.

The chapters included in this book accurately reflect an emerging awareness of the importance of viewing the AT system as a whole, rather than concentrating on just the assistive device. Through discussion of the role of the user (or consumer) and the nature of the tasks (or activities) to be performed and through consideration of the physical and social contexts in which the system is used, the contributors provide a broad view of the state of the art in AT applications. The contributors also recognize the importance of including AT as an integrated part of the system. The inclusion of both hard technologies (e.g., computers, wheelchairs, mouthsticks, other tangible products) and soft technologies (e.g., strategies of use, decision making, training and development of expert users) is representative of current thinking in the AT field.

This book is of benefit to a very diverse audience. The contributors have addressed the most pressing problems in AT development and application, and they have done so from a variety of perspectives. This adds value for the reader. The compilation of chapters in this book is highly recommended reading for anyone interested in assistive technologies and their application.

Albert M. Cook, Ph.D.
Professor and Dean
Faculty of Rehabilitation Medicine
University of Alberta
Edmonton, Alberta, Canada

Preface

This book describes the design and use of assistive technology (AT) by and for people with physical disabilities. These chapters are modified versions of some of the papers presented at a conference entitled "Behavioral Adaptation to the Use of Assistive Technology: Enhancing Human Movement in the 21st Century for People with Disabilities." This conference was sponsored by several organizations, including the National Center for Medical Rehabilitation Research (NCMRR) of the National Institute of Child Health and Human Development at the National Institutes of Health, Paralyzed Veterans of America, The Johns Hopkins University, Kennedy Krieger Institute, and Evan Kemp Associates. The conference was held in Baltimore, Maryland, April 7–9, 1995.

The importance of incorporating AT and environmental modifications into the scope of rehabilitation treatments for people with disabilities cannot be overemphasized. Unfortunately, classification systems used to plan for the lives of people with disabilities are not structured to count the types and numbers of AT devices needed for people with disabilities to maximize their residual function, restore lost functions, or allow old functions to be performed in new ways. Discovering what assistive technologies exist is a difficult task for both the consumer and the professional. As of 1998, matching the best AT device with each individual's needs is more of an art than a science. Many errors are made, resulting in people with disabilities discarding anywhere from 20% to more than 50% of the AT devices provided to them. Discarding or not using AT devices may be the result of a variety of factors. Some people with disabilities feel stigmatized if seen using AT devices. The person's sense of self and the role of AT in her or his life are the key considerations in the equation used to match an AT device with personal needs. Others find that the AT device does not improve their performance. The functions that each person perceives as essential need to be addressed. Single functions that rarely are needed by people with disabilities are likely candidates for low AT use or discard of AT devices. No science of AT prescription is well developed. Health professionals who have responsibilities for requesting payment for AT from third-party payers or in recommending purchase through private funds need to base their recommendations on firmer foundations. Often the improved performance is not sufficient enough to justify the trouble of taking the equipment from place to place or the equipment that worked so well in the showroom or hospital does not fit the person's home, work, transportation, or recreation environments.

In many cases, the root of the disuse problem lies in the design of the equipment. Equipment designed for adults to assist in their work environments has little applicability and use for infants, children, adolescents, and older adults. Chances for acceptance and use by people with disabilities seem to increase when the consumers of AT are consulted at each step of designing, developing, manufacturing, and marketing the product. AT devices designed for multiple uses that appear attractive and may be purchased by large numbers of individuals are the type of equipment that can be supported from idea to marketplace through the usual capitalist system. However, many products that provide a small number of people with severe disabilities significant improvements in essential life functions need to have government funds provided to stimulate development, production, distribution, and education in order for scientists, therapists, and consumers to cooperatively develop a viable project. Protection against product liability, "orphan" products programs (modeled on government and foundation support for orphan drugs), tax code changes, and acceptance of justifications broader than medical necessity for purchase by third-party payers all are factors that need to be addressed. The various chapters in this book provide insights into some parts of the solution to the large, complex puzzle of design, development, provision, and use of AT by and for people with disabilities. The chapters are divided into five sections, an outline of which follows.

SECTION I: CONCEPTS, CLASSIFICATIONS, AND CATEGORIES OF DISABLING CONDITIONS AND ASSISTIVE TECHNOLOGIES

In Chapter 1, Nancy A. Brooks develops the notion that AT needs to be considered within the person's construct of his or her meaning of disability. The person's acceptance or rejection of AT is influenced by his or her culture's understanding of disability. These socially accepted views are based on a variety of models, including medical, economic, political, and minority group models. Although each model has contributed to cultural understanding, these models have been inappropriately extended to cover phenomena beyond the models' conceptual boundaries. When, for example, medical diagnoses define the living arrangements (e.g., nursing homes, group homes) and employment opportunities (e.g., sheltered work, not capable of substantial gainful employment), models may become constricting to personal freedom to choose life activities. The models used by societies to communicate individual needs may set limits on what is considered necessary AT. Although eyeglasses are a commonly used aid for those with visual impairments requiring little justification for third-party purchase, AT that provides mobility, enhanced speech reception, or improved cognitive functions requires extensive justification for consideration prior to purchase. In each of these examples, AT may be an essential component for enhancing the lives of people with disabilities. However, if the models that society uses to communicate the needs of those with disabilities do not reflect the importance of different types of AT, then people with disabilities will be prohibited from living fulfilling lives. AT stands at the critical interface between human biological capacity and human imagination to construct devices to enhance function. Existing models of disability have not captured the meaning of AT to the lives of people with disabilities. Nevertheless, the challenge for rehabilitation professionals is to incorporate AT in their existing conceptual models of disability and provide their clients current information on AT that meets their specific needs. For people with disabilities, learning how to select and use AT is becoming increasingly important for improving the number and quality of life choices.

The second chapter of this volume, by Patrick Fougeyrollas and David B. Gray, places the development and use of AT in the broader context of classification of people with disabilities, their capacity and incapacity (i.e., impairments), ability and inability (i.e., disabilities), and social advantage and disadvantage (i.e., handicaps) related to their impairments. Classifying people and their environments may seem somewhat tangential to a book on AT. However, the market forces influencing purchase and development of AT are driven by third-party payers, including local, state, and national governments as well as health insurance, managed care, and charitable organizations. To a large degree, these entities base their decisions to purchase AT on the numbers of people in need. Thus, some measure of the severity of need for AT is needed. In addition, a justification for purchasing AT must be put in the context of how well the AT assists in maintaining health and returning the person to a productive life. To describe people with disabilities and their need for AT is not an easy task. Chapter

2 provides a framework for understanding the importance of AT in the lives of people with disabilities in the environmental context in which they live. The scope of what is considered AT ranges from devices used by individuals in their daily activities to accessible cities. The authors propose the use of an interactive classification system that has as a focus social participation rather than the static concepts often attributed to impairment and disability. This system makes it clear that the use of AT has societal significance well beyond outcome studies that focus on an individual's capacity to perform a limited number of actions within the controlled environment of a rehabilitation facility.

In Chapter 3, Steven A. Stiens addresses the importance of integrating the use of mobility devices into the lives of people with mobility impairments in the context of their self-concepts. Adjustment can be difficult for those who are injured or have a condition that impairs their mobility after they have developed skills, expectations, and relationships. Rehabilitation goals and programs are described that address issues of people adapting to reduced mobility. Assistive technologies are considered different interfaces with the newly injured person's environment. Assessing the person's history, current capabilities, and plans for future activities can give the rehabilitation team useful insights as they develop suggestions for assistive technologies. The aesthetic and functional aspects of the AT device are of primary consideration in making choices that will result in the person returning to effective interactive relationships with his or her environment.

Chapter 4, by Margaret G. Stineman, uses the *International Classification of Impairments, Diseases, and Handicaps* (ICIDH) as a framework for assessing the mode of action of AT and the difference that AT can make in the outcome of rehabilitation. To assess the need for AT, she details two generic health status measures (the Sickness Impact Profile and the Functional Independence Measure). She presents recommendations for selecting instruments for outcome measurement through the use of device-specific indicators. Finally, a method for measuring subjective quality of daily life (the Cantril Self-Anchoring Striving Scale) is suggested. A three-stage measurement strategy is described. Initially, information from generic instruments is attained from general descriptors of the AT. Next, these findings are supplemented with a battery of technical questions specific to the device. Finally, the specific match of person and device is assessed through an open-ended approach to the personal interpretation of outcome. This approach to fitting personal needs with the characteristics of the AT to enhance function is an important step forward in developing justifications for the purchase of AT. This framework allows payers to extend the rationale for AT purchase beyond a specific health-related problem to the needs of the whole person.

SECTION II: WHEN ASSISTIVE
TECHNOLOGY IS USED AND WHEN IT IS NOT

In Chapter 5, George A. Covington provides an entertaining and insightful story of his response to choosing to use a white cane after many years of functioning without one. His description of the stigmatizing effects of using AT should provide a cautionary note to those who design, prescribe, and advocate the use of AT for solving problems associated with disabilities. Clearly, the use of AT involves a complex set of positive and negative social factors. The constricting influence of models described in Chapter 1 is well illustrated in Covington's experience of being forced to wear eyeglasses in grade school to satisfy the expectations of school authorities, in spite of the fact that they provided no improved vision. Later in his life, he decided to use a cane to guide his mobility. The avoidance responses of people to Covington's use of a cane provide a clear illustration of our society's acceptance of one type of AT (i.e., eyeglasses) and less tolerance of another (i.e., a white cane). For the individual who uses AT, the stigma associated with the device must be factored into designing, developing, marketing, and using the device. When a device that has multiple purposes can be built and can be used by many people with and without disabilities, the stigma associated with the AT can be minimized. He encourages consideration of common characteristics of all people rather than focusing solely on their differences; making people with disabilities neither heroes nor objects of pity allows them to be considered as individuals rather than as members of a separate class of people. Covington advocates using principles of universal design as a framework for the professions involved in designing equipment and environments for people with disabilities.

The meaning of a device to the individual in his or her life may be more important than technical descriptions of the device in improving our understanding of which AT will or will not be incorporated into the lives of people with disabilities. This theme is developed by Jean Cole Spencer in Chapter 6. She postulates three fundamentals of understanding the role of AT in the lives of people with disabilities. AT are tools that are given meaning by the intentions that individuals have for their use, both personally and in the context of their culture. Adapting to the use of AT requires building new skills, developing positive emotional response to the device, modifying one's self-perception in AT use, and incorporating the use of AT into daily activities. Changes in life circumstances require a flexible, individualized approach to considering the selection of AT. Using an approach to the allocation and distribution of AT on the basis of generic qualities of the devices may appear attractive, but it runs the risk of providing the wrong AT at the wrong time to the wrong people. Establishing standards and critical pathways for provision of AT may not be the correct approach. Assessing the individual's needs and willingness to accept AT may be difficult, but the individual's use of an AT device may prove to be the best and most cost-effective way of dealing with disability if the generic approach provides AT that is not used.

In Chapter 7, Marcia J. Scherer warns against assuming that AT will be the solution for people with disabilities who seek to live typical lives. In many cases, the provision of AT may lead the user and his or her community to believe that the problems associated with the disability are solved. The person with a disability who finds that the AT does not solve all of his or her problems may abandon the AT. Those who live and work with the person with a disability may consider abandonment of AT a failure attributable solely to the user. The reality is that the diversity of disabilities, coping strategies, willingness to use AT, skill in use of AT, varieties of AT, and the characteristics of the milieu in which the AT is used all have significant effects on whether AT is optimally used, partially used, or abandoned. Involving the user in AT selection, introducing the AT at the best time during rehabilitation, targeting relevant functional outcomes, and considering the person's past coping strategies are important factors in determining whether AT will be used. Continued use of AT after purchase is based on the consumer's expectations for effectiveness, reliability, durability, comfort, and ease of use. Scherer points out the alarmingly high abandonment and underuse of AT. Her recommendations for matching the person to the most appropriate AT include determining current and desirable milieu or environmental influences on use, knowing the person, and finding the best technology. Achieving optimal matches is a complex and dynamic process that takes skill, dedication, knowledge, and time. Premature introduction of assistive technologies may result in rejection of best fit options or selection of technologies not suited to post-rehabilitation environments. The high rate of new or improved AT being introduced into the marketplace does not allow for awareness or adequate assessment of devices that may maximize function. Thus, therapists who make recommendations for the purchase of AT must not only seek out information on the personal qualities of the client but also remain vigilant in the pursuit of learning how new technologies may be of use to their clients.

Laura N. Gitlin describes in Chapter 8 the acquisition and use of AT by older adults who experience impairments late in life. She cites numerous examples from the literature to demonstrate the increased use of AT by older adults. Three single case reports are used to illustrate the positive and negative aspects of AT use. Older adults with disabilities (all studied had more than one disability) have difficulty in incorporating AT use into their standard behavioral repertoires because they need to adjust to their new condition emotionally, physically, and socially. Introducing the concept of career use of AT, Gitlin makes the point that most older adults are introduced to a multitude (e.g., one person took 21 items home) of AT during their hospital stay but have a short career use when they find that the devices are not suitable for use at home. The decreased home use of AT is attributed to a wide variety of factors. However, much misuse, avoidance of unnecessary purchases, and early warning of needed home modifications or additional in-home AT needs can be best served through home visits by professionals while the person is still in the hospital. AT user careers that begin with successes continue to be AT users even as their needs and environments change. One danger not often discussed in consideration of AT device abandonment is the fatigue associated with use of AT. The balance of the benefits of AT use and the costs of its use (e.g., financial, emotional, physical) are not well captured by standard measures of independence and dependence. Other constructs and associated measures are needed for developing and using AT for older adults.

In Chapter 9, Carolyn M. Baum emphasizes the importance of treating clients as partners in the selection of AT. She provides a case example of a person who had filled an entire living room with mobility devices that had been provided for her use. She chose to use a shopping cart because it fit best with her needs and minimized the social stigma associated with the medical devices. A client-centered model for choosing, learning, and retaining AT is presented as an alternative to the medical necessity approach to the assignment of AT. The outcome of client-centered AT selection is improved consumer satisfaction, reduced limitation in social participation, increased independence, and higher levels of self-reliance. Baum provides a table for use by clients and therapists in their deliberations of the activities that might be enhanced through the use of AT. She includes an interesting option: choosing not to engage in an activity. The consequences of including this option may be a key to reducing AT underuse, misuse, or total abandonment. Another interesting proposal for optimizing provision and use of AT by people with disabilities is to expand the range of decision makers to include families, employers, insurers, and others who provide the essential resources for individuals with disabilities in their quest to live satisfying lives as integral people in their home communities.

SECTION III: SELECTING, DESIGNING, AND DEVELOPING ASSISTIVE TECHNOLOGY FOR USE BY PEOPLE WITH DISABILITIES

Chapter 10, by Rory A. Cooper, elaborates on the importance of involving consumers with disabilities in the design processes used in developing a new AT. He begins by pointing out the lack of statistical information available on the number and types of devices used by people with disabilities. The purchase of AT by those with severe physical limitations consumes a significant portion of their annual income or is provided for in a rapidly decreasing number of government and insurance programs in their attempt to reduce health care costs. Given these restraints, designing and providing AT for people with disabilities require a careful process that may include testing the person's use of AT in a controlled clinical setting prior to purchase. This may help to avoid the cycle of purchase, trial, modification, retrial, further modification, retrial, failure, discarding of the device, and purchase of another AT device for further attempts to meet needs. Other approaches to breaking this costly and ineffective cycle include computer simulations, component part construction, equipment lending programs, shared-equipment pools, and designing unique AT based on specific task requirements of individual consumers. In designing AT, the engineer must consider a host of factors, including cost, human performance requirements, duration of acquisition of skills, safety, reliability, redundancy, durability, robustness, appearance, locus of device control (internal, external, or shared), simplicity in manufacturing, and ease of repair. Cooper advocates the use of total quality control for the purpose of ensuring the best designed and most used AT devices. These devices will provide a basis for third-party payers and consumers with adequate funds to make the decision to purchase AT that will make a difference in the quality of the lives of people with disabilities.

In Chapter 11, Kenton R. Kaufman presents an overview of the design process. Engineering design involves developing a methodology to proceed from concept to final product while knowing which technological resources to use and considering economic factors, timeliness, reliability, safety, and practicality during the design process. The need for AT for use by people with partial or complete paralysis of the lower extremities is identified. Several approaches to assessing and restoring function in individuals with paralysis of the lower extremities is described. Kaufman advocates the use of intramuscular pressure measurements during gait to improve understanding of the relationship of these measures to the timing and intensity of muscle contraction when walking. He is conducting research and development in cooperation with Lawrence Livermore National Laboratory to develop a smaller intramuscular pressure biosensor. These sensors will give designers of AT valuable information on the energy used in walking with newly designed orthoses. Nearly all long-leg braces are rejected by consumers because they require so much energy to use. Kaufman and his colleagues have designed a new knee–ankle–foot orthosis that, in the brace-unlocked configuration, reduces metabolic energy requirements for ambulation. Kaufman describes the high cost of AT in the United States as a barrier to its purchase and a disincentive to its development. A portion of the high cost may be attributable to the frequency of litigation in the United States, the lack of exact methods for determining the safety of AT, and the variety of payment sources for AT. Although the overall goal is to obtain forward locomotion in the most energy-efficient way possible, the design goal must include minimizing overall cost, balancing reliability cost with repair costs, and reducing the consequences of a system failure to near zero.

Assistive technologies are beginning to be used by individuals with mobility impairments for control of their internal and external movements. These devices, neuroprostheses, are implanted within the body for the purpose of controlling body functions through the electrical stimulation of muscles or organs that have been rendered dysfunctional as a result of injury or disease. P. Hunter Peckham describes a new generation of neuroprostheses in Chapter 12. A neuroprosthesis for restoration of hand function provides a user with the ability to open and close his or her hand. These movements are made in response to command signals provided by the user that activate electrical stimulation of arm, wrist, and finger muscles. These hand movements allow the person to perform a variety of tasks that are fundamental to many life activities (e.g., grooming, eating, working, driving). One advantage of the grasp neuroprosthesis is that the user can move from task to task in a natural, fluid fashion rather than adding or removing devices that are designed for specific tasks. A second neuroprosthetic device, the Brindley–Finetech system, allows individuals who are paralyzed to control bladder voiding through electrical stimulation. The neuroprosthetic device stimulates the bladder to contract and the urinary sphincter to open when the user activates a command signal by pushing a switch on a remote controller. Control of the urinary system is one of the most fundamental needs of humans. Without bladder control, infection and kidney damage may occur that can be life threatening. Participating in social activities is limited when external urinary collection devices fail. Use of the hand and bladder neuroprostheses reduces the need for personal assistance in performing activities of daily living, lowers the rate of secondary medical complications, and increases the probability of participation in more life activities by people with mobility impairments. Since the 1960s, scientists have studied a host of problems associated with placing in the body foreign materials that might be used to control muscles and organs through electrical stimulation. Many of the fundamental issues have been resolved; however, developing and deploying neuroprostheses require considerable effort in convincing regulatory agencies, training health care personnel, obtaining third-party payment for installation, and gaining acceptance in the disability community.

The author of Chapter 13, Peter W. Axelson, a wheelchair user, has applied his engineering skills to develop many types of AT that are being used in the home, at work, and for recreation by others with mobility disabilities. He describes the process that he uses in designing AT, focusing on developing technologies that are primarily aimed at preventing functional limitations from keeping people with disabilities from participating in activities of their own choosing. The first step is to look for products with universal design features that are already accessible or can easily be modified by adapting the control or seating interface. If a specific technology needs to be designed, can the technology be used to enhance the person's performance in all situations or is an activity-specific technology needed? Getting to know the consumers provides direction in determining how the AT will be used to establish or reestablish balance in their lives. Focusing efforts on the needs and problems that will affect their life activities most will help select priorities for developing AT devices that will be used. Finally, evaluate individuals' levels of function and their interest related to the specific tasks that they are trying to accomplish. Using this approach will help to avert functional limitations or at least to prevent them from becoming disabilities. Axelson illustrates these principles by describing several projects that he has developed. As an example of personal technology, the Back Support Shaping System was developed for people who use wheelchairs. He explains the need to consider a variety of factors in designing the product, including the height of the support, the amount of skin pressure, the variety of functions improved through its use, the influences of postural changes, and the appearance of the product. Working with wheelchair users was an essential feature in designing prototypes of a back support that is commercially available. A second example of applying engineering to solve problems is provided in Mr. Axelson's description of how he developed a universal trail assessment that can be used by all nature trail users to determine the degree of trail difficulty. Grade, cross-slope, width, obstacles, and the surface of the trail all have an influence on the degree of access for all user groups. Universal Trail Assessment research has developed standards for the construction of new trails and the renovation of existing ones to provide easy, moderate, difficult, and most difficult degrees of access. Recreationalists of all abilities can use this information to help make informed decisions about which trails to hike. A stand-alone trails information kiosk is being designed for use in Yosemite National Park in California.

Stephen Sprigle and Adam Abdelhamied, in Chapter 14, provide a rationale for matching individual differences in capabilities and needs with available AT and in developing new AT. They describe an eight-step prescription process for selecting AT for people with disabilities that includes assessing the consumer's needs, physical abilities, functional performance capacities, and expected outcomes. They illustrate their approach by using several compelling examples. The variety of AT available and the diversity of individual abilities are difficult to map by using manual and observational measures. Use of standard measurement tools offers the promise of improved validity and reliability of data for use in assessing the user's ability to operate selected AT. The provision of the standards for specific devices (e.g., wheelchair reliability, durability, and stability; service factors) can make the selection of AT less of a risk. Standard charts that list performance values and AT requirements; computer programs designed to match device, abilities, functions, and desired outcomes; and expert systems all hold the promise for better AT selection. However, these approaches rely on the quality of the data and algorithms used in compiling the matching rules, which are not well developed. These authors suggest that not every problem can or should be answered by the use of AT. Some problems occur so infrequently that carrying an AT device is more trouble than it is worth. Some devices can be so annoying that they will be discarded. Even when a use of a device is indicated, trade-offs in how and where the AT device can be used must be made. The complex processes involved in determining whether a device is justified and what type of AT will enhance which function is a matter that needs to be addressed by the research community in the very near future. Even now, third-party payers have begun to restrict the purchase of AT in their zeal to streamline reimbursement and reduce costs. Empirical findings are needed to sort those devices that have useful outcomes from those that have little or no influence on the lives of people with disabilities. Sprigle and Abdelhamied suggest several research directions that could improve the design, development, selection, and use of AT.

SECTION IV: INCORPORATING ASSISTIVE TECHNOLOGY INTO CHILD DEVELOPMENT

In Chapter 15, Rosanne Kermoian advocates the provision of assistive mobility technology for young children with physical disabilities based on the underlying assumption that early mobility promotes higher levels of independence and greater integration into society at an earlier age. She reviews the literature on cognitive, perceptual, and emotional development that supports the importance of motor activity for the psychological development of young children. Independent motor activity allows exploration of the infant's environment and increases parents' expectation of the child's beginning to act autonomously. For those children with physical disabilities who experience delays in the onset of independent mobility, the new opportunities and demands associated with locomotion are infrequent and specific aspects of psychological development may be delayed. The importance of motor activity is described for the typical development of many important human characteristics—emotional attachment, sense of autonomy, and person–environment relationships. Locomotion experience improves the infant's sensitivity to objects and events that are out of reach. In addition, locomotion increases the infant's goal-oriented behaviors. Clinical reports of dramatic behavioral change associated with the use of mobility aids by these children support Kermoian's hypothesis. She advocates preventing delays in psychological development through the early provision of independent mobility-enhancing AT. This goal can be reached through provision of inexpensive devices that promote safe environmental explorations by infants and young children with significant physical impairments. In addition, the new generation of AT for children must be designed to accommodate the child's growth and must be easy for the child to learn in his or her physical and social environments. Finally, research is needed to evaluate both the short- and long-term effects of a wide variety of mobility devices for physical and psychological development of children with different diagnoses. Kermoian describes barriers to AT device use by infants, makes suggestions for design features, and provides recommendations for when and how to introduce the use of assistive technologies to infants.

The importance of designing, testing, and using augmented mobility devices to enable infants and young children to participate in family and school activities is clearly set forth by Jean Crosetto Deitz in Chapter 16. She discusses the importance of establishing a positive attitude in parents of infants and children who need augmented mobility devices (e.g., wheelchairs, scooters). Developing age-, activity-, and setting-appropriate devices can reduce negative attitudes of parents, users, and playmates. AT devices that look like toys promote acceptance of the devices and increase the chance of social inclusion for the child. Teaching device use should begin with simple, single-function AT. As the child develops, he or she may progress to more complex, multipurpose AT devices. Deitz illustrates her point by comparing two powered wheelchairs that provide the user with a variety of options. The AT device's designers will be challenged by a series of thoughtful questions that she lists that describe optimal device capacities for enhancing the child's functions. Finally, Deitz addresses the problem of affording and repairing devices by suggesting a new service system that emphasizes modular equipment, exchange of components, repair and exchange clubs, and person–family involvement.

In Chapter 17, Christine Wright-Ott describes the development of an AT device that addresses Kermoian's call for increased attention to motor development of children with disabilities and Deitz's description of the need for AT designed specifically for young children. Wright-Ott was a member of a design and development team that produced an AT device that allows young children to initiate interactions with their environments without compromising their need to engage in therapy. The device, the Transitional Powered Mobility Aid (TPMA), was developed using a consumer-centered approach that involved the children and their parents, therapists, teachers, and third-party payers in determining the need for the device, its uses in differing environments, and its appearance. Wright-Ott describes different ideas for design that came from evaluating the TPMA in both controlled and natural settings. Other influences in developing and marketing the TPMA are instructive for people interested in entering the field of AT. Wright-Ott points out that the success of the TPMA was directly related to changes in legislation that have provided justification for AT devices other than those for medical needs and have built an information-sharing system that improves awareness of product availability. Finally, she makes the point that, in order for new assistive technologies to succeed, old paradigms of medical needs or enhancement of specific motor functions need to be replaced with the new evidence that children need to learn that they can have an influence on their environment (physical and social) for full development of their potential as humans.

SECTION V: SUMMARY

A short summary chapter by David B. Gray, Louis A. Quatrano, and Morton L. Lieberman reviews the major themes in the book. The NCMRR model is used as a heuristic tool for placing AT in five domains of importance to people with disabilities: pathophysiology, impairments, functional limitations, and disability and societal limitations. Some of the major barriers to AT development and use are reviewed. A series of recommendations for future research efforts are made in five general areas: classification, selection of AT, design of AT, acquisition of skills for AT use, and evaluation of AT. Finally, the importance of moving beyond medical justifications for AT provision to the incorporation of AT into the mainstream of life for people with disabilities is advocated.

Acknowledgments

This book is a result of the splendid efforts of many individuals. We deeply appreciate those who made the extra effort to make the conference on design and use of assistive technology (AT) productive, thought provoking, and enjoyable. These people were the support staff of the National Center for Medical Rehabilitation Research: Diane Eagle, Shana Malone, Kerri Purdy, Marika Searle, and Debbie Welty. The chapters were reviewed and formatted by Katherine Weston, who is a research assistant in the Program in Occupational Therapy at Washington University in St. Louis. Her hard work and dedication to this project were essential to the production of this volume. Jennifer Lazaro Kinard of the Brookes staff provided essential encouragement and direction for assembling the contents of this book into a work that contains a healthy balance of views from science and practice, professionals and consumers, and designers and therapists. Those readers who are aided in designing, developing, introducing, or using AT will be the beneficiaries of the persistence, dedication, and skill of those who brought the book to press.

To Margy, who has the courage to modify her life to enable her husband to live a fully productive life, and to three beautiful children, Dave, Beth, and Polly, who learned to use, repair, store, and even enjoy a plethora of assistive technologies, including manual and electric wheelchairs, air-filled and layered urethane wheelchair cushions, orthotic "hands and fingers," adapted vehicles, remote-controlled door and window shade openers, push-button door locks, stand-aids, upper-extremity-powered exercise bikes, hospital beds, leg bags, shower chairs, portable ramps, raised furniture, grabbers, sticky keys for computer keyboards, computers and printers, speaker phones, elevators, "built-up" devices (e.g., shavers, eating utensils, dressing aids), eyeglasses, and a variety of home modifications, all to let their Dad be their Dad

—David B. Gray

Designing and Using
Assistive Technology

CONCEPTS, CLASSIFICATIONS, AND CATEGORIES OF DISABLING CONDITIONS AND ASSISTIVE TECHNOLOGIES

CHAPTER 1

Models for Understanding Rehabilitation and Assistive Technology

Nancy A. Brooks

This chapter offers a view of disability that comes from sociology and some of its specialty areas. This view incorporates the concept of the social construction of reality as it relates to rehabilitation and disability technology, briefly summarizes five contemporary models of disability and assistive technology (AT), and points out how the postindustrial professional–client relationship is changing the world of rehabilitation. The term *assistive devices* as used here refers to mechanical aids specifically intended to assist the physical functions of the human body.

SOCIAL CONSTRUCTIONS OF REALITY

Humans attempt to explain events in their lives by attributing meaning to the salient features of those events as they experience them. For people living with a disabling condition, many of these events are shared with their family members, friends, personal assistants, and professionals who provide services to them. For the person with a disability, constructing a reality that can be shared with others is essential for meaningful communications. The shared definition explains why disability exists and what, if anything, should be done about it. It is the nature of those shared interpretations, or *models*, that is of concern in this chapter.

Whether intimate or formal, all groups develop their own interpretations of reality and work hard to sustain them. Both positive and negative sanctions are applied to sustain group members' alle-

3

giance to the accepted group definition of the situation. The rehabilitation disciplines are like other groups in that way. French sociologist Herzlich (1973) proposed that, within any group that is living with a chronic illness or disability, an unspoken understanding
of what the condition is or will be is constructed. The model they
create becomes almost a "thing," an entity to be managed. Family
members, for example, tend to believe together that the condition
is a monster that has ruined their lives, a blessing that has brought
them closer together, a challenge that is to be analyzed and confronted, or even a liberator from everyday obligations. Any of these
or other constructions can become a guiding model for group beliefs
and actions. In more formal terms, the model can also be called a
paradigm.

MODELS OF DISABILITY

Outwardly, the human body seems to remain rather constant, but
the ways in which a body with disabilities is perceived, evaluated,
labeled, and acted upon are part of a socially dynamic process.
There are three main features of shared models for thinking:

1. Social constructions of reality are held so close to our being
    that we may not notice the direct influence they have on our
    decision making and behavior.
2. Shared models influence what kinds of questions we raise
    about our tasks.
3. Shared models are supported by social arrangements, such as
    social conditions, policies, and laws.

How each group defines and responds to disability realities is
closely linked to the social place of disability technology. According
to historian Mumford (1934), we are *all* defined by our technologies.
That is even more true when disability technology becomes part of
life. Assistive devices have particular effects on social identities and
social relationships because the devices are often intimate to the
user's body and essential to personal functions such as mobility,
sight, and even breathing. In addition, assistive devices are cues for
social interaction because they link the person to formal social systems, such as vocational rehabilitation or medical systems. Furthermore, assistive devices become a social signal because the sight
of a person using AT sends a message that this is not an ordinary
person and that one needs to behave differently around this person.
Assistive devices are cues to social behavior for all parties in the
interaction.

For example, when I first began to use a cane many years ago, my multiple sclerosis (MS) became a public matter. Several times I met people who asked me to my face, "What did you do that was so bad that God gave you multiple sclerosis?" I do not use that particular model for interpreting my MS, so I answered with something flippant, such as, "Gosh, I don't know. There were so many things." The point is, I never received such intrusions into my privacy until I began using a cane.

The members of the rehabilitation team are active participants in the social construction of disability in association with AT. Rehabilitation specialists often demonstrate their collective views through the application or withholding of technology. Then, through interactions with clients and other professionals and working with larger social systems such as Medicare, they make AT a formalized public expression of what disability represents. Assistive technology can represent an ordinary life occurrence or a condition that is associated with multiple disadvantages. Disability technology provides a good focal point for observing the way in which disability is perceived by society because it is a selective and tangible symbol of social values. If disability were a highly desirable characteristic, hearing aids, crutches, and wheelchairs would be highly advertised and socially valued products.

RESEARCH OBSERVATIONS

In 1988, a national survey of 595 scientists and engineers with disabilities was conducted to investigate users' perceptions of AT (Brooks, 1991). The mailing list was drawn from a database of more than 1,200 scientists and engineers with disabilities that is maintained by the American Association for the Advancement of Science. The response rate to the mailed questionnaire was 47%. The results are informative for this discussion of rehabilitation models.

Although the scientists and engineers expressed satisfactory opinions about their AT devices, they were critical of the *systems* that inform consumers about the availability, cost, and methods for distribution of the devices. The social implications of these messages are intriguing. How is access to basic information about AT related to social definitions of disability itself? Should people with disabilities be subjected to some kind of social control through these complex systems? What are the underlying assumptions about the value of the consumers with disabilities? These are important questions.

In the United States, investigations of questions pertaining to disabilities traditionally begin by gathering numerical data on individuals with one or more disabilities. For example, the Institute of Medicine report titled *Disability in America: Toward a National Agenda for Prevention* provides an estimate of the number of people with disabilities as approximately 14% of the total population (Pope & Tarlov, 1991). The use of descriptive statistics and quantitative techniques for data analysis is the basis for one way of understanding the realities of disability. However, the manner in which questions are framed for collection of data to address the question of population size will determine the type of information collected and the set of answers obtained or derived.

As an illustration, in 1979, I had the opportunity to visit Sweden and meet with several people who were active in shaping Sweden's housing policies regarding people with disabilities. When I met with a director of housing policy in the Ministry of Health and Welfare, she told me that Sweden's housing authority had conducted a long-term survey of government-subsidized housing complexes over a 5-year period. In 1972, they found that 60% of the housing controlled by the housing authority was occupied by people who had had disabilities that lasted more than 6 months. In addition to the standard impairment conditions used in U.S. surveys, this survey included women who were pregnant, people with short-term impairments (e.g., broken leg or arm), and people providing care for older adult relatives. The Swedish government based its housing policy for disability on the 60% figure. The findings had convinced authorities that the need for accessible housing was substantial and likely to grow with the aging of the population.

By 1984, Sweden had a federal law requiring that all newly constructed housing be adaptable. Under the Swedish model, housing was seen as a resource that should be available to all. Their working framework, their model for disability, was that anyone can become a member of a disability group. Thus, it would be realistic to acknowledge disability when housing is designed for people in general rather than to ignore disability and retrofit specific housing units one at a time.

The Swedish example shows how application of Swedish definitions and counting procedures resulted in housing plans different from those based on definitions and counting procedures that are usually applied in the United States. A different framework for thinking leads to different questions and, ultimately, to different solutions. Perhaps we can use this case to rethink some of the models we use for distributing AT in the United States.

SELECTED MODELS OF REHABILITATION

There are five models commonly used to frame discussions on disability: the medical model, the psychological model, the rehabilitation model, the minority group model, and the political model. Each of these is discussed in turn in the subsections that follow.

Medical Model

The traditional model used to discuss disability is the medical model. This model assumes that an abnormality exists in the patient's body and that the medical doctor is the appropriate professional for identifying problems of a structural or physiological nature (the disabling condition). The problem to be addressed is placed *within* the person, and the exercise of possible solutions is in the doctor's hands. The traditional medical model has included a passive role for the patient.

In general, physician–patient interaction patterns are changing toward more mutual participation. Physicians have learned that the patient may know a great deal about the best health practices for living with a chronic disabling condition. However, people with disabilities still have difficulties in transactions regarding their medical care. In large part, the continuing dominance of health care professionals in this transactional process is sustained by social policies and financial regulations governing the prescription of pharmaceuticals, admission to hospitals and clinics, and distribution of AT.

The physician is the gatekeeper for all access to services and AT, even when he or she is not the most knowledgeable person in the complex pathway from determination of need for AT to its use by a person with a disability. Acquiring AT is not like typical shopping. The consumer's functional limitations and life circumstances are studied by a variety of specialists. Many evaluations are made prior to ordering an assistive device. Rarely are the devices provided to consumers for a trial period of time prior to purchase. Third-party payers with little or no formal or informal training in AT or disabilities are often the final decision makers.

Psychological Model

Another frequently used model in rehabilitation, the psychological model, emphasizes the emotional and cognitive problems that are associated with many disabilities. These include problems of coping with anger, fear, and feelings of helplessness. Again, the problem to be fixed is identified by the professional and is located within the person who has the disabling condition. A longstanding example of the psychological tradition in rehabilitation is the emphasis given to "motivation"—the individual's motivation, of course.

Rehabilitation Model

The rehabilitation model is a relatively new one on the health care scene. It is characterized by the team approach, in which many specialists and the consumer contribute parts of the rehabilitation process. From the consumer's perspective, this can mean inclusion in decision making or confusion about the whole process. AT is assumed to be a part of the rehabilitation process. Choosing the AT device, obtaining it, and learning how to use it are part of the consumer's role. Ideally, professional and consumer work together, but another component is often added: third-party payers. The consumer may be overwhelmed by the differing authoritative voices and pressures. Acquiring AT may be a visible sign of losing control over one's life and experiencing downward social mobility. Assistive devices may be rejected or adopted very slowly because physical, psychological, and social forces are all at work.

Minority Group Model

An alternative framework, the minority group model for disability, emerged in the mid-1970s (Hahn, 1993). This model shifted attention away from the disabling condition to the social, political, and environmental disadvantages imposed on people with disabilities. The focus shifted from locating the problem within the person to seeing the problem in social or built environments. A good example of the minority group viewpoint appeared on a poster of the time. It showed a young woman seated in a wheelchair in front of a building with many stairs leading to the door. The caption read, "My legs don't keep me out of buildings; stairs do!" The minority group model acknowledges the fact that disability can bring substantial psychological and medical problems but argues that the social, political, and built environments create problems external to the individual that can be modified. This model has been the basis for the development of the independent living and disability rights movements that have evolved since the mid-1970s. The minority group model raises awareness of the high cost and limited choice of essential AT for people with disabilities.

Political Model

The political model is a new framework being used by people with disabilities to address their circumstances both during and after rehabilitation. This model is still under construction, but it does encourage more community involvement and activism than the minority group model does. The political model has been analyzed most by political scientist Hahn (1993), who concentrated on studying patterns of disability discrimination and segregation and proposed a range of possible responses to those conditions. Under this model, the concern is for the restriction of resources experienced by groups who lack power. Having direct access to information about the distribution of AT would be a political matter.

MODELS OF DISABILITY
AND PROFESSIONAL RELATIONSHIPS

Shifts in the guiding models of disability may change the professional–consumer relationship. Partners in these relationships will negotiate which roles they may adopt based on differing models operative at different times during the rehabilitation process. The rehabilitation professional's role has been oriented toward the team approach, but that situation is being strained by the increasing corporatization of the medical professions. Medical sociologist Cockerham (1994) argued that the patient–professional relationship is experiencing several changes; the dispensing of AT is likely to be affected as well.

Sociologist Freidson (1994) wrote in *Professionalism Reborn: Theory, Prophecy, and Policy* that the roles of specialists are changing and so are the models that guide them. A new task for the rehabilitation specialist may be to assist the consumer with information overload, quite a different problem from what was experienced prior to the 1990s. The Information Age is bringing new models for the professional–consumer relationship. Especially since the advent of the Internet, information about AT can be disseminated worldwide on disability-related bulletin boards. Unlike the earlier lay referral networks, a consumer may easily access professional journal articles and make decisions about which AT device to use. Today's rehabilitation professional has the responsibility of monitoring the integrity of information received by telecommunication: Is the information accurate? Is it complete? Does it fit with other information? Does it meet the needs of the consumer? The availability of and ease of access to information can put the professional into an even stronger consulting relationship with the consumer, because the professional can bring order to the avalanche of information. If professionals participate in telecommunication, interact with consumers, and remain accessible to electronic discussions about AT, a new model and a more balanced professional–consumer relationship could emerge.

A timely illustration of this transition was reported in the *Wall Street Journal* (Bulkeley, 1995). The situation concerned the experimental drug neurotonin, a possible treatment for amyotrophic lateral sclerosis (ALS). The drug was being tested in clinical trials, with some ALS patients receiving the drug and others receiving a placebo. Some volunteers in the trial began telecommunicating nationwide and shared information that allowed them to guess who was getting the placebo. Many of those receiving the placebo quit the trials; as a result, the research findings were substantially affected. The rapid transfer of specialized information over great distances to untrained individuals adds a new wrinkle to the professional–consumer relationship. Research procedures are likely to require modification as a consequence.

Rehabilitation may not have a corollary to the neurotonin case, but the incident does send loud signals about the kinds of major changes we can expect to see in this Information Age. The professional–consumer relationship is being affected by the relatively easy availability of specialized information, such as that found in journal articles. A new professional role will be that of preventing a potential information overload by applying to the available data the theories and standards of practice that are judged most appropriate. The control and use of information gathered by telecommunication will make professional–consumer negotiations more interesting, complicated, and balanced in degree of control.

In contrast, there will also be large numbers of rehabilitation consumers who are not computer literate. When the professional wishes to use the computer system with individuals, that computer literacy gap may create new divisions between consumer groups and professionals. In addition, a large proportion of rehabilitation consumers come from the working and lower social classes; class differences require the professional to maintain awareness of the different models of disability that are constructed by different social groups.

These examples underscore the different levels of significance attributed to the acquisition and use of AT for a variety of models of disability. AT stands at the intersection of body and environment while many models of disability roll by. It is time to build a model for evaluating, choosing, purchasing, and learning which AT devices are best for improving specific functions of each person with a disability.

REFERENCES

Brooks, N.A. (1991). Users' responses to assistive devices for physical disability. *Social Science and Medicine, 32*(12), 1417–1424.

Bulkeley, W.M. (1995, February 27). Untested treatments, cures, find stronghold on on-line services. *Wall Street Journal*, p. A1.

Cockerham, W.C. (1994). *Medical sociology* (5th ed.). Englewood Cliffs, NJ: Prentice-Hall.

Freidson, E. (1994). *Professionalism reborn: Theory, prophecy, and policy.* Chicago: University of Chicago Press.

Hahn, H. (1993). The politics of physical differences: Disability and discrimination. In M. Nagler (Ed.), *Perspectives on disability* (2nd ed., pp. 37–43). Palo Alto, CA: Health Markets Research.

Herzlich, C. (1973). *Health and illness: A social-psychological analysis.* London: European Association for Experimental Social-Psychology and Academic Press.

Mumford, L. (1934). *Technics and civilization.* New York: Harcourt Brace Jovanovich.

Pope, A.M., & Tarlov, A.R. (Eds.). (1991). *Disability in America: Toward a national agenda for prevention.* Washington, DC: National Academy Press.

CHAPTER 2

Classification Systems, Environmental Factors, and Social Change

The Importance of Technology

Patrick Fougeyrollas and David B. Gray

In 1980, the World Health Organization (WHO) published the *International Classification of Impairments, Disabilities, and Handicaps* (ICIDH), an experimental classification scheme for assessing and describing the consequences of diseases. Based on the work of British epidemiologist Wood (1980), this innovative classification scheme has been used as a model to attribute cause-and-effect relationships between each conceptual level. Injury leads to functional and organic impairment, which in turn leads to disability in an individual's behavior and activities, which generates a handicap or handicaps, which are disadvantages with respect to survival roles (Figure 1).

The ICIDH was the first conceptual and classification scheme to allow for distinctions among the organic, functional, personal, and—above all—social consequences of disease and trauma. This explains its considerable international influence. The ICIDH conceptual model has stimulated a great deal of research. It has provided a framework for evaluating the need for and effectiveness of a wide variety of medical, social, and economic programs directed toward improving the lives of people with impairments and disabilities. However, since the mid-1980s, activities of advocacy groups,

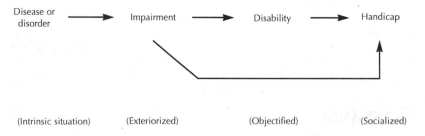

Figure 1. The *International Classification of Impairments, Disabilities, and Handicaps* (ICIDH) model. (From World Health Organization. [1980]. *International classification of impairments, disabilities and handicaps* [p. 30]. Geneva: Author.)

studies by social scientists, technologies designed by engineers, and therapies targeting skill development have contributed to a growing realization that the lives of people with disabilities can be greatly improved by means and methods that fall outside the scope of any classification scheme used by the biomedical community, including the ICIDH.

To clarify terms and concepts for a revised ICIDH, the Québec Committee on the ICIDH has proposed a different conceptual segmentation of impairment (organic anomaly), disability (physical or mental functional limitation), and handicap (life habits depending on individual identity and social context). A positive approach is used when speaking of the components—organic systems, abilities, and life habits replace impairment, disability, and handicap. This chapter develops the rationale for changing the concept of the handicap dimension and introduces environmental factors as a fourth dimension.

THE HANDICAP DIMENSION

The initial perspective illustrated by the linear cause-and-effect conceptual model of the ICIDH was that *handicaps* are defined as social disadvantages. The term *handicap* came to represent what a person was missing. What was missing seemed to be the inevitable consequence of impairments and disabilities. The term *handicap* provided a convenient social label for describing people with disabilities in terms of a specific status that is stigmatizing and reduces the person to a series of negative attributes. However, social changes aimed at ensuring equal opportunity; facilitating the exercise of human rights; and adapting socioeconomic structures, social rules, and the physical environment have led us to question the very notion of a "handicapped" person. Our view now is that *hand-*

icap must always be defined as situational and interactive. That is, the handicap situation is a result of a person's individual characteristics and his or her identified life activities that are set within particular developmental periods, cultural norms, and physical settings. Understanding of the cultural creation of handicap situations demands a conceptual model that takes into account the life activities expected or desired by the person, his or her family, and his or her friends. The model must provide for assessment of the specific context in which that personal life habit is performed.

Since 1986, the Canadian Society for the ICIDH and the Québec Committee on the ICIDH have worked to develop projects and proposals aimed at better meeting the needs of people with impairments or disabilities and people living in handicap situations by promoting, applying, and improving the conceptual framework of the ICIDH. In keeping with the positions taken by Disabled People International and the views set out in *On Equal Terms* (Office des Personnes Handicapées du Québec, 1984), the Québec government policy for social integration of people with disabilities, the Québec Committee, has concentrated on critically reviewing the concept of *handicap* (Fougeyrollas, St.-Michel, & Blouin, 1989). Specifically, it has focused on the consideration of environmental factors that facilitate or inhibit social participation by people with disabilities— in other words, a study of the handicap creation process. This emphasis on the social and physical environment is characteristic of the Canadian and Québec perspective and activities. Its aim is to better define, analyze, study, and evaluate obstacles to the integration of people whose bodies or functional capabilities are different. In part, this work will clarify the definition and structural cohesiveness of a classification of the consequences of disease and trauma. However, the main purpose of such endeavors is clear. Social change is advocated and fostered from a multisectoral and multidisciplinary standpoint. These efforts are made to identify obstacles to the social participation of people with disabilities and transform them into facilitators that compensate for disabilities. This approach promotes the emergence of an accepting social context that is adapted to or respects individual differences. Most important, it ensures that people with disabilities are directly involved in making decisions and determining their own life choices.

Community values and attitudes associated with impairments and disabilities can, depending on the circumstances, become obstacles that lead to a process of stigmatizing and excluding people with disabilities from social participation. This handicap creation process can be examined by means of systemic analysis. Some very interesting research is being done in Québec that has examined the resistance encountered in some residential areas when efforts have been made to establish group homes for people with severe mental or physical limitations. These studies illustrate the usefulness of making a social and environmental analysis of obstacles to inclusion of people with disabilities in residential communities. In Québec, many failures have occurred in attempts to establish community homes for people who have been deinstitutionalized. No attempt was made to determine which residents of a particular neighborhood would accept people with functional and behavioral differences living in their midst. Knowing this type of information provides useful guidelines for adjusting conditions to improve the probability of successfully establishing a group home. Additional information on the accessibility of neighborhood buildings, availability of assistive technologies, possibilities for employing personal assistants, and *affordability* of social and health services contributes to making recommendations for the best location for establishing a group home in a specific area. This example illustrates the importance of assessing environmental factors in planning to provide equal opportunity for people with disabilities to participate in social activities. This type of information is useful in adjusting strategies for changing the conditions that create handicaps, such as failed attempts to locate a group home where the neighboring residents will tolerate people with differences participating in social events.

ADDITION OF AN ENVIRONMENTAL DIMENSION

Documenting environmental factors for preventing the handicap creation process provides an extension and expansion of the ICIDH model. The challenge is to devise a classification that can reflect the richness of human environments in social and ecological terms while maintaining a complementary relationship to the concepts of impairment and disability. Included in this new concept of environment are all social, cultural, and physical dimensions that determine the organization and context of a society (see Table 1). These factors can either become obstacles or facilitators to individual social participation. The new dimension of environmental factors permits us to identify and act on environmental obstacles that interact with organic and functional characteristics to create inequality of opportunity, discrimination, or exclusion in a specific social situation. This addition moves the model from a biomedical basis toward an interactive one that includes a broader range of variables

Table 1.   Taxonomy of environmental factors

Social factors	
Socioeconomic organization	Family structure
	Political system and government structures
	Legal system (services)
	Economic system (work, income, etc.)
	Health care and social services system
	Education system
	Public infrastructure services (transportation, communications, housing, etc.)
	Community organizations (associations, support network, etc.)
Social rules	Law
	Values and attitudes
Ecological factors	
Nature	Geography
	Climate
	Time
Development	Architecture
	Land development
	Technology

From Fougeyrollas, P., & St.-Michel, G. (1991). Proposal of a revised nomenclature of environmental factors: QCICIDH. *ICIDH International Network, 4*(1-2), 21–22; reprinted by permission.

that contribute to the handicap creation process because there is nothing that can be said about the phenomenon of handicap that is not relative. This expanded model provides room for study of the relative contribution of environmental factors to social consequences and the life habits of people with different abilities (Figure 2) (Fougeyrollas, St.-Michel, Bergeron, & Cloutier, 1991).

Using at least three broad dimensions for analysis of environmental factors makes it possible to discover obstacles or facilitators to participation in society by people with impairments and disabilities. These dimensions are referred to as macrosystemic, mesosystemic, and microsystemic. They must be analyzed by means of reading a grid that contains a variety of environmental factors. Each system's dimension may contribute multiple obstacles that singly or in combination create handicap situations. The presence and severity of the obstacles are assessed for each category in the taxonomy. The choice of which dimension within the environmental taxonomy to analyze depends on the needs of the user and the way the ICIDH is being applied. Like Bronfenbrenner (1979), researchers

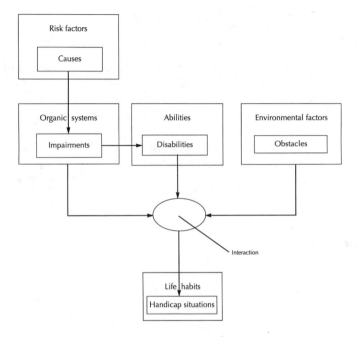

Figure 2.   The handicap creation process. (From Fougeyrollas, P., St.-Michel, G., Bergeron, H., & Cloutier R. [1991]. The handicap creation process: Analysis of the consultation: New full proposals. *ICIDH International Network*, 4[1-2], 17; reprinted by permission.)

can identify the contributions of the individual's impairments and disabilities in differing environments to determine the most effective manner in which to improve social participation of people with disabilities (Figure 3) (Fougeyrollas, 1993, 1995a). Fougeyrollas and colleagues are using this approach in their research on the handicap creation process. These studies will allow the reliability and validity of their interaction model to be improved. The results will be used in contributing to the ongoing ICIDH revision process coordinated by the WHO and specifically the North American Collaborating Center on ICIDH. At this point in the development of the model, only general descriptors of each category of environmental determinants of handicap situations are available. These are provided here for general consideration.

Macrosystemic Analysis

A macrosystemic level of analysis provides basic reference documentation that is essential in studying a target population as a part of society as a whole. This perspective is especially valuable for

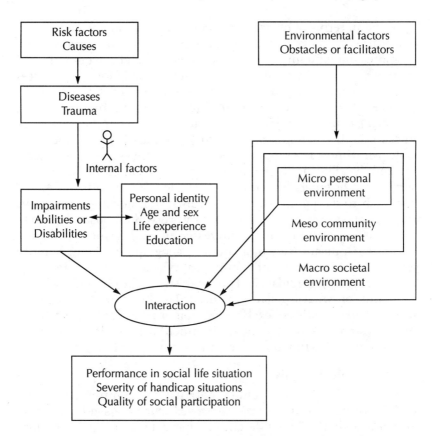

Figure 3.   The individual and environmental determinants: Components of the interaction model for the ICIDH. (From Fougeyrollas, P. [1995a]. Documenting environmental factors for preventing the handicap creation process: Québec contributions relating to ICIDH and social participation of people with functional differences. *Disability and Rehabilitation,* 17[3-4], 151. Copyright © 1995 by Taylor & Francis Ltd.; reprinted by permission.)

population surveys. The meaning and impact of statistics-based studies analyzing solely impairments and disabilities cannot be translated for use in planning programs and policies to avoid creating handicap situations. To begin to achieve macrosystemic levels of analysis, each country needs to describe general socioeconomic systems as they apply to social participation of people with disabilities. Implicit in this approach is a review and codification of the formal rules contained in the country's laws, economic policies, and religions. The cultural values and beliefs regarding people with disabilities must be spelled out. Welfare, charitable, advocacy, and business programs operating throughout a country should be included in the database. Geographic and climatic factors should be analyzed in terms of obstacles to social participation by people with disabilities. Results of surveys on national programs that require, promote, and fund improved access to natural and person-built environments should be cataloged and made available for use in assessing the effects these programs have on the lives of people with disabilities. Assistive technology (AT) resources for removing barriers to social participation, including reference to universal design guidelines for built environments, should be well documented and accessible. Multimodal communication systems are essential for accessing and distributing information regarding technology, health, and service sector programs relevant to people with disabilities. As this approach to data collection and organization develops, macrosystemic analysis can be performed for a variety of purposes. For example, legislators and planners interested in facilitating inclusion of people with disabilities in a country, geographic region, homogeneous subculture, or specific municipality could turn to a macrosystemic analysis for guidance. This analysis might provide useful information on what legislation is needed and how to craft it to best fit the characteristics of each population or region of interest. These macrosystem-based maps of environmental obstacles will change very slowly and will require nothing more than periodic review.

Mesosystemic Analysis

Mesosystemic analysis includes detailed and community-specific reviews of many of the same categories that are used for a macrosystemic analysis. The difference is that data are collected on local factors that reflect national laws or that are specific to the community. The data collected at this level might include data on factors related to national policies on requiring access, civil rights, health care, or employment. The focus here should be a description of the person's local environment, such as his or her neighborhood and the places he or she frequents in the course of carrying out social activities or fulfilling social roles. For example, in the category of environmental obstacles and facilitators in the person-built environment, a mesosystemic analysis would include data on numbers of accessible buildings, sidewalk curb cuts, and recreational sites. The category of economic facilitators would include employment opportunities, income from community programs, and support by local charities. Legal codes could be analyzed for regulations that facilitate or hinder social participation. For example, residential zoning ordinances, driver's license regulations, tax codes, and health care eligibility restrictions give local planners valuable information on boundary conditions for developing programs. Surveys of community attitudes, beliefs, and mores give an indication of where and how much change can be accepted within the community. Local resources for purchase and maintenance of assistive technologies are included at the mesosystemic level. The availability of captioning facilities, braille printing services, visual icon-based communication boards, audiotapes, and other assistive technologies to enhance or substitute for communication functions must be assessed. Analysis of these types of environmental factors allows officials responsible for administering programs aimed at improving social access for people with impairments and disabilities to use their facilities and programs in a maximally efficient manner. This type of analysis is vital in setting realistic and appropriate objectives in the areas of rehabilitation and support for participation in society of people with disabilities.

Microsystemic Analysis

A microsystemic analysis involves examination of the immediate environment of the person using many of the same categorical distinctions of facilitators and obstacles set forth in macro- and meso-level analyses. Data are collected on factors of specific relevance to the individual's need for employment, education, training, housing, health care, technology, transportation, and food. For example, the microsystemic analysis would include home, work, and recreational site accessibility for an individual's particular abilities and for the assistive devices he or she uses or might purchase. A bathroom may have to be modified quite differently for use by a person who uses an electric wheelchair versus one who uses leg braces and arm crutches. Communication devices that are mass produced may have to be modified for the unique needs of the individual being studied.

This level of analysis is actually the dimension over which rehabilitation professionals have the most control and influence, the one that most allows them to effect change in order to attenuate the handicap situation of the person concerned, the consumer. Identifying specific personal needs is not an unfamiliar activity for clinical, community, and home care professionals. However, the professional making the assessment at the microsystemic level will need to cross-check the other two levels of analysis of environmental factors in order to determine eligibility for programs such as the allocation of hours of housekeeping services or assistive devices. Rehabilitation professionals should make much use of all three levels of analysis to set realistic objectives for effective intervention. Provision of these services in the places where individuals live, in their actual activities, and with their families and friends makes it possible for them to participate in activities that have meaning for them.

APPLICATION OF THE INTERACTION MODEL

Since the early 1990s, Fougeyrollas has conducted applied anthropological research at a day center of the Centre François-Charon in Québec City (Fougeyrollas, 1995b). This center provides a clinical intervention environment in which the standard consumer profile is a person with a level of disability requiring ongoing guidance or support to live in the community. These individuals come to the center as outpatients and thus live in private homes within the general boundaries of the Québec metropolitan area. From case studies drawn from this population, the focus here is on interrelationships between walking disabilities and access to assistive devices. All of the individuals studied had walking disabilities. Each consumer had to use a substitute for walking to be mobile. The interaction of environmental factors and assistive technologies in facilitating or inhibiting social participation by people with walking disabilities is illustrated in the following portion of this chapter. The example of the use of the interaction model provided therein is but a sample of the variables that could have been examined at each level of environmental analysis.

Macrosystemic Analysis—Economic System

Québec social and health policies provide people a manual or motorized wheelchair according to a professional assessment of their individual ability and circumstances requiring mobility. These case studies did not indicate any particular difficulty in obtaining this AT. Thus the economic system (fiscal) and the health and social services systems (assistive devices and rehabilitation programs) work together well to provide needed technology for people with motor disabilities. This is good evidence that Québec's socioeconomic policies play a crucial role in preventing handicap situations through coordination of different social support systems.

In countries in which this kind of program does not exist, people with the same walking disabilities as those living in Québec are unlikely to obtain a wheelchair and thus are extremely restricted in participating in life activities that require mobility. Therefore, these people would be, in current ICIDH terminology, more handicapped. In this case, the cause is the economic system. To reduce the handicap situation, the person would have to buy a wheelchair. The cost of this AT device varies from inexpensive to very expensive, depending on the complexity of the device. Thus, the person's level of social participation would be more or less severely restricted as a function of his or her income and the cost of AT. Clearly, the laws governing provision of AT for people with disabilities influence the degree of social participation they have. If the law stipulates that people with walking disabilities shall be provided with AT, then the level of the walking disability does not determine the level of social participation. The sophistication of the technology available becomes a prime factor in facilitating performance of activities of interest to the person with a walking disability.

Mesosystemic Analysis: Geographic and Architectural Factors

Many individuals at the day center use tricycles or electric wheelchairs to travel in their communities. The development of improved models of motorized wheelchairs and more sophisticated controls (e.g., operated with the head or foot) has enabled people who were previously completely immobilized to go shopping by themselves, visit accessible public places, travel to the movie theater, and even go out of their homes to work independently.

However, limitations in mobility for people using even these improved wheelchairs exist in the built and natural environments. Not all sidewalks have curb cuts. Many buildings have no access ramps, automatic doors, or elevators. All of these factors contribute to reduced social participation. A survey of accessible sites provided people with walking disabilities with information about where they could attend social events, reducing the handicap situation.

A variation of creating handicap situations would be to put those people who are unable to walk in a country setting. In natural settings, when activities involve traveling on unpaved roads and nature trails, obstacles such as uneven and unstable surfaces often prevent social participation. Even the most accommodating AT for mobility would have limited success in these types of topography. A systemic analysis of nature trails would at least provide people with different walking disorders who use assistive technologies information on which to base their decision on entering into activities conducted in the mapped geographic areas. Just such an effort is under way in the United States: Axelson (see Chapter 13) is making detailed trail maps from the perspective of people with walking or visual disabilities or both.

Microsystemic Analysis

Although assistive technologies are provided by Québec province for its citizens with walking disabilities, the exact specification of the technologies comes from assessments made by rehabilitation professionals. These specialists match the individual's capacity for function with the technical capabilities of assistive devices. If analysis shows that the person needs to control his or her electric wheelchair through hand, mouth, head, or voice control, the range of options of existing technologies is explored. The individual is given the opportunity to try to learn to use the device in optimal conditions. The consumer tests those devices that remain as options after the trial period as he or she performs tasks of everyday living within his or her local environments—home and work. Demands made in gaining access to local buildings and traveling on neighborhood sidewalks and streets are assessed. When all of these factors have been examined, the availability, reliability, and cost of the mobility devices remaining as options are considered. Finally, the equipment is ordered, delivered, and put in use. This careful, step-by-step microsystemic analysis of a variety of environmental variables has allowed us to provide people in Québec with AT that matches their needs and allows them to participate very well in society.

Conclusions Regarding the Interaction Model

This illustration of the relationship between the inability to walk and varying factors in physical and sociopolitical environments demonstrates that it is quite inadequate to consider only the dimension of a person's physical functional capacities in order to deduce or project their social consequences. The person's life history must also be analyzed. His or her self-identity is influenced by the onset of impairment and the impairment's influence on his or her ability to perform activities of choice. The social and situational contexts at the macro, meso, and micro levels must be considered in order to determine to what extent they facilitate or hinder the participation of the person in social activities and roles. The handicap situations of people with functional differences can be understood only in the light of a complete environmental analysis in terms of socioeconomic organization and ecological factors.

IMPACT OF CLASSIFICATION CHANGES ON SOCIAL CHANGE

Our purpose in seeking to understand the cultural handicap creation process is to contribute to potential changes in it. The fact is that handicaps do not exist in isolation, and there is no such thing as the "status" of "handicapped" people. There are only life situations in which the interaction between functional differences and the context leads to a discrepancy with the norm, with what would have happened in the same situation if the person did not have these differences. Without an evaluation of environmental factors, there can be no ecological approach to creating handicap situations, no oriented social change, no transformation of what in anthropology is called the *social normative creation process*. This is a major shift in approach to the classification of the consequences of disease and trauma, which had been characterized primarily by its biomedical roots and individual-centered perspective. The revision process has created new opportunities for participation by people with disabilities in the development of a classification system that will have direct effects on their lives. With the application of the interactive conceptual model, Fougeyrollas and colleagues intend to develop a methodology that will enable a planner, a clinician, or a person functioning differently to analyze the environment to assess its capacity to respond to the functional characteristics of a person or population.

Several categories of environmental obstacles are normally involved in creating a handicap situation. Thus, adding a fourth dimension of environmental factors requires the construction of standardized databases for each level of environmental analysis. Assessment instruments and methodologies for data collection are required. Organization and access routes for the use of the data need to be developed. Documenting the environmental factors associated with a handicap situation will involve not only health and rehabilitation specialists but also urban planners, economists, jurists, political scientists, sociologists, anthropologists, engineers, environmental experts, and many others. A methodological guide for use by each interested consumer will make it possible to increase the involvement and participation of experts and decision makers from a variety of disciplines. This strategy will enable us to draw up profiles of environmental barriers, compile standard profiles, and actually map obstacles unique to each society based on the broad categories of impairment with their associated functional disabilities. It is precisely this type of information that is needed by organizations dedicated to promoting the rights of people with disabilities and organizations that work to prevent handicap situations.

Scientific literature shows a definite interest in applying the tenets of ecological and environmental models to the study of the activities of people with impairments and disabilities. This underscores the burgeoning of new linkages among discipline- and sector-based perspectives that prior to the early 1990s were isolated from one another. This paradigm shift calls for cooperation among specialists in rehabilitation, social integration, education, and employment for people with disabilities. New studies will make their inquiries regardless of the cause or severity of the impairment or disability. Single-purpose administrative systems that have maintained separate processes for treatment, education, compensation, and access to other services are beginning to consider the benefits of the person–environment interaction model both for their programs and for the people they serve.

The recognition, proliferation, and benefits of applying the interaction approach to understanding what is important in the lives of people with impairments and disabilities are being acknowledged. This is especially evident in Québec, where the new conceptual model is being applied to interdisciplinary intervention as well as to policy and program planning. Another example is that the United Nations' standard rules on equal opportunity use the context of the activity in describing practices that produce social participation on equal terms. In the new preface to the ICIDH, the WHO (1993) recognized the importance of adopting an interactive person–environment model.

This approach raises exciting possibilities for adapting socioeconomic structures and transforming the built environment for increased use by people with impairments and disabilities. Changes will have to be made in urban planning, land use, and access to technologies. To facilitate this transition, the concepts of universal accessibility and barrier-free design must be embraced in their social context by architects, urban planners, engineers, economists, jurists, sociologists, policy planners, and politicians. The findings of studies based on the interaction model will be directly linked to the development of general multisector policies applicable to the entire process of preventing impairments, disabilities, and handicap situations. Formulation of national and local laws, policies, procedures, and regulations will be done with a better understanding of how they facilitate or inhibit the social participation of people with disabilities in the activities covered by the policy under consideration. This approach will make it possible to meet the expectations not only of organizations of people with impairments and disabilities but also of private and public partners collectively involved in the prevention of social and ecological obstacles to participation in society by such individuals.

Finally, this model will generate the type of information that can be used as a basis for international comparative studies of different sociocultural environments and their relationship to creating or preventing handicap situations. These studies will identify factors in culturally and geographically diverse environments that foster optimum participation in society by people with impairments and disabilities. This is the goal those in the disabilities field would like to reach. With the development of an international research and information network on environmental determinants of handicap situations and social participation of people with disabilities, the goal is attainable.

An intersectoral approach based on respect for individual differences will shatter the traditional, narrow view of people with disabilities as a social minority. Indeed, it is a clarion call for a complete transformation of our societies. New concepts of health as physical and social well-being will be formulated. Quality-of-life definitions will be centered on personal satisfaction in performing social life habits, day-to-day activities, and typical social roles in each cultural context. The main principles of the independent living movement will form the cornerstones of the plan to rebuild our societies. The transformed societies will engage people with impairments and disabilities as equal partners in decision making, provide for free and informed choice of life goals, reinforce self-reliance and participation in social activities, and promote access to and provision of services and technology that meet their individual needs.

REFERENCES

Bronfenbrenner, U. (1979). *The ecology of human development: Experiments by nature and design.* Cambridge, MA: Harvard University Press.

Fougeyrollas, P. (1993). *Applications of the concept of handicap of ICIDH and its nomenclature.* Strasbourg, France: Committee of Experts on the Applications of ICIDH, Council of Europe.

Fougeyrollas, P. (1995a). Documenting environmental factors for preventing the handicap creation process: Québec contributions relating to ICIDH and social participation of people with functional differences. *Disability and Rehabilitation, 17*(3-4), 145–153.

Fougeyrollas, P. (1995b). *Le processus de production culturelle du handicap: Contextes socio-historiques du développement des connaissances dans le champ des différences corporelles et fonctionnelles [The cultural handicap creation process: Sociohistoric contexts of the development of knowledge in the area of bodily and functional differences].* Québec, PQ, Canada: Québec Committee of the ICIDH.

Fougeyrollas, P., & St.-Michel, G. (1991). Proposal of a revised nomenclature of environmental factors: QCICIDH. *ICIDH International Network, 4*(1-2), 21–22.

Fougeyrollas, P., St.-Michel, G., Bergeron, H., & Cloutier, R. (1991). The handicap creation process: Analysis of the consultation: New full proposals. *ICIDH International Network, 4*(1-2), 8–37.

Fougeyrollas, P., St.-Michel, G., & Blouin, M. (1989). Consultation: Proposal for revision of the third level of the ICIDH: The handicap. *International ICIDH Network, 2*(1), 8–32.

Office des Personnes Handicapées du Québec. (1984). *On equal terms: Proposal of policy on prevention and social integration of persons with disabilities.* Québec, PQ, Canada: Les Publications du Québec.

Wood, P.H.N. (1980). The language of disablement: A glossary relating to disease and its consequences. *International Rehabilitation Medicine, 2*(2), 86–92.

World Health Organization (WHO). (1980). *International classification of impairments, disabilities, and handicaps* (ICIDH). Geneva: Author.

World Health Organization (WHO). (1993). *International classification of impairments, disabilities, and handicaps* (ICIDH). Geneva: Author.

CHAPTER 3

Personhood, Disablement, and Mobility Technology

Personal Control of Development

Steven A. Stiens

Sometimes rehabilitation/habilitation is like surgery from the skin . . . out.

(Shamberg, Stiens, & Shamberg, 1997, p. 86)

Mobility has a profound effect on who we are and who we become. Mobility offers two basic capabilities: travel through the environment and manipulation of the environment. Particular limitations in these capabilities as experienced by individuals offer unique problems potentially solved with assistive technology (AT).

This chapter presents a concept of the person that emphasizes his or her unique mobility needs. The importance of mobility in the relationship of the person with the environment is modeled. Next, the model is utilized to relate prescription of AT to patient-centered goals in the process of rehabilitation. Finally, the effect on the community of the successful integration of AT into the life of a person to increase his or her effectiveness is described.

The person is the focus of the rehabilitation process (Stiens, O'Young, & Young, 1997). When an individual's particular capabilities

The author would like to thank Karna McKinney and the author's daughter Hanna for rendering some of the figures in this chapter to clarify the concepts discussed in the text. As always, the author thanks Debra Roberts for word processing of the manuscript and seeking out references that relate the message to the good work of so many others.

are considered as a subject for rehabilitation intervention or evaluation, such capabilities must always be considered as related to the goals and activities of that person. The person is a particular living human being with characteristic genetic, physical, mental, social, and spiritual dimensions. The person is guided by past experiences, changes through development, and is consequently self-determining through life decisions made with free will. Personal behavior and development occur within the environment (Shamberg, Stiens, & Shamberg, 1997). Mobility therefore is fundamental to personhood because it provides the active link between the person and the environment. The environment as it has an impact on the person is the physical interface that presents barriers or accessibility and the social interface that presents prejudice or acceptance. The person therefore represents the real self as the subject of rehabilitation intervention within his or her environment and presents her or his vast resource of previous experience in world exploration to the rehabilitation team.

Therefore, personhood is the dynamic process of being and becoming the self. Awareness of the person's self-understanding is critical to the rehabilitation process because no one with a new injury comes to rehabilitation de novo (i.e., without a past history). Even the habilitation process for a disability apparent at birth begins with parental aspirations. A person's past mobility capability and his or her utilization of such capability is critical information for the interdisciplinary team. The person has the right of choice in problem solving and is the essential contributor to health goal setting. The person develops through adaptation. *Adaptation* may be defined simply as a change in the capabilities of the person as a result of interaction with the environment. This interaction could include communication, education, adaptive technology acquisition, prosthetic body part replacement, orthotic body support, environmental control, or environmental modification as part of the rehabilitation process. Mobility devices are enabling catalysts in this process. Persons act as patients when they ally with physicians as members of the interdisciplinary rehabilitation team.

PERSONAL DISABLEMENT:
THE BIOPSYCHOSOCIAL EFFECTS OF MOBILITY

To intervene on the person's behalf by enhancing mobility capability, it is necessary for members of the treatment team to have foci for intervention as well as a global perspective for the anticipated outcomes of such interventions. Engel (1980) has defined the relationships between biological systems with the biopsychosocial model (see Figure 1).

Event	Hierarchy of natural systems	Intersystem effects	Mobility intervention
	Biosphere	Spacecraft accessibility	Weightlessness and disability research
	↕	Airline accessibility	Redesign of aircraft
	Society–Nation	Discrimination, handicap	Achieve equal motor capacity with adaptation; social inoculation: Example in society
	↕	Disability attitudes	Demonstrate personal effectiveness to others
	Culture–Subculture	Religion participation	Redesign church architecture
	↕	Accessibility, vocation	Modification of streets, public buildings
	Community		
	↕	Role reorganization, recreation	Role-based task modification
	Family		
	↕	Sexuality	
	Two-Person		Positioning, adapted transfers, movement option
	↕	Psychological adjustment, depression risk	Minimize impairment, maximize environment exposure; reestablish control of manipulation of and in environment
	Person		
		Neuroplasticity	Support, facilitate self-initiated movement
	Nervous System	Spasticity, hyperreflexia	Position to minimize
	↕	Muscular atrophy	Promote use
	Organs/Organ Systems		
	↕	Decubiti	Minimize pressure and shear forces
	Tissues		
	↕	Denervation supersensitivity	Promote reinnervation
	Cells	Transsynaptic degeneration	Promote voluntary movement
	↕		
	Organelles		
	↕	Inflammatory mediators	Stabilize, minimize reinjury
	Molecules		
	↕		
	Atoms	Osteoporosis	Promote weight bearing

Nervous injury ↑ ↑ ↑ ↑

Figure 1. Intersystem effects of interventions to enhance personal mobility. (Nervous system injury secondary effects and interventions to improve mobility are related to the hierarchy of natural systems as outlined by Engel. Intersystem effects that could result from a severe nervous system injury or rehabilitation interventions are listed in the column in the middle. In the far right column, interventions at various system levels that would enhance personal mobility are listed. Mobility impairments as secondary effects from many potential causes prevent the achievement of personal goals. Intersystem effects must be a consideration in evaluating patient's mobility status. The results of such interventions must be interpreted with pertinent data that relate to the person along the entire axis of the systems hierarchy.) (↕, effect of systems on one another.) (Hierarchy of natural systems column from Engel, G. [1980]. The clinical application of the Biopsychosocial Model. *American Journal of Psychiatry, 137*[5], 537. Copyright © 1980 by the American Psychiatric Association. Reprinted by permission.)

31

The hierarchy of natural systems is a continuum of discrete organizational levels that illustrates the relatedness of interacting systems. These various systems provide targets for rehabilitation intervention and foci for assessment of outcome (Stiens, Haselkorn, Peters, & Goldstein, 1996). The person is entwined with interdependent relatedness to this hierarchy, necessitating a broad view when assessing the impact of interventions to enhance personal mobility (Stiens et al., 1996).

Particularly germane to rehabilitation are classification systems for disablement, such as the *International Classification of Impairments, Disabilities and Handicaps* (ICIDH) of the World Health Organization (1993). This framework categorizes the consequences or secondary effects of a disease or injury into the organ level (impairment), whole-person level (disability), and societal level (handicap) and has been succinctly reviewed by Badley (1993). This topology has been further modified to distinguish between functional activities and task-based, whole-person activities (Figure 2) (National Center for Medical Rehabilitation Research, 1993).

The term *disablement* is a summary term for all of these consequences of injury, disease, or abnormality on the person (Badley, 1993). Peters (1995, 1996a, 1996b) has argued that the subjective experience of the person in disablement is as valid for clinical research and theory development as it is for the clinical process of interdisciplinary rehabilitation. Disablement can be modeled using a framework that includes the organ, person, and societal levels as experienced by the person in disablement (insider), the outsider, and the interventionist (rehabilitation discipline) (Peters, 1996a). Furthermore, these consequences of disease can be sorted by system level as outlined in the hierarchy of natural systems (i.e., impairment–organ, disability–person, handicap–community). It should also be clear that people have capabilities and advantages at these multiple system levels that serve to compensate for and overcome many of the secondary effects of disease as well. For example, options for community mobility are associated with reduced handicap in people with mobility disabilities (McDonough, Badley, & Tennant, 1995). Therefore, a person's formulation of mobility goals must be carefully integrated into the rehabilitation plan because these individual mobility goals project into life goals of the person as related to the world.

Quantification of the contribution of interventions to improve personal mobility requires broad assessment of the far-reaching effects. Many researchers are investigating associations among reduction in the secondary effects of injuries, the cost of treatment

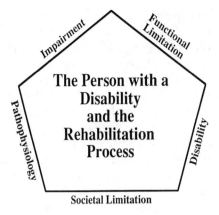

Figure 2.   The domains of science relevant to medical rehabilitation. Five domains that have an impact on the function of the person have been identified by the National Center for Medical Rehabilitation Research as areas for inquiry and assessment. The individual with a disability must simultaneously resolve or adapt to problems within all five domains. (From National Center for Medical Rehabilitation Research. [1993]. *Research plan for the National Center for Medical Rehabilitation Research* [NIH Publication No. 93-3509] [p. 34]. Bethesda, MD: National Institutes of Health.)

(Batavia, 1992), and health policy (Frattali, 1993). In addition, there are person-centered models of assessment and intervention that emphasize derivation of unique goals as defined by the individual and the rehabilitation team. Success can also be quantified with goal attainment scaling (Kiresuk, Smith, & Cardillo, 1994) through ordinal scoring of the degree of attainment of a variety of patient-specific goals. The fullest perspective must include data regarding the effects of mobility at each of the system levels that surround and make up the person (see Figure 1) (Stiens et al., 1996).

PERSONAL MOBILITY: MULTIPLE PERSPECTIVES ON THE MULTIPLE EFFECTS OF INTERVENTION

There are a number of perspectives that illustrate the varied effects of mobility on these various interacting systems. Mechanical interventions to reachieve functional movement may contribute to motor recovery as well. This is the perspective of *restorative neurology*, which attempts to promote neuroplastic motor recovery. This discipline focuses at the nervous system level of the hierarchy of natural systems (see Figure 1). Advances in the understanding of the nervous system have demonstrated that anatomical distinctions between sensory and motor areas are not as hard and fast as previously imagined. This mix of sensory and motor neurons at the anatomical level has provided a rationale for developing therapeutics at the functional level. In a motor cortex stimulation and recording study with a grid of electrodes applied to the cortex, Uematsu and colleagues showed that the primary motor and sensory cortices are actually anatomically intertwined (Nii, Uematsu, Lesser, & Gordon, 1996; Uematsu et al., 1992). Because sensory and motor function are therefore inseparably intertwined and interdependent, sensory stimuli may affect motor recovery.

Devices that enable spontaneous mobility have been demonstrated to reduce the severity of motor impairments after stroke by producing a paradigm for interaction with the environment that facilitates repeated use of recovering motor capabilities and sensory cues for gait recovery (Nugent, Schurr, & Adams, 1994). These findings have been replicated with interventions that provide weight-supported movement to enable spontaneous mobility and locomotor recovery after stroke (Hesse et al., 1995). Therapies that stress repeated use of recovering motor capabilities and sensory cues can contribute to sensorimotor development (Sporns & Edelman, 1993) and improve motor recovery. Such interventions not only produce changes at the level of the nervous system but also reinforce a healthy relationship with the environment. The patient integrates the perception that there is hope for recovery and the potential for meeting his or her personal goals in spite of impaired mobility (MacDonald, 1971).

Another perspective is that of phenomenology, which focuses on the immediate experience of the person. Phenomenology, initially described by Husserl (1954), is a branch of philosophy that breaks with the long-held concept of Cartesian dualism that splits the person into mind and body. Phenomenologists question the philosophical completeness of natural science. They also seek to rewrite quantitative science with personal life experiences and to explore the relationship between the abstract world of the sciences and the concrete world of human experience (Baron, 1985). *Medical phenomenology* is therefore the philosophical study of the lived experience of the body: "embodiment." From the phenomenological perspective, mobility is part of the person, a way of being and acting within the environment. The "person with body" experience of the self is a developmental process that begins in infancy with exploration of sensory awareness boundaries. As a child matures, experimentation with the animated body within the environment provides cues to the developing and adapting nervous system. Other systems adapt as well; for example, the musculoskeletal system adapts to upright standing and the strength demands of activity.

These "person with body in environment" experiences are essentially operant experiments that confirm or refute the person's perceived world impact and capacity to independently meet his or her physical needs in the environment. The study of the body–environment experiences in rehabilitation requires interdisciplinary research that emphasizes analysis of multiple simultaneous systems contributions to the effects of therapeutics and devices that are intended to improve mobility (Redford, 1993; Spencer, Young, Rintala, & Bates, 1995; Stiens et al., 1996).

The clinical understanding of the person as interacting with the environment through mobility must come through interviews, with an emphasis on understanding the person's unique experience and needs. Provision and trial of an AT device as an intervention to adapt the person–environment interaction must include a discussion of the person's perspectives on the experience of interacting with the environment with the device. A kinetic analysis of adapted activity to demonstrate greater efficiency with mobility tasks is only part of the rehabilitation process to achieve personal adaptive mobility. The person's experience of mobility with the AT device in multiple environments must be elicited and analyzed. Mobility devices are often experienced as extensions of the body and certainly catalyze the relationship of the body to the environment.

The lived experience of embodiment can be simply modeled (Figure 3) with representations of the person interacting with the environment. Analysis of this interaction comes from examination of stimulus-and-response characteristics as originated from the person as well as aspects of the environment.

Yet another perspective, that of *interdisciplinary research*, emphasizes multiple simultaneous analyses of the effects of mobility at varied system levels (Figure 1) as perceived by various specialists. The trend toward interdisciplinary research emphasizes multiple simultaneous systems analyses of the effects of mobility at varied system levels. Inclusion of varied disciplines in the continuum of research allows for broad conceptualizations of the needs of the user. Such groups present challenges for the communication of perspectives and for a consensus that will guide AT and rehabilitation projects from restrictive problem definitions to wholistic solutions (Orpwood, 1990).

Often engineering approaches are similar to that of the medical model: diagnosis and solution. Such restrictive views that confine perspectives to a single system or disablement domain (e.g., impairments, disabilities) are less likely to lead to devices that will fully complement the person and enhance effects up and down the hier-

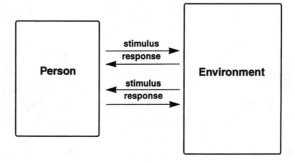

Figure 3.   The person schematically illustrated interacting with the environment. The person represents a unique invidividual in a particular place in space and within society. The environment represents all of the physical and psychosocial effects having an impact on the person at the current place and time. The person presents stimuli to the environment that may evoke a response. Simultaneously, the environment presents stimuli to the person that may take the form of physical barriers, accessibility, discrimination, or social acceptance.

archy of natural systems. Alternatively, the broad interdisciplinary expert representation allows for immediate consideration of the wide repercussions of devices, minimizing side effects and recognizing spin-off advantages that may be built into the design. These considerations maximize personal and societal acceptance and promote compatibility of the device as an adaptive tool at all person–environmental interfaces and system levels.

Finally, the perspective of *participatory action research* emphasizes the role of the consumer as end user for the final product (i.e., the device or intervention). Inclusion of consumers in the process of needs assessment (Prior, 1990), study design, and prototype development and testing allows for feedback as to their expectations and the actual effect of the AT devices on their lives (Batavia & Hammer, 1990; Kejlaa, 1993). Consumers test the assistive device as whole persons in real-life activities within their real world, producing perceptions that feed back into the iterative device development process (Orpwood, 1990). This approach requires consumer input on the dimensions of practicality, device demand, use, and maintenance of AT. Batavia and Hammer (1990) summarized consumer-based criteria for evaluation of assistive devices. They used the Delphi technique to come to a consensus on factors for consumer satisfaction, which included (in order of importance) effectiveness, affordability, operability, dependability, portability, durability, compatibility (with other AT devices and the environment), flexibility, ease of maintenance, securability, learnability, personal acceptance, physical comfort, supplier repair, customer repair, and ease of assembly.

PERSON-CENTERED REHABILITATION: INTERVENTIONS TO RESTORE MOBILITY

As part of a comprehensive program, the rehabilitation team must integrate these many perspectives to the extent that they include therapeutics focused on enhancing personal mobility. In contrast to classical medical therapeutics, which emphasizes diagnosis and treatment directed against the pathological process, rehabilitation orchestrates multiple simultaneous interventions addressing both the cause and the secondary effects of illness (Stiens et al., 1997). Traditionally, medical science has emphasized diagnosis to explain illness in terms of biology, physiology, or anatomy and has directed treatment at the cause of disease. This reductionistic technique leads to the neglect of the secondary effects of illness as therapeutic foci. The very nature of rehabilitation includes assessment of the individual's personal task capacities and life aspirations. Mobility objectives must be closely linked to a patient's life goals and objectives in areas such as typical development (Butler, 1986; Butler, Okamoto, & McKay, 1983, 1984), independent living, and vocation. Human capacities serve the person when they are exercised in chosen tasks that meet the life goals of the individual. Such activity as carried out is self-creative and developmental.

   Rehabilitation has been defined as the development of a person to his or her fullest physical, psychological, social, vocational, avocational, and educational potential consistent with his or her physiological or anatomical impairment and environmental limitations (DeLisa, Martin, & Currie, 1993). Mobility goals must be prioritized to allow for higher-level education and vocational goal attainment. Comprehensive rehabilitation can be further considered to require five necessary and sufficient subcomponents (Table 1) (Stiens et al., 1996). Priorities for mobility must be established early in rehabilitation through interdisiplinary planning in order to permit the patient's fullest participation in the overall rehabilitation program (Stiens et al., 1997).

REHABILITATION OF THE PERSON: THE PROCESS

The process of rehabilitation includes multiple simultaneous interventions from many perspectives. As a result, there are many con-

Table 1.   Conditions for comprehensive rehabilitation

- Unique patient-centered plan is formulated by the patient and the rehabilitation team.
- Goals are derived and prioritized through an interdisciplinary process.
- Patient participation is required to achieve the goals.
- Plan results in an improvement in the patient's personal potential.
- Outcomes demonstrate reductions in impairments, disabilities, and handicaps.

cepts of this process (Stiens et al., 1997). Many of them are directed primarily toward the restoration of mobility, although many others are dependent on successful achievement of mobility solutions for the patient. First, the age-old concept of rehabilitation as a convalescent period of rest for natural recovery from acute illness should not be underestimated because a significant amount of spontaneous recovery is routinely observed after injury to the nervous system.

A second concept of the rehabilitation process includes the familiar approach of impairment restoration to remediate limitations in functional capacity—for example, strengthening or prosthetic replacement of the damaged part. A third concept is task reachievement or refinement of skills, which provides compensatory or modified techniques for achievement of goals. This involves modification of residual skills through teaching the person with disabilities to compensate or modify actions using a device to achieve mobility goals. Application of orthotics or tools as solutions for carrying out activities is a component of the task enhancement and impairment restoration concepts.

Performance of complex activities is accomplished through adaptation of behaviors associated with learning to use a new mobility-enhancing device. A third concept, successful acquisition of disability-appropriate behaviors, is reinforced, and disability-inappropriate behaviors are extinguished. This concept of the process clarifies rehabilitation as adaptation of the individual with disabilities to his or her unique situation in disablement through use of residual capabilities.

The concept of environment modification—adaptation of environment to the person as he or she is—has become a more common approach utilized in rehabilitation (Shamberg et al., 1997). Such changes reduce handicap by reducing barriers to performance through changing a person's experienced environment (Stiens & Stiens, 1993). Aspects of the environment include physical (e.g., doors, curb cuts, ramps), psychological (e.g., attitudes, prejudice, discrimination), and social (e.g., culture, laws, rituals) factors.

Finally, rehabilitation can be conceptualized as patient self-actualization, which is essentially improvement of personhood through increasing the individual's personal effectiveness. AT can contribute to desired personal independence and vocational options (Hammel, 1995; Hammel, Van der Loos, & Perkash, 1992). It is necessary to approach the person with mobility impairment as an individual who is attempting to self-actualize by using a changed and different body that is enabled through AT.

In actuality, each person's rehabilitation process is based on many of these concepts and includes many subroutines. The fullest understanding of the rehabilitation process comes with the experience of how these concepts converge. An immediate goal of rehabilitation is the enhancement of independent mobility. This restores the dynamic relationship between the person and the environment that allows continued self-initiated development through person–environment interaction. Improving personhood after injury or chronic disease requires the development of new personal skills that are effective in managing person–environment interactions. Each rehabilitation perspective includes many subroutines, but all are directed at restoring this dynamic relationship. When the person with a disability is able to self-initiate actions that enhance his or her independent mobility, then a primary goal of rehabilitation has been achieved (Bailey, 1994; Platts & Fraser, 1993).

Person–Environment Interactions:
Adaptive Environmental Enhancement.

No discussion of the process of requisition of personal mobility would be complete without exploration of the relationship of the person to the environment (Shamberg et al., 1997). Even before people sought to occupy heaven, environmental modification was a characteristic of the human race, for better or for worse. The environment as related to the person can be divided into sectors. There has been a drive to modify, craft, and assemble the *immediate* (i.e., in direct physical contact with the person [e.g., wheelchair]), *intermediate* (i.e., personal space at home or at work), and *community environments* (i.e., spaces modified for public use) as part of becoming and being. There are strong associations between our capabilities and the characteristics of the environments in which we function. This human creation process is critically important when the unique capabilities of individuals with disabilities are considered. Adaptive environmental enhancement is yet another rehabilitation intervention to minimize the effects of impairment, disability, and handicap on the person. Such enhancement facilitates the presence of the person to the environment while maximizing personal capabilities, facilitating evolving skills, and magnifying the impact of the person's efforts. These experiences reinforce the presumption that the person can act through the environment to meet his or her needs (Partridge & Johnston, 1989; Stickland, 1978).

Essentially, behavior is carried out and played out against or through the medium of the physical environment. Mobility is crucial for development (Butler, 1986; Butler et al., 1983, 1984). The human maturation process requires physical interaction with the environment to develop functional mobility and to facilitate physical adaptation. The variety of physical capabilities acquired in this interaction defines the freedom to move about and modify the environment to personal specifications. These experiences of mastery are internalized as self-discovery and development. Mastery becomes a behavioral pattern that is successful and is acted out in relationship to the world. It is uniquely human to adapt to the environment and adapt the environment to our specifications.

Immediately after a catastrophic illness or injury, the experience of the lived body is radically different, which produces a new relationship between the person and the environment. Person–environment interactions are altered by both a changed body (e.g., paralysis) and a changed environment (e.g., hospital). The body image may be altered as a result of new limitations in perception, sensation, or motor performance and loss of body parts. Environmental perception may be altered as a result of sensory impairment or neglect. This situation is compounded by the depersonalization of hospitalization. The person with a newly acquired injury loses his or her identity (e.g., father, teacher, movie star) and becomes a patient. The person is separated from the immediate environment of clothes and personal objects and confined to a bed in a horizontal position.

The relationship of the patient to the environment is often determined in the interaction of patient pathophysiology with the medical institution. Communication as a means to share personal identity and to alter the physical environment frequently dominates this interaction. Repeated requests for assistance and communication can put significant demands on staff time. Patients may be labeled as "problems" if attention is not given to the radical change in their physical capabilities and the necessary adaptation process. Comprehensive rehabilitation intervention is useful to establish a bridge that maintains a rudimentary capability for environmental manipulation by the patient. This can be as simple as modified call light switches, telephone modifications, page turners, modified drinking straws, and mouth sticks. Reengineering of the immediate environment contributes to the rehabilitation outcome by putting the patient in control. These experiences confirm the patients' belief in their capacity to meet their own needs (MacDonald, 1971).

This situation of a person in a new body struggling to adapt to the hospital environment can be compared with that of an infant in a crib testing the environment (Shamberg et al., 1997). This testing and modifying of the environment through verbal and physical interaction is crucial for beginning the problem-solving process and eliminating potential barriers to independence. The new relationship must be recultivated through physical interaction in the changed body. The patient carries memories, impressions, attitudes, and fantasies about his or her new physical state into this reality. Patients' projections regarding their capability to continue as persons in the world in spite of their new state of paralysis often affect their decisions to pursue further medical care and even to go on living (Rodgers, Field, & Kunkel, 1995). Early experiments of environmental interaction in the new state confirm or refute such impressions and color the person's future expectations. The ongoing process of adaptation is an operant process that is facilitated by multiple repetitions, spontaneous activities, and a variety of perceptual and physical interactions.

Rehabilitation professionals should facilitate the patient's articulation of feelings and memories of satisfaction with past physical prowess through experiences with the physical world in their lived bodies. After injuries that produce mobility impairments, the patient's experience changes radically. These dialogues help the practitioner to identify patient expectations and plan interventions to reestablish successful interaction with the environment. Alterations in the person's immediate and intermediate environment enables the person to reachieve an ongoing expression of personhood and successfully interact with the physical environment. The patient moves toward achieving self-feeding, dressing, and using and manipulating environmental controls (e.g., bed, call light, television, telephone). Independent transfers and mobility to and from the bed are achieved as soon as possible. The goal is for the individual to rediscover a healthy interaction with the environment that he or she can generalize to the achievement of his or her personal goals for the future. This may require the demonstration of solutions offered through technology or environmental design early in the rehabilitation process.

The full capabilities of the patient are difficult to predict early in the rehabilitation process. Emphasis must initially be placed on the team knowledge of the person's activity in environments before the injury. The lived experience of embodiment can be simply modeled with representations of the person interacting with the environment (Figure 3). Analysis of the interaction comes from examination of stimulus-and-response characteristics as originated from the person as well as aspects of the environment.

Knowledge of patient activity from the recent past can be elicited through retrospective sociobehavioral mapping (i.e., review of a typical 1-week period for patient location, activity, and companionship). The chronology of the rehabilitation process from the perspective of the environment can be understood as a continuum that starts with the design of the person's immediate environment (e.g., braces, wheelchair) and progresses to the intermediate environment (e.g., their home and work) and then to the community and natural environments (Figure 4) (Shamberg et al., 1997). Decisions must be very tentative, and the rehabilitation process must be physically participative. Assessment of the home environment can include floor plans, photographic or videotaped depictions, or home visits. The progression homeward must include experimentation and interaction with the environment after physically entering it (e.g., therapeutic leave of absence, pass, predischarge home visits, outings in the community). Kinetic exploration and experimentation with interventions is essential. In essence, the goal is to progressively design an environment that enhances personhood and reflects the characteristics and goals of the individual and others living in the home.

Person–Device–Environment
Interactions: Personal Impact of Assistive Technology

An adaptive mobility device becomes a part of the person's immediate environment (Figure 4). The device occupies a position as an intermediary between the person and the greater environment. The installation of an adaptive mobility device into the person–environment interaction precipitates a new series of stimulus–response sets that occur at the person–device, device–environment, and person–environment interfaces (Figure 5). At the person–device interface there are issues of comfort, device control, and personal acceptance. When using the device over time, it is often absorbed into the body image (i.e., the mind's picture of one's own body) of the user. At the device–environment interface, there are issues of physical compatibility and the perception of the device by others (persons and animals) within the environment. Ideally, the user of the assistive device has the most control over the activity at these interfaces. However, the device itself may trigger the curiosity of

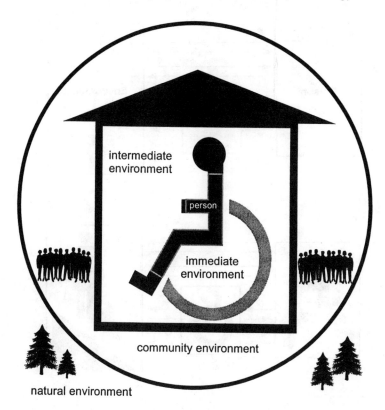

Figure 4.   The person and sectors of the environment. The diagram relates the person who experiences disablement to adaptive equipment and to his or her environment. The *environment* is that which is outside the person. The *immediate environment* is directly in contact with the person and moves with the person (e.g., clothes, adaptive equipment). The *intermediate environment* is the personal living space (i.e., home) and work space (i.e., office). The *community environment* is the space modified for public use. The *natural environment* is the space that has been minimally changed or left unaltered.

observers and act as a lightning rod for questions and comments. Living in society as a perceived curiosity requires the development of adaptive social skills in addition to those for mobility (Braithwaite, 1991). For example, the presence of a mobility impairment offers challenges to typical development and socialization in children with disabilities (Honeyman, 1977).

An adaptive device should ideally magnify personhood and certainly not eclipse the person. The device must not be confused with the user in spite of the intimate contact between the device and the user's body (Figure 6). The device itself presents with the person and should support the intent of the person through nonverbal com-

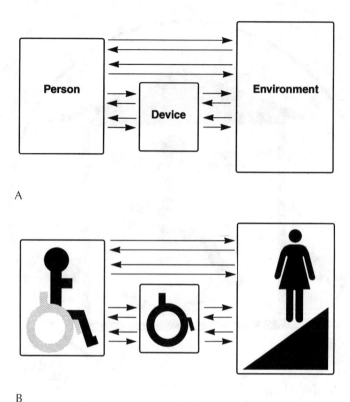

A

B

Figure 5.   Person–device–environment interactions. A) The diagram represents the person as related to the total environment. The arrows represent stimulus–response pairs as explained in Figure 3. The person generates stimuli that affect the environment and elicit a response. The environment also generates stimuli for the person requiring a personal response. The device itself generates stimuli and responses that must be considered in its design and use as an intervention. B) A representation of the considerations that exist in the use of a wheelchair to provide adaptive mobility to a person with spinal cord injury. The box at the left represents the person requiring a wheelchair for mobility. The wheelchair that acts as the adaptive device is shown interacting with the user as well as the persons and physical characteristics within the environment. This situation evokes a variety of stimulus–response sets that gauge the success of the adaptive fit of the device to the circumstances of the user.

munication (Deegan, 1977). People within the environment should receive from the person *and* the device an image that most fully represents who the user is. Personal style is an important mechanism of self-expression through design and choice to fill the person's immediate environment. The market provision of a variety of colors, designs, and sizes of some assistive devices offers the user

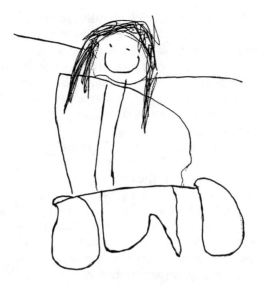

Figure 6.   Pen drawing of the author of this chapter by his daughter Hanna (4 years old). When drawing her father, a T2 complete paraplegic, Hanna depicted his animate parts (upper extremities). The lower limbs are one with the wheelchair: The person and the chair are continuous. Although the author and the wheelchair may be perceived as one by the author's daughter, thankfully the "wheelchair part" has been received positively and compared to a stroller or bicycle by many young observers.

the opportunity to choose them as his or her own. Personal choice of a device that reflects the self in its appearance is often a user's first consideration.

In addition, the functionally enhancing characteristics of the device should meet with the life goals of the person. Bozzacco (1993) explored the experience of adaptively compensated persons with spinal cord injury living in the community. As they recounted their experiences of mobility after spinal cord injury, three predominant themes emerged: Paralysis increases the time necessary to achieve movement, mobility requires more planning, and the seating position affects communication. An adapted mobility device should enable the person to project him- or herself effectively in interpersonal interactions. The device should also facilitate communication, enabling gesture and positioning for ideal mutual perception of communicated meanings during interaction.

Successful user–device combinations should also present examples to society of the unique solutions to mobility impairments of a particular person. The device should illustrate how the particular user uniquely compensates for disability. Through experience and interactions with these effective persons as users of adaptive devices, society will grow in appreciation of the contribution of AT to adaptation to mobility impairments. This is expected to produce even greater openness of people to those individuals with adapted mobility. An effective person visibly adapted with a technological device provides an example to society of the usefulness of the device in enhancing personhood. An individual who successfully projects his or her personhood by performing in his or her role and interacting with and acting on the environment with adapted mobility will therefore function as a *social inoculum* against society's negative images. People who encounter such an individual will spread new attitudes, resulting in greater openness and genuine positive interest in others who utilize adapted mobility devices.

Evaluation of device effectiveness should be primarily focused on the remediation of impairments and disabilities of the consumer. Evaluation should begin in the hospital with patient and staff responses (Dijkers, deBear, Erlandson, & Kristy, 1991) and extend to the family and community (Brooks, 1991). Patient and family expectations as well as experience using the device in the field must be explored through interview and discussion. However, the objectives for the design of the device must consider all interfaces between the user, the device, and the environment. The biopsychosocial model offers a checklist of system-level categories that allow for consideration of scenarios exploring intended effects and side effects within each system sphere. In conclusion, effective device interventions should ultimately enhance personhood; catalyze the adaptation process at all relevant system hierarchy levels; minimize impairment, disability, and handicap; and aim for consumer satisfaction and maximum acceptance (Batavia & Hammer, 1990; Brooks, 1991).

REFERENCES

Badley, E. (1993). An introduction to the concepts and classifications of the *International Classification of Impairments, Disabilities and Handicaps. Disability and Rehabilitation, 15*(4), 161–178.

Bailey, D. (1994). Technology for adults with multiple impairments: A trilogy of case reports. *American Journal of Occupational Therapy, 48*(4), 341–345.

Baron, R.J. (1985). An introduction to medical phenomenology: I can't hear you while I'm listening. *Annals of Internal Medicine, 103*, 606–611.

Batavia, A. (1992). Assessing the function of functional assessment: A consumer perspective. *Disability and Rehabilitation, 14*(3), 156–160.

Batavia, A., & Hammer, G. (1990). Toward the development of consumer-based criteria for the evaluation of assistive devices. *Journal of Rehabilitation Research, 27*(4), 425–436.

Bozzacco, V. (1993). Long-term psychosocial effects of spinal cord injury. *Rehabilitation Nursing, 18*(2), 82–87.

Braithwaite, D. (1991). Just how much did that wheelchair cost? Management of privacy boundaries by persons with disabilities. *Western Journal of Speech Communication, 55*, 254–274.

Brooks, N.A. (1991). Users' responses to assistive devices for physical disability. *Social Science and Medicine, 32*(12), 1417–1424.

Butler, C. (1986). Effects of powered mobility on self-initiated behaviors of very young children with locomotor disability. *Developmental Medicine and Child Neurology, 28*, 325–332.

Butler, C., Okamoto, G., & McKay, T. (1983). Powered mobility for very young disabled children. *Developmental Medicine and Child Neurology, 25*, 472–474.

Butler, C., Okamoto, G., & McKay, T. (1984). Motorized wheelchair driving by disabled children. *Archives of Physical Medicine and Rehabilitation, 65*, 95–97.

Deegan, M. (1977). The non-verbal communication of the physically handicapped. *Journal of Sociology and Social Welfare, 4*, 735–748.

DeLisa, J., Martin, G., & Currie, D. (1993). Rehabilitation medicine: Past, present, and future. In J. DeLisa (Ed.), *Rehabilitation medicine: Principles and practice* (2nd ed., pp. 3–24). Philadelphia: J.B. Lippincott.

Dijkers, M., deBear, P., Erlandson, R., & Kristy, K. (1991). Patient and staff acceptance of robotic technology in occupational therapy: A pilot study. *Journal of Rehabilitation Research and Development, 28*(2), 33–44.

Engel, G. (1980). The clinical application of the Biopsychosocial Model. *American Journal of Psychiatry, 137*(5), 535–544.

Frattali, C. (1993). Perspectives on functional assessment: Its use for policy making. *Disability and Rehabilitation, 15*(1), 1–9.

Hammel, J., Van der Loos, H.F.M., & Perkash, I. (1992). Evaluation of a vocational robot with a quadriplegic employee. *Archives of Physical Medicine and Rehabilitation, 73*, 683–693.

Hammel, J.M. (1995). The role of assessment and evaluation in rehabilitation robotics research and development: Moving from concept to clinic to context. *IEEE Transactions on Rehabilitation Engineering, 3*(1), 56–61.

Hesse, S., Bertelt, C., Jahnke, M., Schaffrin, A., Baake, P., Malezic, M., & Mauritz, K. (1995). Treadmill training with partial body weight support compared with physiotherapy in nonambulatory hemiparetic patients. *Stroke, 26*(6), 976–981.

Honeyman, A. (1977). *Sam and his cart.* St. Paul, MN: EMC Publishing.

Husserl, E. (1954). *The crisis of European sciences* (D. Carr, trans.). Evanston, IL: Northwestern University Press.

Kejlaa, G. (1993). Consumer concerns and the functional value of prostheses to upper limb amputees. *Prosthetics and Orthotics International, 17*, 157–163.

Kiresuk, T., Smith, A., & Cardillo, J. (Eds.). (1994). *Goal attainment scaling: Applications, theory and measurement.* Hillsdale, NJ: Lawrence Erlbaum Associates.

MacDonald, A. (1971). Internal–external locus of control: A promising rehabilitation variable. *Journal of Counseling Psychology, 18*(2), 111–116.

McDonough, P., Badley, E., & Tennant, A. (1995). Disability, resources, role demands and mobility handicap. *Disability and Rehabilitation, 17*(3-4), 159–168.

National Center for Medical Rehabilitation Research. (1993). *Research plan for the National Center for Medical Rehabilitation Research* (NIH Publication No. 93-3509). Bethesda, MD: National Institutes of Health.

Nii, Y., Uematsu, S., Lesser, R., & Gordon, B. (1996). Does the central sulcus divide motor and sensory functions? Cortical mapping of human hand areas as revealed by electrical stimulation through subdural grid electrodes. *Neurology, 46,* 360–367.

Nugent, J.A., Schurr, K.A., & Adams, R.D. (1994). A dose–response relationship between amount of weight-bearing exercise and walking outcome following cerebrovascular accident. *Archives of Physical Medicine and Rehabilitation, 75*(4), 399–402.

Orpwood, R. (1990). Design methodology for aids for the disabled. *Journal of Medical Engineering and Technology, 14*(1), 2–10.

Partridge, C., & Johnston, M. (1989). Perceived control of recovery from physical disability: Measurement and prediction. *British Journal of Clinical Psychology, 28,* 53–59.

Peters, D. (1995). Human experience in disablement: The imperative of the ICIDH. *Disability and Rehabilitation, 17*(3-4), 135–144.

Peters, D. (1996a). Disablement observed, addressed, and experienced: Integrating subjective experience into disablement models. *Disability and Rehabilitation, 18*(12), 593–603.

Peters, D. (1996b). Expanding rehabilitation medicine's research repertoire: A commentary. *American Journal of Physical Medicine and Rehabilitation, 75*(2), 144–148.

Platts, R., & Fraser, M. (1993). Assistive technology in the rehabilitation of patients with high spinal cord lesions. *Paraplegia, 31,* 280–287.

Prior, S. (1990). An electric wheelchair mounted robotic arm: A survey of potential users. *Journal of Medical Engineering and Technology, 14*(4), 143–154.

Redford, J. (1993). Seating and wheeled mobility in the disabled elderly population. *Archives of Physical Medicine and Rehabilitation, 74,* 877–885.

Rodgers, C., Field, H.L., & Kunkel, E.J. (1995). Countertransference issues in termination of life support in acute quadraplegia. *Psychosomatics, 36*(3), 305–308.

Shamberg, S., Stiens, S., & Shamberg, A. (1997). Personal enablement through environmental modifications. In B. O'Young, M. Young, & S. Stiens (Eds.), *Physical medicine and rehabilitation secrets* (pp. 86–93). Philadelphia: Hanley & Belfus.

Spencer, J., Young, M., Rintala, D., & Bates, S. (1995). Socialization to the culture of a rehabilitation hospital: An ethnographic study. *American Journal of Occupational Therapy, 49*(1), 53–62.

Sporns, O., & Edelman, G. (1993). Solving Bernstein's problem: A proposal for the development of coordinated movement by selection. *Child Development, 64,* 960–981.

Stickland, B. (1978). Internal–external expectancies and health-related behaviors. *Journal of Consulting and Clinical Psychology, 46*(6), 1192–1211.

Stiens, D., & Stiens, S. (1993). Environmental modifications and role function: Redesign of a rowhouse for a family with a paraplegic father. *Journal of the American Paraplegia Society, 16*(4), 278–279.

Stiens, S., Haselkorn, J., Peters, J., & Goldstein, B. (1996). Rehabilitation intervention for patients with upper extremity dysfunction: Challenges of outcome evaluation. *American Journal of Industrial Medicine, 29,* 590–601.

Stiens, S., O'Young, B., & Young, M. (1997). The person, disablement and the process of rehabilitation. In B. O'Young, M. Young, & S. Stiens (Eds.), *Physical medicine and rehabilitation secrets* (pp. 1–4). Philadelphia: Hanley & Belfus.

Uematsu, S., Lesser, R., Gordon, B., Hara, K., Krauss, G., Vining, E., & Webber, R. (1992). Motor and sensory cortex in humans: Topography studied with chronic subdural stimulation. *Neurosurgery, 31*(1), 59–70.

World Health Organization. (1993). *International classification of impairments, disabilities, and handicaps.* Geneva: Author.

CHAPTER 4

The Spheres of Self-Fulfillment

A Multidimensional Approach to the Assessment of Assistive Technology Outcomes

Margaret G. Stineman

This chapter describes existing classifications for studying people with ongoing medical conditions and how they might be applied to the use of assistive technology (AT). Linkages are provided between classification schemes used to describe factors influencing the lives of people with disabilities and various AT devices used to increase the effectiveness of person–environment interactions. Measurement tools are proposed for quantifying AT influences on the capacity of people to perform activities.

Assistive technology can be defined broadly as any technical application inside (intrinsic), outside (extrinsic), or distant from the body that enhances the person's ability to move about and function within the environment. The mode of action of AT is the way in which it operates (i.e., mechanism of action) and the level at which it operates (i.e., impairment, disability, or handicap). AT can be designed either to increase a person's physical functioning or to re-

This chapter was supported in part by the National Institutes of Health under Grant KO8 AG00487 from the National Institute on Aging and under Grant RO1 HS07595 from the Agency for Health Care Policy and Research. The opinions and conclusions expressed herein are those of the author and do not represent the views of the sponsoring agencies or the U.S. government.

duce the environmental factors that impede the achievement of personal goals. Thus, within this context and depending on its design, AT can enhance function (i.e., have a more intrinsic mode of action), reduce barriers (i.e., have a more extrinsic mode of action), or both. The appropriate prescription of AT can increase an individual's independence, employment opportunities, and life satisfaction (O'Day & Corcoran, 1994), but about 50% of devices issued at hospital discharge are quickly abandoned (Gitlin, 1995). High rates of abandonment and the economic implications of such waste, in light of a real potential for benefit, highlight the need to address AT outcomes in a standard way within the functional and sociocultural contexts of people's lives. The outcome of AT is the degree to which an AT device has an impact on the capacity of a person to achieve fulfillment within the physical or social environment. Outcomes may relate to changes in impairment, disability, or handicap.

Survival for a person with disabilities living in the community is dependent on

1. Physical functioning (i.e., physical ability)
2. Presence of environmental factors that aid or impede the achievement of personal goals
3. Psychosocial factors and self-reliance
4. Availability of environmental resources (Nosek & Fuhrer, 1992; Nosek, Fuhrer, & Howland, 1992)

These factors are frequently reciprocal in nature in that, as physical functioning increases, the individual becomes more able to withstand a harsher environment and requires fewer environmental resources for adaptation.

The experiences and abilities of each person are dependent on his or her physiological and mental capacities and the environment in which he or she lives, as illustrated by the self-fulfillment spheres shown in Figure 1. This model shows the intersections among four spheres—two that are intrinsic and relate to the body and mind and two that are extrinsic and relate to the physical world and society. The greater the overlap among these spheres, the better the person is able to integrate self and environment. In this model, AT serves as a catalyst to enhance the person's access to the environment.

Dimensions within the World Health Organization's (1980) *International Classification of Impairments, Disabilities and Handicaps* (ICIDH) can be represented by various overlapping portions of these spheres. *Impairment* is defined by the ICIDH as "any loss or

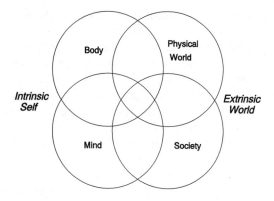

Figure 1.   The sphere of self-fulfillment: Modeling the relationship between self and world.

abnormality of psychological, physiological, or anatomical structure or function" (p. 47). Within the context of the self-fulfillment spheres, a person's impairment (or capacity) is intrinsic and is represented by the intersection between the spheres of mind and body. *Disability* is defined as "any restriction or lack (resulting from an impairment) of ability to perform an activity in the manner or within the range considered normal for a human being" (ICIDH, p. 143). Disabilities (related to physical and mental abilities) are both intrinsic and extrinsic because expression depends both on abilities of the person and on the surroundings in which the person functions. Physical abilities are represented at the intersection between the spheres of the body and the physical world. Psychosocial and cognitive abilities are represented at the intersection between the spheres of the mind and society. *Handicap* is defined as "disadvantage for a given individual, resulting from an impairment or a disability, that limits or prevents the fulfillment of a role that is normal (depending on age, sex, and social and cultural factors) for that individual" (ICIDH, p. 183). Handicap is extrinsic and is represented as the intersection between the physical world and society. The degree to which the person achieves self-fulfillment or self-actualization (Maslow, 1987) is seen as the overlap among all four spheres.

AT is intended to enhance the interface between the person (intrinsic) and the environment (extrinsic) in which he or she lives. The person–environment interface describes the manner and degree to which the individual is able to gain access to, operate within, move through, or have an impact on his or her physical and social environments. Thus, the spheres of self-fulfillment are particularly well suited to the description of AT modes of action and outcomes. In its efforts to enhance the person–environment interface, a particular device can have its primary mode of action at one or multiple spheres and can lead to outcomes in the dimensions of impairment, disability, or handicap. Thus, AT can have an intrinsic, mixed, or extrinsic mode of action, with resultant reductions in impairment, disability, or handicap. The degree to which AT enhances self-fulfillment is the outcome of overriding importance, but the construct of self-fulfillment can be approximated only through status in other, more concrete dimensions (e.g., impairment, disability, handicap).

ASSESSING THE MODES OF ACTION AND OUTCOMES OF ASSISTIVE TECHNOLOGY

Modes of Action of Assistive Technology

An AT device that has an intrinsic mode of action operates inside the body, generally at the level of impairment. A device with an extrinsic mode of operation is completely outside the body and is used to change or manipulate objects surrounding the person and distant from him or her. An AT device with a mixed mode of action operates close to but outside the body, like a tool. It is generally worn on the body, sat in, or leaned on, often operating at the level of disability. The surgical plating of a fractured femur is completely intrinsic, a wheelchair is mixed, and a computerized environmental interface unit that allows a person to control the environment remotely is completely extrinsic in its mode of action. Those devices that are most purely intrinsic affect impairment directly and, in turn, feed forward to reduce disability and handicap. Those that are mixed affect disability most directly and, in turn, feed forward to reduce handicap. Those that are most purely extrinsic affect handicap directly by reducing social or physical barriers or both, but rarely feed back to affect either disability or impairment. In general, the more intrinsic the mode of action, the more likely its outcome will be global across all ICIDH dimensions.

Table 1 illustrates modes of action for several impairment–assistive technology (I–AT) pairs, focusing, for purposes of simplicity, primarily on mobility outcomes. Mobility outcomes include the ability to walk through, move through, or gain access to the physical environment. Within this framework, certain technologies directly restore walking ability, others substitute an alternate mode of mobility, and still others reduce need for mobility by adapting the environment.

Table 1.   Alternate strategies of assistive technology viewed within the ICIDH framework

Impairment–AT pair	Capacity (impairment)	Ability (disability)	Interface (handicap)
Multiple fractures of femur—surgical stabilization and plating	**Direct; substitution for fractured bone**	Direct; restoration of walking ability	Invisible internal aid
Lower-limb amputation— prosthesis	Direct; substitution for lost limb	**Direct; restoration of walking ability**	Invisible external aid
Lower-limb amputation— wheelchair	Indirect; compensation for lost limb	**Direct; substitution for walking**	Visible external aid; requires an accessible environment
Quadriplegia— environmental interface unit	Indirect; compensation for lost capacities	No substitution; reduces need for walking through environmental adjustment	**Environmental adaptation; restricted to small physical space**

Note: The bold type represents the main dimension at which the AT device operates (mode of action) and thus where expression of outcome is expected to be greatest.

Surgical plating saves the leg by stabilizing bone and, by its intrinsic mode of action, increases capacity and reduces impairment. Provision of a prosthesis also has its primary mode of action at the impairment dimension because it represents direct substitution for a lost anatomical structure. In contrast, provision of a wheelchair has its primary mode of action at the disability dimension because it enhances mobility without having a direct impact on impairment. Wheelchair mobility represents an indirect compensation for lower-limb loss by substitution of wheeling for walking. The computerized environmental interface unit, or robotic device, has its primary mode of action at the handicap dimension because it allows the individual to control his or her environment without moving from one place to another. Mode of action has an impact on the individual's outcome (Table 2), which can also be analyzed within the contexts of the self-fulfillment spheres and the ICIDH dimensions of impairment, disability, and handicap.

Outcomes of Assistive Technology

Impairment-Related Outcomes   At the level of impairment, AT outcome results in either increased or decreased capacity. The more intrinsic the mode of action, the more direct the physiological

Table 2.   Examples of short- and long-term outcomes of assistive technology

AT device	Capacity (impairment)	Ability (disability)	Interface (handicap)
Surgical stabilization and plating	• Mortality • Osteomyelitis • Mechanical failure • Acute discomfort • Reduced pain	• Walking • Stair climbing • Endurance	Determine extent to which AT allows person to achieve vocation and avocation consistent with his or her desires
Prosthesis	• Skin breakdown • Safety risk (i.e., falling) • Component failure • Endurance	• Walking • Stair climbing • Endurance	Same as above
Wheelchair	• Patterns of joint stress • Component failure	• Mobility (i.e., wheelchair) • Endurance • Ability to go up and down grades	Same as above
Environmental interface unit	• Component failure	• Determine extent to which adaptation ameliorates need for mobility	Determine extent to which environment fits person and enhances vocational and avocational potential

risks imposed (i.e., the potential cause of increased impairment or pathology). For example, of all the I–AT pairs listed in Table 2, surgical stabilization and plating of the fractured limb is the most directly life threatening because of the potential for perioperative complications such as death or long-term osteomyelitis. In contrast, use of a prosthesis can lead to skin breakdown, which is annoying but usually not life threatening, yet ambulation with a prosthesis may place the person at greater risk of falling, which can be secondarily life threatening. Prolonged use of a wheelchair or crutches will cause unusual patterns of stress on the smaller upper-extremity joints not intended for weight bearing, thus placing the user at increased risk for overuse and degenerative joint disease. Use of an environmental interface unit poses the least direct physiological risk because it is fully extrinsic and its operation is distal to the person.

Disability-Related Outcomes   At the level of disability, AT enhances or reduces the ability of the individual to undertake usual or basic activities of daily living. The disability dimension represents the content of most functional status instruments and is the dimension for which outcome is most commonly measured in rehabilitation. AT reduces disability by providing the individual with an adaptive strategy or tool for functioning. Because the results of any adaptive strategies depend on the environment in which the individual functions, outcomes in the disability dimension have both intrinsic and extrinsic determinants.

Handicap-Related Outcomes   At the level of handicap, AT outcome is more extrinsic and less easily measured because its main focus is the influence of the environment and social attitudes surrounding the individual. If a person adapts well to walking with a prosthesis following amputation of a leg, it can seem so effortless that the prosthesis is no longer visible to the casual observer. Compared with a person without the prosthesis, the person with it has greater potential for interaction with the physical and social environments and thus can realize greater reduction of handicap. Wheelchairs are visible and socially stigmatizing and require environmental accessibility. People without disabilities show social strain around people using wheelchairs, manifested as short interaction times, excessive physical distance, and negative self-talk (Bates, Spencer, Young, & Rintala, 1993). The environmental interface unit, or robotics device, increases the capacity of the person to gain access to the physical and social environments without moving through them, thus enabling the individual to manipulate objects in the environment indirectly.

People without disabilities often find the gadgetry of environmental interface units intriguing rather than stigmatizing, perhaps because those devices often incorporate systems that they would also find useful, such as automatic garage door openers or other remote control units. If one takes a broad view, then automobiles are as much devices of assistive technology as are wheelchairs. It is this type of broad thinking that could ultimately remove the stigma from those devices so necessary for the optimal functioning of people with disabilities.

SELECTING INSTRUMENTS FOR
MEASURING ASSISTIVE TECHNOLOGY OUTCOMES

Knowledge about the mode of action of an assistive device makes it easier to select appropriate instruments for the measurement of AT outcomes. The following factors should be addressed in selecting such instruments:

1. Breadth and depth (generalizability and specificity)
2. Assessment vantage point
3. Objectivity and subjectivity
4. Validity
5. Reliability
6. Responsiveness to change
7. Method of scaling (Guyatt & Jaeschke, 1990; Nunnally, 1978; Wilkin, Hallam, & Doggett, 1992)

There are trade-offs in the selection of outcome measures between *breadth* and *depth* of assessment. *Breadth* refers to comprehensiveness of the instrument, whereas *depth* refers to its precision or details of measurement. Instruments with a great deal of breadth are often generic, meaning that they can be applied to a broad range of disease states or therapeutic approaches. In general, the greater the breadth, the more the instrument will be applicable to a wide range of AT approaches and the more it samples the complete spectrum of disability and distress relevant to quality of life (Guyatt & Jaeschke, 1990). In contrast, the more in depth the measure, the more specific the information obtained and the more tied it will be to a limited number of assistive technologies. In-depth instruments are best when answering highly technical and specific questions about a particular technology.

The *vantage point* of assessment refers to the viewpoint and method of assessment. Clients and clinicians may have very different views of status and goals. These differences highlight the need for mutual respect, communication, and assessment that spans several points of view. Outcome assessment can address client perceptions (e.g., satisfaction, perceived status, self-concept) or clinician perspectives (e.g., performance, examination, prognostication).

Objective measures describe particular constructs in a standard way across all people tested and thus can be used to generalize across populations. *Subjective* or *qualitative measures* allow for personal interpretation, are open-ended, and therefore may be more valuable when attempting to understand the unique concerns of the individual.

Validity refers to accuracy and the extent to which the instrument is expressing what it is intended to express. There are three types of validity: predictive, content, and construct (Nunnally, 1978). The *predictive validity* of an instrument is important when attempting to predict some form of behavior or outcome that is external to the instrument. This external behavior is referred to as the *criterion*. If a clinician or researcher wanted to identify people with paraplegia who are good candidates for an orthosis, the criterion might be the achievement of household ambulation by some later date. An instrument would have good predictive validity if it accurately classified people into categories associated with increasing probability of later achieving household ambulation. *Content validity* refers to the degree to which an instrument measures what it is intended to measure within a range appropriate to the population and questions under study. It relates to direct measurement rather than prediction. To determine whether a measure has appropriate content for describing the outcome of a given assistive device, it is necessary to determine the types of outcomes expected based on its mode of action. Once content is specified, range of measurement becomes important. This involves ruling out the presence of floor or ceiling effects or both in the instrument. *Floor effects* occur when large numbers of people get the lowest score, suggesting a need for a less challenging instrument. *Ceiling effects* occur when large numbers of people get the highest possible score, suggesting a need for a more challenging instrument. *Construct validity* describes the extent to which component items within an instrument measure some underlying dimension. Constructs are abstract, but the individual items used to form them are more concrete. The dimensions of impairment, disability, and handicap are examples of constructs. The person's need for help with eating, bathing, and dressing are examples of component items that might make up the disability dimension within an instrument. The performance levels for items contained within any dimension should statistically correlate with one another.

Reliability refers to the extent to which measurements can be repeated or reproduced on different occasions or by different researchers. There are two sources of measurement error: systematic bias and random error (Nunnally, 1978). *Systematic bias* would occur with use of a strain gauge that is being read precisely but that always registers 3 pounds too heavy. *Random error* would occur if the strain gauge were registering correctly but the read-out scale was so small that many clinicians could not read it precisely. High reliability does not imply high validity. One might seek to measure walking ability by quantifying muscle strength in some reliable manner; but, if the person were unable to walk because of severe proprioceptive loss, muscle strength would not constitute a valid measure.

Responsiveness to change refers to the instrument's capacity to detect clinically important differences in status over time (Guyatt & Jaeschke, 1990). To be responsive, the instrument must be reproducible, assuming that no change has occurred, but must register change in the event that true status improves or deteriorates.

The *method of scaling* refers to the ways in which the instrument is scored. This may include Guttman scaling, Likert scaling, category scaling, equal-appearing interval scaling, and equal interval scaling (Wilkin et al., 1992). A Guttman scale is a rank order or ordinal scale. Likert scales usually consist of combinations of ordinal variables that relate to a single dimension. The responses on related items are then summed, assuming appropriate internal consistency. Category scaling implies no numerical ranking. In equal-appearing interval scales, experts (or consumers) are asked to sort items within any dimension by their relative importance. The items are then weighted by perceived degree of importance. Equal interval scales produce true numbers, such as pounds.

Table 3 shows health status and functional status instruments placed within the context of the self-fulfillment spheres and the ICIDH. Three of these instruments—the Functional Independence Measure (FIM^{SM}) (Hamilton, Granger, Sherwin, Zielezny, & Tashman, 1987; Keith, Granger, Hamilton, & Sherwin, 1987; State University of New York at Buffalo, 1995), the Sickness Impact Profile (SIP) (Bergner, Bobbitt, Carter, & Gilson, 1981), and the Cantril Self-Anchoring Striving Scale (Campos & Johnson, 1990)—are highlighted here. The FIM and SIP were selected because of their common use, their demonstrated validity and reliability (Bergner et al., 1981; Hamilton, Laughlin, Fiedler, & Granger, 1994), and the wide range of health status dimensions encompassed. The SIP is a global measure of perceived health status that is sufficiently sensitive to detect changes or differences in status over time or between groups (Bergner et al., 1981). In contrast, the FIM is a more specific performance-based instrument that describes functional status in greater depth. Table 4 contrasts the FIM and SIP based on the instrument selection criteria described previously. The Cantril Self-Anchoring Striving Scale was selected as an example of a subjective instrument that can allow for a more personal expression of AT outcome by imposing no culture-specific standards on assessment.

Table 3.   General health status measures potentially applicable to AT outcomes

Spheres of impact and ICIDH dimensions	Instrument	Description
Impairment (intrinsic)	Objective Measures of Lower Extremity Function (Guralnik, Ferrucci, Simonsick, Salvie, & Wallace, 1995)	Physical performance tests, including such activities as standing balance, timed walk, getting up and down
	Folstein Mini-Mental State (Folstein, Folstein, & McHugh, 1975)	Screening instrument for mental status
Disability (mixed)	Barthel Index (Mahoney & Barthel, 1965)	Includes ADLs and mobility
	Functional Independence Measure (Granger, Hamilton, Keith, Zielezny, & Sherwin, 1986; Hamilton, Granger, Sherwin, Zielezny, & Tashman, 1987; Keith, Granger, Hamilton, & Sherwin, 1987)	Includes ADLs, mobility, communication, global cognitive functioning, and social interaction
Handicap (extrinsic)	Craig Handicap Assessment and Reporting Technique (CHART) (Whiteneck, Charlifue, Gerhart, Overholser, & Richardson, 1992)	Quantifies handicap in individuals; primarily used in spinal cord injury
Multiple and global	Sickness Impact Profile (Bergner, Bobbitt, Carter, & Gilson, 1981; Bergner, Bobbitt, Pollard, Martin, & Gilson, 1976)	Multidimensional health status measure developed to express the perceived impact of chronic disease
	Medical Outcomes Study 36-Item Short Form Health Survey (SF-36) (Ware & Sherbourne, 1992)	Multidimensional health status measure developed for evaluating patients with chronic disease
	Measure of Health-Related Quality of Life (Erickson, Wilson, & Shannon, 1995)	Two-dimensional health status measure developed for large population studies that includes activity limitation and perceived health status
	Cantril Self-Anchoring Striving Scale (Campos & Johnson, 1990)	A subjective measure in which the patient defines quality of life based on his or her own perceptions

ADLs, activities of daily living.

Table 4.   Comparing the Sickness Impact Profile (SIP) and Functional Independence Measure (FIM) across the key attributes

Attribute	SIP	FIM
Breadth and depth	More breadth: Includes disability and handicap	More depth in area of specific disabilities
Generalizability and specificity	More generalizable: Can be used across chronic disease with and without associated disabilities	Still generic but more specific to disability and care burden
Assessment vantage	Client perspective	Clinician perspective
Objectivity and subjectivity	More subjective because it relates to perceived health status	More objective because functional performance is observed
Validity	Depends on application: Valid across a broad range of inpatient and outpatient settings	Depends on application: Valid for inpatient rehabilitation setting; few other settings have been tested
Reliability	Found reliable in multiple settings	Reliable in the inpatient rehabilitation setting
Sufficiency of range	Appropriate for those with less severe disabilities; includes instrumental activities	Appropriate for those with more severe disabilities; limited to more basic abilities
Response to change	Depends on application: Will be responsive as an outcome measure when expecting a change in perceived quality of life across many dimensions	Depends on application: Will be responsive as an outcome measure when expecting a change in functional status
Scaling	Equal-interval appearing (weighted)	Likert

Sickness Impact Profile

The SIP represents a multidimensional measure of perceived health status that includes information spanning the physical, emotional, and social spheres. It permits direct comparison between people who do and people who do not have disabilities, and it is intended to be broadly applicable across different types and severities of illness and demographic or cultural subgroups. Test–retest reliability and internal consistency were shown to be high ($r = .92$ and $r = .94$, respectively), based on a random sample consisting of rehabilitation outpatients, rehabilitation inpatients, people with chronic health problems, and enrollees in a health plan who were not ill (Bergner et al., 1981).

The SIP includes 136 items and takes 20–30 minutes to complete. It can be either self-administered or administered by an interviewer. The individual is asked to check only those items that describe his or her status on a given day. The individual SIP questions are dichotomous in structure and thus do not express range of severity within each item. The items are organized into 12 categories that can be grouped into a psychosocial dimension (Table 5) and a physical dimension (Table 6). Scores for these two dimensions can be calculated, but scores for the remaining categories that do not fit one of these two dimensions (Table 7) must be calculated separately. In addition to the dimension and category scores, an overall score for the SIP can be determined.

Because this chapter focuses on the effect of AT on mobility, the mobility and ambulation categories within the physical dimension of the SIP are most relevant for discussion (Tables 8 and 9). Analysis of the content of the SIP shows its calibration for individuals with fairly high functioning. Of particular relevance is its inclusion of mobility within the home and beyond, in addition to the more specific descriptions of walking. Community mobility may be particularly important in assessing the degree to which AT allows the individual to function beyond his or her home.

Functional Independence Measure

In contrast to the SIP, the FIM includes a smaller number of items that are limited to the disability dimension and are rated in more detail by type and amount of assistance required. The FIM score is expected to reflect burden of care (i.e., the economic and social costs of disability). The FIM was developed in 1983 by a task force

Table 5.   Psychosocial dimensions of the Sickness Impact Profile

Category	Example item in category
Social Interaction	I am doing fewer social activities with groups of people.
Alertness Behavior	I have difficulty reasoning and solving problems (e.g., making plans, making decisions, learning new things).
Emotional Behavior	I laugh or cry suddenly.
Communication	I am having trouble writing or typing.

Adapted from Bergner et al. (1981) and Bergner, Bobbitt, Kressel, et al. (1976).

Table 6.   Physical dimensions of the Sickness Impact Profile

Category	Example item in category
Ambulation	I walk shorter distances or stop to rest often.
	I do not walk at all.
Mobility	I stay within one room.
	I stay away from home only for brief periods of time.
Body Care and Movement	I do not bathe myself at all but am bathed by someone else.
	I am very clumsy in body movements.

Adapted from Bergner et al. (1981) and Bergner, Bobbitt, Kressel, et al. (1976).

following review of 36 published and unpublished functional status measures and was intended to measure function in a standard way. The FIM was calibrated primarily for use in the inpatient rehabilitation setting, but within that setting it was designed to be broadly applicable across a wide range of impairments and resulting disabilities. It can also be used in the clinic, nursing facility, or home. Analysis of content indicates that the FIM is suited to populations with severe disabilities. Because it involves direct observation of performance, ideally over time, the time required to complete the FIM depends on the severity of the person's disability.

The FIM is organized into six sets of closely related items, including six that describe self-care, two that describe sphincter control, three describing transfer mobility, two that describe locomotion, two describing communication, and three that describe social cognition (Table 10). These sets of items can be combined to produce dimensions that describe physical disability (the motor FIM) and those that arise as a result of cognitive, communication, and so-

Table 7.   Independent dimensions of the Sickness Impact Profile

Category	Example item in category
Sleep and Rest	I sit during much of the day.
Eating	I am eating no food at all. Nutrition is taken through tubes or intravenous fluids.
Work	I am not working at all.
Home Management	I am not doing any of the maintenance or repair work around the house that I usually do.
Recreation and Pastime	I am going out for entertainment less.

Adapted from Bergner et al. (1981) and Bergner, Bobbitt, Kressel, et al. (1976).

Table 8.   Sickness Impact Profile mobility subscale items

1.   I am getting around only within one building.
2.   I stay within one room.
3.   I am staying in bed more.
4.   I am staying in bed most of the time.
5.   I am not now using public transportation.
6.   I stay home most of the time.
7.   I am only going to places with restrooms nearby.
8.   I am not going into town.
9.   I stay away from home only for brief periods of time.
10. I do not get around in the dark or in unlit places without someone's help.

Adapted from Bergner et al. (1981) and Bergner, Bobbitt, Kressel, et al. (1976).

cial interaction problems (the cognitive FIM) (Linacre, Heinemann, Wright, Granger, & Hamilton, 1994). The FIM has been shown to be reliable and valid for assessment in the inpatient rehabilitation setting (Dodds, Martin, Stolov, & Deyo, 1993; Hamilton et al., 1994; Stineman et al., 1994). Intraclass correlation coefficients have been shown to be .96 for the motor FIM and .91 for the cognitive FIM (Hamilton et al., 1994). Cronbach's alpha ranged from .89 to .98 for 18 different categories of impairment (Stineman et al., 1994). Each item within the FIM is ranked on a 7-level scale. The scale first distinguishes among those who require no help (Levels 7 and 6) and

Table 9.   Sickness Impact Profile ambulation subscale items

1.   I walk shorter distances or stop to rest often.
2.   I do not walk up or down hills.
3.   I use stairs only with mechanical support, for example, handrail, cane, or crutches.
4.   I walk up or down stairs only with assistance from someone else.
5.   I get around in a wheelchair.
6.   I do not walk at all.
7.   I walk by myself but with some difficulty, for example, limp, wobble, stumble, or have stiff leg.
8.   I walk only with help from someone.
9.   I go up and down stairs more slowly, for example, one step at a time, and stop often.
10. I do not use stairs at all.
11. I get around only by using a walker, crutches, cane, walls, or furniture.
12. I walk more slowly.

Adapted from Bergner et al. (1981) and Bergner, Bobbitt, Kressel, et al. (1976).

Table 10. Functional Independence Measure items and performance levels

Items

Self-care
- A. Eating
- B. Grooming
- C. Bathing
- D. Dressing—Upper Body
- E. Dressing—Lower Body
- F. Toileting

Sphincter control
- G. Bladder Management
- H. Bowel Management

Mobility/Transfer
- I. Bed, Chair, Wheelchair
- J. Toilet
- K. Tub or Shower

Locomotion
- L. Walk/Wheelchair
- M. Stairs

Communication
- N. Comprehension
- O. Expression

Social cognition
- P. Social Interaction
- Q. Problem Solving
- R. Memory

Levels

Independence
- 7. Complete Independence (Timely, Safely)
- 6. Modified Independence (Device)

Modified dependence
- 5. Supervision
- 4. Minimal Assist (Subject = 75%+)
- 3. Moderate Assist (Subject = 50%+)

Complete dependence
- 2. Maximal Assist (Subject = 25%+)
- 1. Total Assist (Subject = 0%+)

Adapted from State University of New York at Buffalo (1995).

those who require help (Levels 5, 4, 3, 2, and 1). Once this distinc-tion is made, the performance of people scoring below 6 is rated by the amount of help required. Thus, compared with the SIP, the FIM provides more detailed and specific information about the explicit level at which the person is performing a given activity. The rela-tive depth of assessment of the FIM (compared to the SIP) is illus-trated by comparing definitions of performance levels for the Trans-fers: Bed, Chair, Wheelchair item (Figure 2) to the sample SIP questions (Tables 8 and 9).

MEASURING OUTCOMES
SPECIFIC TO ASSISTIVE TECHNOLOGY

Instruments such as the FIM and SIP are important because they can be used to contrast status across a wide range of diverse popula-tions. However, neither was designed specifically with AT in mind, and thus both are missing important elements. Depending on the research or clinical questions being asked, it may be prudent to add

---

I TRANSFERS: BED, CHAIR, WHEELCHAIR: Includes all aspects of transferring to and from a bed, chair, and wheelchair, or coming to a standing position, if walking is the typical mode of locomotion. Performs safely.

No Helper

7 Complete Independence
   If walking, individual approaches, sits down on, and gets up to a standing position from a regular chair; transfers from bed to chair. Performs safely.
   If in a wheelchair, individual approaches a bed or chair, locks brakes, lifts foot rests, removes arm rest if necessary, and performs either a standing pivot or sliding transfer (without a board) and returns. Performs safely.

6 Modified Independence—Individual requires adaptive or assistive device, such as a sliding board, a lift, grab bars, or special seat or chair or brace or crutches; takes more than reasonable time or there are safety considerations. In this case, a prosthesis or orthosis is considered an assistive device if used for the transfer.

Helper

5 Supervision or Setup—Individual requires supervision (e.g., standing by, cu-ing, coaxing) or setup (e.g., positioning sliding board, moving foot rests).
4 Minimal Contact Assistance—Individual performs 75% or more of transfer-ring tasks.
3 Moderate Assistance—Individual performs 50% to 74% of transferring tasks.
2 Maximal Assistance—Individual performs 25% to 49% of transferring tasks.
1 Total Assistance—Individual performs less than 25% of transferring tasks.

Figure 2.   Sample definitions for a single FIM item. (Adapted from State University of New York at Buffalo [1995].)

a supplemental battery of element sets containing questions specific to the technology being analyzed, thus enabling greater precision in testing specific hypotheses and outcomes. These element sets include pain, endurance for activities, safety, equipment durability, functional status, transportability, image, vocation or avocation, consumer satisfaction, costs, machine–biological system interface, and machine–person interface. They may be classified as contributing primarily to the intrinsic or extrinsic spheres, depending on whether they directly affect the person or the manner in which the environment is affecting the person. Many element sets are loosely linked to the ICIDH. A summary of these elements follows (with relevant questions to highlight each).

Pain (Intrinsic)   Does the device increase or decrease pain? If an orthosis or prosthesis fits poorly or is inappropriately prescribed, it can increase pain in the short term and cause deterioration in joints and soft tissues over the long term. If pain indicates ongoing pathology, then it most closely relates to impairment; otherwise, it can cause an increase in disability.

Endurance for Activities (Intrinsic)   Does the device allow for more prolonged periods of movement? The choice of materials for and ergometric design of wheelchairs and prosthetic limbs can affect the energy required for operation. At the same time, heavier devices are more suited to rugged outdoor terrain and tend to be more stable. Thus, there is often a compromise between designs that conserve user energy and environmental demands. Endurance relates most closely to capacity (impairment).

Safety (Mixed)   Does the device increase or decrease safety? Sometimes a device that enhances function also introduces greater risks (e.g., falling). At times, safety can be compromised by inappropriate efforts to increase function.

Equipment Durability (Extrinsic)   What are the safety issues should the device fail? How durable is it?

Functional Status and Performance Measures (Mixed)   How much does the device improve mobility and other functional activities? These measures describe the individual's ability to perform various activities of daily living (e.g., eating, dressing). In addition to more traditional expressions of functional status, it is important to include performance measures such as maximum distance walked, balance, and the ability to change direction. Functional status elements form the disability dimension. Performance measures relate to functional limitation and are intermediate between impairment and disability (Marino & Stineman, 1996).

Transportability (Extrinsic)   How tied is the device to accessible or specific environments? Does the device enable or inhibit travel? Seating systems may be important to comfort and positioning for people with severe musculoskeletal disabilities, but they are often bulky and heavy, making transport difficult. Need for transportability must be balanced with need for adaptations that add weight or bulk. Ideally, an individual will have several devices for different settings—for example, a light wheelchair to travel and a sturdier one for everyday use. Transportability relates most closely to handicap because it determines entrance into the physical world.

Image (Extrinsic)   Does the individual perceive that use of the device changes the way people see and relate to him or her? How does the device actually change the way in which society relates to the individual? The more intrinsic the device, the more it is invisible and the less impact it has on image—the way in which the device changes the manner in which the person is perceived either by oneself or by society. Extrinsic devices such as wheelchairs are visible and socially stigmatizing. However, social stigma can be reduced by an elegant design. Wheelchairs built with racing-bike technology and attention to style present a more positive image than the strictly utilitarian versions. AT should be seen as an accessory, as a tool, or as a machine, rather than as a prop or expression of physical limitation. Image is most closely aligned with handicap.

Vocations or Avocations (Extrinsic)   How does the AT device affect the capacity of the person to work and play? The impact on vocational and avocational interests correspond to handicap.

Consumer Satisfaction (Intrinsic)   How well does the AT device meet the consumer's expectations? An open-ended, qualitative approach to assessment is important in determining consumer satisfaction.

Costs (Extrinsic)   What are the costs of equipment purchase, maintenance, and failure? The costs of equipment failure are both economic and noneconomic. Greater sophistication can lead to greater costs because of difficulty in getting parts.

Machine–Biological System Interface (Mixed)   How well does the mechanism supplement and fit the person's biological systems? This has to do with *technical parameters* and often relates to the assessment of engineering standards or the more specialized aspects of the clinical assessment. Taking the assessment of prosthetic lower-limb replacement as an example, such parameters include the individual's gait and the technical operation of the prosthesis. Gait parameters include evenness of stride; the presence of abnormalities, such as lateral whip or pistoning; and the general fit between the person and the prosthetic limb. Technical operation of the prosthetic limb must include assessment of its static and dynamic alignment (Sanders, 1986). Specific gait deviations or poor prosthetic alignment will have an impact on outcome over the long term. Table 11 shows some examples of such technical problems coupled with their probable long-term outcomes.

Machine–Person Interface (Mixed)   How optimal is the match between the person and the machine? What, if any, compromises were made among function, cosmesis, and safety? Is the device used all the time, part of the time, or not at all? How does the technology change the way the user relates to the world? How does the device change the way that society relates to the person? Does the person have a creative or resentful approach to its use? This more abstract construct refers to the interface between the machine and the individual's concept of self within the physical and social worlds. It describes the degree to which AT meets the needs of the person and changes the way he or she can relate to the world. Within the context of the self-fulfillment spheres (Figure 1), it represents the extent of overlap among the body, the mind, the physical world, and society, with AT serving to catalyze the link between the intrinsic and extrinsic spheres. This overriding construct relates to the effect of AT on the individual's sense of self-fulfillment and overall well-being. Because it cannot be directly measured, it is only inferred. The machine–person interface is all encompassing in that it includes all aspects of the person, the machine, and the environment in which it is used. Many of the other sets of elements can be seen to feed into it.

Table 11.   Example items for clinical assessment in above-knee prosthesis wearers

Symptom	Prosthetic cause	Possible long-term outcome
Paresthesia in femoral nerve distribution	Excessive pressure on scarpas triangle	Chronic pain and paresthesias
Knee instability	Heel on shoe too high for alignment	Risk of falling
Pain over the adductor longus tendon	Channel for adductor tendon in prosthesis is inadequate	Skin breakdown
Adductor roll with inability to maintain a level pelvis when weight bearing	Insufficient adduction of femur in the socket	Excess wear on pelvis

A STRATEGY FOR SUBJECTIVE MEASUREMENT

Although objective measures are of paramount importance to science, their content is based on researchers' and clinicians' opinions about relative importance. Thus, objective measures may reflect bias on the part of the people who developed them. Some argue that it is difficult to design objective instruments of relevance to all people and that quality-of-life outcome measurement should be subjective (Levine, 1990). Such an argument is particularly relevant when viewing constructs such as the machine–person interface or consumer satisfaction. The Cantril Self-Anchoring Striving Scale represents a subjective measurement strategy with certain quantitative properties. It allows patients to define quality of life based on personal perceptions, aspirations, culture, and values. The scale can be used to elicit subjective responses about specific aspects of life, such as health, functioning, housing, and AT outcomes. To administer the scale, the researcher or clinician shows the person a ladder with 10 rungs. The top rung represents the best or most, and the bottom rung the worst or least; phrases are completed or altered to yield general statements such as the best possible treatment outcome or the most satisfactory device. The questions should be open-ended so that they elicit maximally personal responses. The person is asked to show where on the ladder he or she was at some time in the past, is currently, and expects to be in the future. The person is then asked to explain why he or she chose that particular ladder position. Quantitative change scores can be computed to evaluate the impact of any interventions on quality of life. Content, cluster, or domain analysis of responses can be undertaken to determine common reasons people place themselves at certain rungs. The Cantril Self-Anchoring Striving Scale has been applied to study patients' quality of life following bone marrow transplantation (Baker, Curbow, & Wingard, 1991) and might be used to determine how users' perceptions about AT outcomes differ from those of physicians, therapists, or bioengineers.

CONCLUSIONS

The spheres of self-fulfillment in conjunction with the ICIDH provide a conceptual framework for viewing the impact of AT on client outcomes. Through the interlocking of these spheres, AT is viewed as a catalyst that can change the relationship of the person to the environment. The ICIDH is viewed within the self-fulfillment model. It provides the dimensions of impairment, disability, and handicap through which the modes of action of various AT devices can be visualized, along with their resulting outcomes. The most comprehensive approach to analyzing assistive technology outcomes includes a three-stage assessment:

1. A generic health status measure
2. A supplemental battery of AT-specific indicators
3. A subjective or qualitative assessment

The generic measure enables comparisons across different populations, different assistive devices, or both. The supplemental battery focuses on the biological, functional, and sociological impacts specific to the technology. The qualitative approach will be highly personal and directed to the values, perceptions, and cultural attitudes of the individual.

REFERENCES

Baker, F., Curbow, B., & Wingard, J.R. (1991). Role retention and quality of life of bone marrow transplant survivors. *Social Science and Medicine, 32,* 697–704.

Bates, P.S., Spencer J.C., Young, M.E., & Rintala, D.H. (1993). Assistive technology and the newly disabled adult: Adaptation to wheelchair use. *American Journal of Occupational Therapy, 47,* 1014–1021.

Bergner, M., Bobbitt, R.A., Carter, W.B., & Gilson, B.S. (1981). The Sickness Impact Profile: Development and final revision of a health status measure. *Medical Care, 19,* 787–805.

Bergner, M., Bobbitt, R.A., Kressel, S., Pollard, W.E., Gilson, B.S., & Morris, J.R. (1976). The Sickness Impact Profile: Conceptual formulation and methodology for the development of a health status measure. *International Journal of Health Services, 63,* 93–415.

Bergner, M., Bobbitt, R.A., Pollard, W.E., Martin, D.P., & Gilson, B.S. (1976). The Sickness Impact Profile: Validation of a health status measure. *Medical Care, 14,* 57–67.

Campos, S.S., & Johnson, T.M. (1990). Cultural considerations. In B. Spilker (Ed.), *Quality of life assessment in clinical trials* (pp. 163–170). New York: Raven Press.

Dodds, T.A., Martin, D.P., Stolov, W.C., & Deyo, R.A. (1993). A validation of the functional independence measurement and its performance among rehabilitation in-patients. *Archives of Physical Medicine and Rehabilitation, 74,* 531–536.

Erickson, P., Wilson, R., & Shannon, I. (1995). Years of healthy life: Healthy People 2000. *Statistical Notes, 7,* 1–14.

Folstein, M.F., Folstein, S.E., & McHugh, P.R. (1975). Mini-Mental State: A practical method for grading the cognitive state of patients for the clinician. *Journal of Psychiatric Research, 12,* 189–198.

Gitlin, L.N. (1995). Why older people accept or reject assistive technology. *Generations, 19,* 41–46.

Granger, C.V., Hamilton, B.B., Keith, R.A., Zielezny, M., & Sherwin, F.S. (1986). Advances in functional assessment for medical rehabilitation. *Topics in Geriatric Rehabilitation, 1,* 59–74.

Guralnik, J.M., Ferrucci, L., Simonsick, E., Salvie, M.E., & Wallace, R.B. (1995). Lower-extremity function in persons over the age of 70 years as a predictor of subsequent disability. *New England Journal of Medicine, 332,* 556–561.

Guyatt, G.H., & Jaeschke, R. (1990). Measurement in clinical trials: Choosing the appropriate approach. In B. Spilker (Ed.), *Quality of life assessment in clinical trials* (pp. 37–46). New York: Raven Press.

Hamilton, B.B., Granger, C.V., Sherwin, F.S., Zielezny, M., & Tashman, J.S. (1987). A uniform national data system for medical rehabilitation. In M.J. Fuhrer (Ed.), *Rehabilitation outcomes: Analysis and measurement* (pp. 137–147). Baltimore: Paul H. Brookes Publishing Co.

Hamilton, B.B., Laughlin, J.A., Fiedler, R.C., & Granger, C.V. (1994). Interrater reliability of the 7-level Functional Independence Measure (FIM). *Scandinavian Journal of Rehabilitation Medicine, 26,* 115–119.

Keith, R.A., Granger, C.V., Hamilton, B.B., & Sherwin, F.S. (1987). The Functional Independence Measure: A new tool for rehabilitation. In M.G. Eisenberg & R.C. Grzesiak (Eds.), *Advances in clinical rehabilitation* (pp. 6–18). New York: Springer-Verlag.

Levine, R.J. (1990). An ethical perspective. In B. Spilker (Ed.), *Quality of life assessment in clinical trials* (pp. 153–162). New York: Raven Press.

Linacre, J.M., Heinemann, A.W., Wright, B.D., Granger, C.V., & Hamilton, B.B. (1994). The structure and stability of the Functional Independence Measure. *Archives of Physical Medicine and Rehabilitation, 75,* 127–132.

Mahoney, F.I., & Barthel, D.W. (1965). Functional evaluation: The Barthel Index. *Maryland State Medical Journal, 14,* 61–65.

Marino, R.J., & Stineman, M.G. (1996). Functional assessment in spinal cord injury. *Topics in Spinal Cord Injury, 1,* 32–45.

Maslow, A.H. (1987). *The hierarchy of needs* (3rd ed.). New York: Harper & Row.

Nosek, M.A., & Fuhrer, M.J. (1992). Independence among people with disabilities: I. A heuristic model. *Rehabilitation Counseling Bulletin, 36,* 1–20.

Nosek, M.A., Fuhrer, M.J., & Howland, C.A. (1992). Independence among people with disabilities: II. Personal independence. *Rehabilitation Counseling Bulletin, 36,* 21–36.

Nunnally, J.C. (1978). *Psychometric theory* (2nd ed.). New York: McGraw-Hill.

O'Day, B.L., & Corcoran, P.J. (1994). Assistive technology: Problems and policy alternatives. *Archives of Physical Medicine and Rehabilitation, 75,* 1165–1169.

Sanders, G.T. (1986). *Lower limb amputations: A guide to rehabilitation.* Philadelphia: F.A. Davis.

State University of New York at Buffalo. (1995). *Guide for the Uniform Data Set for Medical Rehabilitation (Adult FIM^SM), version 4.0.* Buffalo: Author.

Stineman, M.G., Escarce, J.J., Goin, J.E., Hamilton, B.B., Granger, C.V., & Williams, S.V. (1994). A case mix classification system for medical rehabilitation. *Medical Care, 32,* 366–379.

Ware, J.E., & Sherbourne, C.D. (1992). The MOS 36-Item Short Form Health Survey (SF-36): I. Conceptual framework and item selection. *Medical Care, 30*, 473–483.

Whiteneck, G.G., Charlifue, S.W., Gerhart, K.A., Overholser, J.D., & Richardson, G.N. (1992). Quantifying handicap: A new measure of long-term rehabilitation outcomes. *Archives of Physical Medicine and Rehabilitation, 73*, 519–526.

Wilkin, D., Hallam, L., & Doggett, M.A. (1992). *Measures of need and outcome for primary health care*. Oxford, England: Oxford University Press.

World Health Organization. (1980). *International classification of impairments, disabilities and handicaps (ICIDH)*. Geneva: Author.

WHEN ASSISTIVE TECHNOLOGY IS USED AND WHEN IT IS NOT

CHAPTER 5

Cultural and Environmental Barriers to Assistive Technology

Why Assistive Devices Don't Always Assist

George A. Covington

In 1991, a Harris poll found that 58% of people without disabilities who were interviewed reported that they felt anxious, uncomfortable, or embarrassed in the presence of a person with a disability. Forty-seven percent of those interviewed reported that they actually felt fear (Harris & Associates, 1991). The percentage of those reporting fear may have been higher had they not been embarrassed to make that admission. This fear factor is the reason why most assistive technology doesn't work in the way its designers intend. My personal experience with a universally recognized assistive device illustrates my point.

THE STIGMA OF A STICK

Many people have wondered why I did not use a white cane until my late 40s. In grade school, I was constantly asked by teachers and other adults why I didn't wear glasses. I explained time and time again that glasses could not correct my vision enough to make a difference. I was an extremely active child, and I realized that glasses didn't allow me to see a printed page, the blackboard, or an incoming softball any better and that in the latter case I could be left with a face full of glass. It was automatically assumed that, because my family was poor, we simply couldn't afford glasses. This was my first encounter with an institution that refused to substitute reason for stigma.

A few months into the first grade, my mother received a telephone call from the school principal. She was told that if we could not afford glasses, the school staff would attempt to take up a collection. My mother told him that we didn't need their charity and that she would buy me glasses if that would make the staff feel better. The family ophthalmologist, who said he was willing to write a note stating that glasses would not help, prescribed the necessary glasses, which provided only a slight assistance. Luckily, the glasses did not look like the bottoms of soda bottles. He knew that in order to make the major corrections necessary, the glasses would be extremely thick and heavy and still would not correct my poor eyesight. I kept these glasses in my pocket most of the time. This seemed to placate most of my teachers. I realized, even as a 6-year-old, that this was a total sham, but it was a way of avoiding grief.

At the beginning of each school year, it was not too tactfully suggested to my mother that perhaps I should be sent to the school for the blind in Austin, Texas, where they could better deal with my "half-blindness." "He can learn to use a cane and use braille," my mother was told. Luckily, the family ophthalmologist believed that most of my problems with school were not visual, and he repeatedly told my mother that if I were sent to the school for the blind, I would be warehoused and would never learn to compete in society. I think his theory was that if I could survive Grim Elementary School (yes, that was the school's name) and the rest of the public school system of Texarkana, Texas, I could survive anywhere. He was right.

A white cane was never forced on me, for two reasons. First, every teacher from the first to the sixth grades would have been leery at seeing me enter a classroom or playground with a potential weapon. Second, I was constantly in motion. A cane would have been an intrusion and an impediment, not an aid to my travel. I always had an excuse, even after substantial vision loss as an adult, not to use a cane. I told myself that the cane would make me less alert and dull my reflexes. I believed that the cane might make my eyesight become weaker if I didn't rely on my eyesight as my primary survival tool. A friend who came to blindness as an adult told me that the first time he bought a cane it didn't make it past the garbage chute in his mother's apartment. Two additional canes met the same fate before he felt comfortable enough to be seen in public.

In the mid-1980s, I finally made a partial surrender to the white stick. My capitulation was the result of air travel. Although I could maneuver throughout most of Washington, D.C., with ease, I found that airports are laid out by people who want to keep the air traveler in a state of constant confusion. In addition, airport security staff become nervous when an individual is standing under a 2-foot sign that has "Gate 15" printed on it asking, "Where is Gate 15?" If I have a white stick, they know why I'm asking. Without a white stick, they assume I'm drunk, drugged, or just crazy.

My cane of choice was a collapsible aluminum one that was easily hidden. These canes are lightweight, inexpensive, and easy to store in an attaché case. In those days, I would whip the cane out when needed, tap violently on the marble floor of the terminal, and start asking passing blurs, "Where's Gate 15?" The minute I was at my gate, the cane was hidden away in my luggage.

Looking back, I realized that I should have started using the cane full time several years earlier. I would have avoided dozens of banged shins and other unnecessary bruises and abrasions. Why didn't I? I hated the white stick because of its terrible stigma. To me, it meant a total loss of independence; it meant a total surrender and an admission that I didn't want to make. I did not want to provoke the pity and condescension that I always had heard in the voices of most sighted people talking to blind people.

An education I give my sighted friends involves walking down the street with me and my white cane. They are amazed to see that some people will spot the white cane at 10 or 15 yards and step into the street to avoid any possible contact. It's as though a certain part of society assumes the white cane causes blindness! In the early days, one of my only amusements with my new stick was to watch blurs spinning, whirling, and jumping out of my path.

Studies showed that people actually rank their fear of disability based on the visibility of the impairment (Abroms & Kodera, 1978; Siller, 1986; Westbrook, Legge, & Pennay, 1993). Polls indicated, before acquired immunodeficiency syndrome (AIDS) became prevalent, that blindness was the second most feared physical condition in the United States, second only to cancer. The fear is based on the same stigma that I tried to avoid for so many years. Another reason I avoided using a white cane was that there were a number of individuals in the disability rights movement who would chide me as unwilling to accept my disability because I would not use a cane. These were the individuals who live, breathe, and drink disability. Their whole life is their disability. Without it, they would simply be colorless creeps trying to meet their mortgage payments like everybody else.

The month I left the White House was the time when I started using my cane full time. My eyesight had continued to slowly deteriorate in the 4 years I'd served on the White House staff, and I decided enough was enough. I broke three canes in 3 months. The short cane-travel course I had taken in the mid-1980s had given me the skills I needed to be safely mobile (for myself and other pedestrians), but I had not practiced since then. Using a cane on the smooth marble floor of an airport terminal is not the same as using a cane on the sidewalks. The tip of my cane found every crack and crevice. Usually, the contact resulted in the cane flying out of my hands. When I would try to grip the cane to prevent this action, the usual result was the cane snapping at the first joint. Nothing is so pathetic as a guy walking down the street holding a cane with the first section dangling at a 90-degree angle to the ground. I looked more like a mine sweeper than a blind man trying to get home.

Less than a month after I started using the cane full time, I began to accept and appreciate what the cane could do. I found it to be an enhancement to my independence, not a barrier. I still have some resentment on rainy days when I'm trying to carry an attaché case, an umbrella, and a white cane. After two or three soakings, I bought an attaché case with a shoulder strap, a minor adjustment.

I still hear a great many condescending and patronizing voices during the day, but I've learned to switch off the resentment. Most of these people simply want to help, and maybe there is no need to analyze their motives.

I once addressed a large group of people who had come to blindness after the age of 50. There were approximately 70 people who were legally blind, but only three white canes, in the room. When I asked "Why not use the cane?" I got back the same answers I would have given years before. I realized that the stigma was still strong and alive. Fear was still at work.

THE FEAR FACTOR

Fear Among Sighted People

There are a number of ways to explain the fear factor among individuals without disabilities. Perhaps the primary one is that, from the dawn of history, most cultures destroyed or left to die those who were identified at birth as different, deformed, or disabled. The tribe had no use for individuals who could not help guarantee the overall survival of the tribe.

Generally, the women were blamed. The priests, shamen, or witch doctors told them that they had violated a taboo, had displeased the gods, were being punished for something they had done in a previous life, or any number of other creative excuses. If a disability was discovered in childhood or if an adult came back from battle or hunting too disabled to contribute, the hunter-gatherer cultures left them behind to be dealt with by the fates.

For countless millennia, history shows a slow evolution in attitudes toward people with disabilities. Well into the 19th century, ecclesiastical writings of both the Catholic and Protestant theologians spoke of many groups with disabilities as spawn of the devil or cursed by God. Demonic possession was also high on the charts. These facts explain why anthropologists have found, in almost every culture on this planet, that during pregnancy women will have at least one dream of having a monster.

In the latter part of the 19th century and into the 20th, society turned from considering people with disabilities as monsters to viewing them as creatures who could be cured by modern medicine. The belief that they could be cured led to medical experiments of such a horrific nature that they almost defy description. During this period, the philosophy of Social Darwinism and the medical model's emphasis on cure were combined to create a school of thought that held that if people with disabilities could not be cured, then they should be removed from society's gene pool (Sloan & Stevens, 1976). This culminated in the Nazi program known as Action T-4, in which between 200,000 and 300,000 people with disabilities perished between 1939 and 1945. In the United States between the 1920s and the 1950s, more than 60,000 individuals diagnosed as having mental retardation were sterilized. It is now believed that many of these people may have been misdiagnosed (Gallagher, 1995).

The fear factor is also part of an attitude of "there but for the grace of God go I." I once had a discussion with a friend who is African American. She said, "Many of you white folks had a fear of us in the early days of our civil rights movement, but we proved that that fear can be overcome." I explained that there was a big difference. I could go hear a speech by Jesse Jackson and leave the hall knowing I would not become African American. However, he could leave one of my speeches, and a drunk driver or a mugger could make him an individual with a disability.

Fear Among People with Disabilities

The negative images, stereotypes, and myths have persisted because of the fear factor. The demonstration of their power is manifest in the situation that develops when adults acquire or develop a disability. Often the inability to accept the disability drives the person to withdraw from society and in many instances become a recluse (Wright, 1960).

I remember two similar situations in which middle-age individuals suddenly developed a visual problem that resulted in their becoming legally blind in a relatively short period of time. They were both highly successful business executives who developed a degenerative eye condition. Both men, in their early 50s, took disability retirement. Both refused to seek help, refused to leave their houses, refused to socialize with former friends, and fell into deep depression. They had allowed their lack of 20/20 vision to rob them of their abilities and perceived social status. All of their lives they had believed the negative images of people with disabilities, and they applied those negative images to themselves.

Both of these men had more eyesight than I was born with, and modern technology could have allowed them to continue in their careers and in their lives. Organizations of blind people and people with visual impairments have told me that there are hundreds of thousands of people in similar situations across the country. Reaching these people is extremely difficult because, like the 58% in the Harris poll, they feel uncomfortable, anxious, and embarrassed in their own presence (Harris & Associates, 1991).

Another element of the fear factor is the concept of people with disabilities as victims. U.S. culture has deemed that the proper reaction to a victim is pity. When people develop a disability in later life, they apply pity to themselves because they believe that all people with disabilities fall into the victim or pity category. No one wants the pity of their peers (Kemp, 1981; Shapiro, 1993).

For years, disability advocates have tried to forge alliances with the major organizations for older adults. They were told, "It's difficult enough dealing with the stigma of old age without having to deal with the stigma of disability also." These older adults state that many people consider them to have a disability just because of their age. They do not want to reinforce this misconception by being openly associated with groups of people with disabilities.

THE MEDIA AND THE MESSAGE

Modern society views its culture through a prism called the media. Information is the light on which the prism acts to create a clear image of that culture. Too often the media's information about people with disabilities consists of images distorted by negative attitudes, myths, and stereotypes. The media claim to be neutral, but they forget that a prism can enlarge and multiply an image.

For most of my adult life, I have explained disability issues in a style that has often been called brisk or blunt. Because of society's media-driven misconceptions about disability, the need for education is never-ending. The first principle is, *People with disabilities can lie, cheat, and steal just like people without disabilities do.* People with disabilities can be fools, fakes, and frauds just like people without disabilities. Individuals who cannot accept these statements cannot truly accept the concept that people with disabilities are just like everyone else, except that they have disabilities. A disability becomes a handicap only when structural or attitudinal barriers make it so.

Some people with disabilities are charming, witty, and highly intelligent; some are not. The disability doesn't determine which are sexy and which are sexist. A disability gives the individual a different perspective, not a different personality. Some people with disabilities get married, have children, and live happily ever after, and some get divorced (not necessarily in that order). Some never leave home; most do.

Some people with disabilities have reached a comfort level that allows them to debate semantics and determine that the terms *crippled* and *handicapped* are no longer acceptable. Others are still debating whether the term *disabled people* should be replaced with *people with disabilities*. This latter debate is generally restricted to the "gurus" with disabilities living inside the Washington, D.C., beltway. However, many people with disabilities prefer not to describe themselves as "visually challenged," "physically challenged," or, if short, "vertically challenged." When the obstacles are removed, so are the challenges. People with disabilities are as different and diverse as everyone else in the world. They simply have a disability. They are part of humanity.

The second principle is, *The road to Hell is paved with good intentions.* The media have always approached disability issues with the best of intentions, but good intentions are not enough. The power of the media is such that its descriptions of people with disabilities and their issues can be devastating. Although the news articles and feature stories are well intentioned, in many cases they have served to perpetuate stereotypes and negative attitudes held by the general public. A good example of the problem with the news media is the following excerpt:

> And he said that those who claimed special rights would also adjust. "There are groups, like the disabled, or parents of the disabled, who will oppose change," he said. But he believes

that most "will gladly give up their so-called rights" because
they understand that in one-on-one disputes, rights become a
"license for extortion." (Howard, 1995, p. A33)

The excerpt is part of an interview with Philip K. Howard, author of
the best-selling book, *The Death of Common Sense* (1994). Disre-
garding the fact that Mr. Howard used several disability horror stories to illustrate his point in the book (stories that were later proved
to be erroneous), his quote in *The New York Times* interview
demonstrates the problem. By allowing Mr. Howard to use the
phrase *so-called rights* unchallenged, *The New York Times* demonstrated the media's unwillingness to look at disability issues as civil
rights issues.

Images of Disability in Print and on Television

In the 1990s, news articles and features have tended to divide individuals with disabilities into two categories: the poor, pitiable, pathetic creature of charity or the heroic, undefeated "Supercrip." It is
not uncommon to find stories that begin with the first image and
culminate in the second.

The individual with disabilities as an object of charity is an image as old as recorded history. Until the 1990s, the news media often wrote of these individuals as though they were characters from
a Gothic horror novel. People with disabilities were "struck down
in their prime," "afflicted with . . . ," "victims of . . . ," "doomed to
a life of . . . ," or "confined or bound to a wheelchair." I have told
hundreds of journalists over the years, "If you ever use the term
bound to a wheelchair, you had better be talking about kinky sex."

Part of the modern image of the person with disabilities as an
object of charity was created by organizations attempting to raise
money for their causes. These organizations, with the assistance of
the news media, have caused generations of Americans to see people with disabilities as poor, defenseless children in need of pity and
charity (Kemp, 1981). Most of these organizations were directed and
managed by people without disabilities. Although they raised hundreds of millions of dollars, they did little to improve the image of
people with disabilities. In the 1990s, a number of these organizations have begun to bring people with disabilities into decision-
making positions (Milam, 1993).

The concept of *Supercrip* has been around since the penny
newspaper, but in the 1990s this image has been the favorite of the
mass media. Supercrip is a character, usually struck down in
the prime of life, who fights to overcome insurmountable odds to

succeed as a meaningful member of society. Through strength of will, perseverance, and hard work, the individual with disabilities usually achieves a "normal" life. Depending on the news organization, this scenario might also include mother, God, country, and the active intervention of UFOs or Bigfoot. Supercrip was born for television. The television industry loves blind Supercrips because they don't have to make the sets accessible.

Perhaps the most troubling aspect of the Supercrip character is that the news media herald as "superhuman" an achievement in the life of a person with a disability that would be considered routine and completely unnewsworthy in the life of a person without a disability. Too often, the news media treat an individual with disabilities who has attained success in his or her field or profession as though he or she were one of a kind. Although this one-of-a-kind aspect might make for a better story angle, it perpetuates in the mind of the general public how rare it is for the citizen with disabilities to succeed (Russell, 1993; Shear, 1986; Zola, 1985).

Another problem with the media is the "I have a handicapped friend" syndrome. It sometimes seems that every member of the media has one acquaintance with disabilities who, by virtue of the disability, is the sole authority on all matters of disability. This friend is quoted as an authority on any matter that involves a disability issue. A person with a mobility impairment may not, however, be an expert on mobility and access problems. One blind person may be an expert on technology, whereas another blind person may have no interest in the subject and thus no knowledge of the issue.

The problem is a circular one. It is as young members of the general public that men and women of the news media form their attitudes about people with disabilities. As a former journalism professor, I know that the images and stereotypes of such people are not left at the front door of the journalism school but remain to become a part of the psyche of the working reporter. With the appearance of these reporters' news stories, the cycle begins again.

BARRIERS BY DESIGN

Good intentions with bad results are not restricted to the press. Too often in the past, individuals without disabilities and groups came up with projects and products that they knew "would be great for handicapped people." They never bothered to ask such people for input. Their enthusiasm was great, but their idea or product was a disaster. They were more interested in a warm and fuzzy concept than they were in a substantive idea. Often their feelings were hurt when people with disabilities threw the cold water of reality on what had been the warm glow of poorly directed good intentions. It is too late to ask for input after the concrete has been poured and the last nail has been driven. Tens of millions of dollars have been wasted on projects for people with disabilities. People without disabilities must learn to ask those individuals if they need it, want it, or can afford it—and then listen to the responses. The closer we get to the goal of a barrier-free world, the less people with disabilities will need AT that is "special." For them, *special* usually means separate and different.

Of equal power to members of the media are those who design the products, places, and services that determine the ability of individuals with disabilities to be part of American culture. The designers are as diverse as people with disabilities, and some of them have disabilities themselves. I have spent the last 5 years trying to convince them to adopt a new concept called *universal design* (Mace, Hardie, & Place, 1991).

The concept of universal design is a Trojan horse that will allow people with disabilities past the gates of prejudice and fear. The concept is intended to be inclusive, not exclusive, in nature. Why do the 48.9 million U.S. citizens with disabilities need a Trojan horse? Because designers are people, and people fear citizens with disabilities. The goal of universal design is to create a product, place, or service that can be used by the widest range of individuals possible. If the product, place, or service can be used by both an 8-year-old and an 80-year-old, it is close to reaching the goal of universal design. Within this 8–80 age range, most, but not all, people with disabilities will fit.

Universal design is, at its best, seamless and invisible. One cannot look at something constructed using universal design and say "That's designed for. . . ." Adhering to universal design does not mean that all people will be able to use the end product. Some individuals with severe disabilities will need specific modification for use; however, with universal design, fewer and less costly modifications will be needed. By understanding universal design from a disability perspective, it is also a concept that can broaden domestic markets and aid the United States in global competition.

To get past the gates of fear, designers, like the media, must understand that people with disabilities are not one mass of creatures that can be designated by a single label. Designers must understand that such people are just like everyone else, except that they have disabilities. Any individual disability becomes a handicap only when a barrier is encountered. Designers, not God, created most of the barriers people with disabilities face. Ramping a building is easier than ramping the human heart and mind. People with disabilities can destroy the fear by educating designers. If they can't educate, then they can terrorize the bastards.

As a Fellow of the International Design Conference in Aspen, Colorado, I once said to several hundred famous designers: "If you designers will stop creating a world of barriers that constantly 'challenge' us, we poor crips will stop 'inspiring' you with how we manage to overcome the challenge of your bad designs. Inspiration is such a burden." Isn't it ironic that it takes a blind man to make the designers and the media see a world where nearly 49 million Americans live?

REFERENCES

Abroms, K.I., & Kodera, T.L. (1978). Expectancies underlying the acceptability of handicaps: The pervasiveness of the medical model. *Southern Journal of Educational Research, 12,* 7–21.

Gallagher, H.G. (1995). *By trust betrayed: Patients, physicians and the license to kill in the Third Reich.* Arlington, VA: Vandamrer Press.

Harris, L., & Associates. (1991). *Public attitudes toward people with disabilities.* Washington, DC: National Organization on Disability.

Howard, P.K. (1994). *The death of common sense.* New York: Random House.

Howard, P.K. (1995, April 7). Author, a hot political commodity, hints at how he'd repair the system. *New York Times,* p. A33.

Kemp, E.J. (1981, September 3). Aiding the disabled: No pity please. *New York Times,* p. 19.

Mace, R., Hardie, G., & Place, J. (1991). Accessible environments: Toward universal design. In W.F.E. Preisler, J. Vischer, & E.T. White (Eds.), *Design intervention: Toward a more humane architecture* (pp. 309–311). New York: Van Nostrand Reinhold.

Milam, L.W. (1993). *CripZen: A manual for survival.* San Diego: Mho & Mho Works.

Russell, M. (1993, March). Hollywood and disability, doing the wrong thing. *Mainstream,* 24–27.

Shapiro, J.P. (1993). *No pity: People with disabilities forging a new civil rights movement* (pp. 142–210). New York: Times Books.

Shear, M. (1986, November/December). No more supercrip. *New Directions for Women,* 10.

Siller, J. (1986). The measurement of attitudes towards physically disabled persons. In C.P. Herman, M.P. Zana, & E.T. Higgins (Eds.), *Physical appearance, stigma, and social behavior* (pp. 245–280). Hillsdale, NJ: Lawrence Erlbaum Associates.

Sloan, W., & Stevens, H.A. (1976). *A century of concern: A history of the American Association on Mental Deficiency, 1876–1976.* Washington, DC: American Association on Mental Deficiency.

Westbrook, M.T., Legge, V., & Pennay, M. (1993). Attitudes towards disabilities in a multicultural society. *Social Science and Medicine, 36,* 615–623.

Wright, B.A. (1960). *Physical disability: A psycho-social approach.* New York: Harper & Row.

Zola, I.K. (1985). Depictions of disability—metaphor, message & medium in the media: A research and political agenda. *Social Science Journal,* 22(4), 5–17.

CHAPTER 6

Tools or Baggage?

Alternative Meanings of Assistive Technology

Jean Cole Spencer

The intent of this chapter is to foster consideration of alternative meanings of assistive technology (AT). The proposition is that meaning is at least as powerful an influence as skill in determining whether a device will be incorporated by an individual as a useful tool or discarded as excess baggage. In examining the issue of meaning as being fundamental to the adaptation process, three premises are addressed:

1. Tools are meaningful objects as instruments of human intention.
2. Sources of meaning are both personal and cultural.
3. Adaptation to AT involves not only increasing skill in the use of devices but also incorporating personal and cultural meanings of technology into one's daily life routines and into one's identity.

After considering each premise, implications of an individualized, meaning-centered view of AT for research and for clinical practice

The author's ways of thinking about AT have been strongly influenced by discussions with Sara Bates, M.A., OTR, a former student and collaborator at Texas Woman's University who at this writing is a doctoral student in medical anthropology at the University of California in San Francisco. I am grateful to my husband, Dr. William Spencer, for his assistance in preparing the figure for this chapter and for the larger gift of inspiring my interest in the lives of people with disabilities.

are examined. Consideration is given to whether an individualized approach is possible in an era of increasing pressure for standardization of service provision.

TOOLS AS MEANINGFUL OBJECTS

Can AT devices be considered, not as physical devices designed to solve technical problems, but as objects that are inextricably associated with particular activities or occupations and with the contexts in which these occupations are performed? If one is asked to provide a description of the use of a common type of AT device, will the narrative be a technical essay on the design features and capabilities of the device? Or will people provide comments on the meaning, purpose, and context of where, how, when, and with whom the device is used in their lives? For example, when people are asked to describe how they prepare coffee, few describe the coffee-making apparatus. For most people, the images brought to mind are of the entire setting and rounds of activity in which coffee is made and consumed rather than the technical details of the coffee-making device. Perhaps these reflections include the kitchen of one's home, where the automatic coffee maker starts the morning routines; the kitchen of the house in which one grew up, where family and friends gathered for socialization over a pot of coffee; social settings in which espresso accompanies the conversation following a meal; or restaurants and coffeehouses, in which the technology takes on a ceremonial function far beyond the requirements of producing a concrete outcome.

At one level, using a controlled experimental method, one can evaluate each of these assistive devices for its efficiency and effectiveness in making coffee in terms of quality of outcome produced, time requirements, and human effort demands. However, limiting the examination to these factors seems to miss something fundamental about the occupation of making coffee in various contexts and the tools used for this purpose. Somewhat paradoxically, although technology may be designed to be generically useful for multiple purposes in a mass market, for the individual it is always employed to accomplish specific purposes that are valued in a particular local world and thus are invested with meaning through use in everyday life.

SOURCES OF MEANING

The meanings of tools and the occupations for which they are used have often been disregarded in research on AT as messy, in that they lack quantities that are measurable, or as confounding variables (Bates, 1992). Often the effects of such factors are eliminated by involving enough subjects in the research sample to wash out qualitative differences among individuals. Although this strategy offers some definite advantages, it also means adopting a view of humans as standardized, interchangeable multiples of ourselves, a view that ignores human capacities for intention and interpretation of meaning (Bruner, 1990). One cost of this approach is the frequent surprise of designers or providers of technology when individuals with disabilities do not share the professionals' opinions of how wonderful a particular device is.

This problem was illustrated in a qualitative study that examined ongoing changes in adaptive processes of a young man during initial rehabilitation after spinal cord injury through daily interviews with the young man and weekly interviews with key staff members (Bates, Spencer, Young, & Rintala, 1993; Spencer, Young, Rintala, & Bates, 1995). A comparison of perspectives revealed that, whereas staff saw initiation of wheelchair sitting as an opportunity to increase mobility and sitting tolerance, Russell saw his wheelchair as a dreaded symbol of disability. In his words, "You might as well stick me in a damn closet. That wheelchair just makes me think of how helpless I am."

Russell's views of the wheelchair were shaped in part by his personal life story, in which ability to take off in his pickup truck was highly valued. In contrast to his past easy mobility, the wheelchair was a very laborious way of getting around. Russell worked in construction and enjoyed woodworking in his free time, giving him an appreciation for how things are made. He regarded his first, rather ancient, wheelchair from the stock at the rehabilitation facility as "a piece of junk from World War I." In addition to his criticisms of the wheelchair based on previous personal experience with technology, Russell's views were also shaped by cultural use of the wheelchair as a universal symbol of disability. He considered becoming a person with a disability to be a very threatening and limiting prospect. In his words, "Wouldn't be fair to my son, having a cripple for an old man." Although Russell's opinions about becoming a person with a disability changed to some extent during rehabilitation, he brought with him a view that is probably quite common in the local world of his construction job, where physical prowess is highly valued. Losing these abilities meant losing an important part of who he was.

The meaning of his wheelchair for Russell was thus shaped both by his life story, which many health care researchers now study in such individuals through use of narratives (Frank, 1984;

Kleinman, 1988; Mattingly, 1991; White & Epston, 1990), and by his local world, which is a way of examining cultural settings at the level of the individual's personal territory (Kleinman, 1992; Rowles, 1991). Personal sources of meaning include the individual's history of tool use, the meaning of specific occupations to the individual, and the symbols associated with particular tools by the individual. Cultural meanings include the kinds of tools routinely used in relevant local worlds, the meaning of occupations in these local worlds, and the cultural meanings associated with particular tools. Appreciation of the individual's story can help us understand people like the woman who found it too fatiguing to use a mouthstick to operate her computer, a task for which she was trained during rehabilitation, but who valued this simple piece of AT highly after returning home because it allowed her to pet her cat. Appreciation for the importance of the culture of local worlds can help us understand people like the adolescent who liked her new purple sports wheelchair, not so much for its performance characteristics but because her friends referred to it as a "punk wheelchair."

ADAPTATION AS A PROCESS OVER TIME

Having examined a meaning-centered view of tools, the focus turns to the question of how to conceptualize and study adaptation to AT. In one sense, adaptation occurs at a behavioral level that is represented by increasing skill in use of technology by the user, a process that usually occurs over relatively short periods of time if it is going to occur at all. Such skill or capacity can be measured in fairly straightforward ways in laboratory settings by performance measures such as accuracy or efficiency in completing preselected standardized tasks. In the study of Russell, this was labeled *pragmatic adaptation.*

It can be argued, however, that the process of incorporating new technology into one's daily life routines involves much more than skill acquisition, which can be taught in a laboratory or clinical setting. Encouraging and teaching the use of AT involves rethinking what activities or occupations are most valued in the individual's life and considering alternative ways in which these might be performed that are most congruent with the personal life story of the individual and with the meanings of occupations and tools in the person's local world. The process of reorganizing one's occupational routines around technology can involve a complex orchestration of many factors. Figure 1 illustrates the circumstances of a young man who had developed a disability as a result of a spinal

cord injury during adolescence and documents how living arrangements, transportation options, and major productive activities outside the home shaped the use of AT devices, including the use of
manual versus electric wheelchairs. This individual moved to a sequence of new local worlds after completion of medical rehabilitation, including his parents' home, a nursing facility near the university, an independent living project with shared support services, and
his own apartment. Each move involved reorganization of many aspects of life, including attendant assistance, social support, transportation, and use of technology that he acquired and discarded as
circumstances made various items useful or superfluous.

In addition to reorganization of life routines, the process of
adaptation to AT often includes recognition of new or increasing
disability and incorporation of a new image of oneself. In an account of his own adaptation to progressive disability resulting from
a spinal cord tumor, anthropologist Murphy (1990), in his book *The
Body Silent*, spoke of his life being divided into two periods that he
called *prewheelchair* and *postwheelchair*. More important than
changes in his daily routines was the fact that becoming a wheelchair user meant taking on a very different social identity. This aspect of the adaptive process, which in the study of Russell was
called *emotional adaptation to technology*, may be a much more
complex and lengthy process than pragmatic adaptation marked by

| | Years since onset of spinal cord injury | | | | | | | | | | | |
	1	2	3	4	5	6	7	8	9	10	11	12
Living arrangements	Parent's home		Nursing facility near university		Independent living project with shared support services			Single apartment				
Productive activities	Completion of high school		University with large campus		University with large campus			Accounting job				
Transportation options	Van with ramps driven by father		Van service provided by volunteers		Project van with lift			Own car with hand controls		Own van with hand controls and lift		
Mobility technology	Manual wheelchair pushed by friends or father		Electric wheelchair loaded into van with assistance		Electric wheelchair loaded into van with assistance			Manual wheelchair with quad rims loaded into car without help		Electric wheelchair loaded into van without assistance		

Figure 1.   Choices of mobility technology influenced by living arrangements, productive
activities, and transportation.

skill acquisition. The long-term nature of this process may be seen, for example, in the lives of people with postpolio syndrome, who may find it difficult to return to assistive devices, such as wheelchairs or respirators, that they had given up years ago (Scheer & Luborsky, 1991). McCuaig and Frank (1991) described a similar long-term adaptive process of a 53-year-old woman with cerebral palsy who used a communication device as well as other forms of AT.

The emotional adaptation process may be marked by particular landmark experiences. An individual with a spinal cord injury told of an incident when he first began using an electric wheelchair. He was shopping in a department store when a child seized his wheelchair control and drove the chair through several racks of hanging clothes, scattering people and clothing in all directions. He recognized an important change in his life when he first was able to laugh about this experience that had initially aroused both anger at his loss of control and great embarrassment because of public attention to what at the time seemed to be a disaster. Viewing his disability and problems with AT with a sense of humor took several years, but, once achieved, he regarded the use of humor as an important adaptive strategy in many areas of life.

IMPLICATIONS FOR RESEARCH AND CLINICAL PRACTICE

Recognition of the powerful significance of meanings associated with AT has several important implications for how to study the adaptation process and for how to collaborate with individuals in practice settings to help them select and learn to use AT:

1. A holistic view of the adaptation process must be adopted that includes not only skill acquisition and behavior change in task performance but also reorganization of daily life routines in the community and emotional incorporation of new aspects of one's identity. These are the pragmatic and emotional aspects of adaptation.

2. The significance of the local worlds of individuals with disabilities must be assessed for how AT devices are viewed and used in a daily life context as tools for positively influencing the adaptation process for the individual. The concept of local worlds directs attention to shared ways of life at the level of neighborhood, workplace, or leisure settings and avoids the overgeneralization and stereotyping that can occur when cul-

ture is considered at the broad level of ethnic group or social class.

3. Methods are needed that recognize and value individual differences in adaptation to technology that complement group comparison methodologies in which members of the group being studied are presumed to be homogeneous (Batavia & Hammer, 1990; Brooks, 1991). Rather than assuming that a finding will generalize to a larger population of similar individuals based on sampling procedures, careful examination should be made of the experience of various individuals. Then empirical investigations can be made of similarities and differences between types of individuals for factors important in influencing the use of AT.

4. A longitudinal perspective is needed to capture how various aspects of the adaptation process evolve over time. The concept of narratives or life stories allows an examination of changes in an integrated way from the insider's perspective of the person with a disability (Frank, 1984; Kleinman, 1988; Mattingly, 1991).

Advocating an individualized and holistic view of adaptation to AT runs against some strong trends, both in research and in service provision. Large-scale quantitative studies have greater credibility in many arenas than either small-population time-series methods for examining individual differences in response to interventions, which have been advocated in various clinical fields (Ottenbacher, 1986), or qualitative studies that can address issues of meaning and change through a life history or narrative perspective (Frank, 1984; Kleinman, 1988). In health care and other service settings, there is great pressure to standardize service provision through mechanisms such as common treatment protocols or critical pathways, often with the rationale that such standardization will reduce costs. However, costs have not been reduced if great efficiency is achieved in selecting and teaching use of devices that people with disabilities regard as baggage and choose not to use when they return home. Listening to people tell about their life stories and local worlds can be woven into other aspects of the interactions of consumers and professionals without requiring ponderous methods and inordinate amounts of time. As Bruner (1990) noted, people will tell us about their experiences in the form of meaningful stories if they are not interrupted with too many questions and are not expected to respond in terms of scientifically constructed categories.

Attention to an individualized, holistic, and meaning-centered view of adaptation helps to provide a better understanding of why some people use technology to what is considered its maximum potential and why others prefer adaptive alternatives that seem to be less efficient and a lot more trouble. With such understanding, one can be prepared to collaborate more effectively with users of AT to imagine future possibilities for their lives rather than assuming that they share the perspectives of the provider. A meaning-centered view can remind one that, for most people, technology is a means to an end rather than an end in itself.

REFERENCES

Batavia, A., & Hammer, G. (1990). Toward the development of consumer-based criteria for the evaluation of assistive devices. *Journal of Rehabilitation Research, 27,* 425–436.

Bates, P.S. (1992). *Cultural differences in relating to electronic adaptive equipment: Occupational therapists, engineers, and persons with spinal cord injury.* Unpublished master's thesis, Texas Woman's University, Denton.

Bates, P.S., Spencer, J.C., Young, M.E., & Rintala, D. (1993). Assistive technology and the newly disabled adult: Adaptation to wheelchair use. *American Journal of Occupational Therapy, 47,* 1014–1021.

Brooks, N.A. (1991). Users' responses to assistive devices for physical disability. *Social Science and Medicine, 32*(12), 1417–1424.

Bruner, J. (1990). *Acts of meaning.* Cambridge, MA: Harvard University Press.

Frank, G. (1984). Life history model of adaptation to disability: The case of a congenital amputee. *Social Science and Medicine, 19,* 639–645.

Kleinman, A. (1988). *The illness narratives: Suffering, healing, and the human condition.* New York: Basic Books.

Kleinman, A. (1992). Local worlds of suffering: An interpersonal focus for ethnographies of illness experience. *Qualitative Health Research, 2,* 127–134.

Mattingly, C. (1991). The narrative nature of clinical reasoning. *American Journal of Occupational Therapy, 45,* 998–1005.

McCuaig, M., & Frank, G. (1991). The able self: Adaptive patterns and choices in independent living for a person with cerebral palsy. *American Journal of Occupational Therapy, 45,* 224–234.

Murphy, R. (1990). *The body silent.* New York: W.W. Norton.

Ottenbacher, K. (1986). *Evaluating clinical change.* Baltimore: Williams & Wilkins.

Rowles, G. (1991). Beyond performance: Being in place as a component of occupational therapy. *American Journal of Occupational Therapy, 45,* 265–271.

Scheer, J., & Luborsky, M. (1991). The cultural context of polio biographies. *Orthopedics, 14,* 1173–1181.

Spencer, J., Young, M., Rintala, D., & Bates, S. (1995). Socialization to the culture of a rehabilitation hospital: An ethnographic study. *American Journal of Occupational Therapy, 49,* 53–62.

White, M., & Epston, D. (1990). *Narrative means to therapeutic ends.* New York: W.W. Norton.

CHAPTER 7

The Impact of Assistive Technology on the Lives of People with Disabilities

Marcia J. Scherer

We continue to be so fascinated with the potential benefits of assistive technology (AT) that we often fail to fully consider the quality of life of the individuals who will use AT devices. An illustration is provided by Jim, one of the individuals who shares personal experiences with and perspectives on AT in *Living in the State of Stuck: How Technology Impacts the Lives of People with Disabilities* (Scherer, 1996a). At birth, Jim was diagnosed with cerebral palsy and mental retardation. His parents were advised to institutionalize him because he would need permanent custodial care. However, Jim learned to feed himself at age 19 and to drive at age 21. At age 25, he was hired as an accountant for a major insurance company.

At the time I met Jim, he was becoming a reluctant user of assistive technology because he preferred to look "normal" and do things without assistive devices, but his nonuse led to him "getting run down and worn out physically." Jim was caught in a dilemma. The rehabilitation services he received trained him for a job that he likes and in which he has had success. His co-workers treated him as both a colleague and friend and tried to help and further socialize him. He tried very hard to form an identity as, he said, "a normal person." Yet Jim's prior socialization did not prepare him for such possibilities and opportunities. His striving to be "like everyone else" and physical exhaustion took an emotional toll on him to the point where he seemed frustrated, insecure, and depressed. Jim's speech therapist commented on his situation as follows:

Compared to persons in sheltered work situations, Jim gets along beautifully. But when he's out in the community, people are not comparing him to people in sheltered workshops; they're comparing him to his [colleagues without disabilities]. . . . Often, by increasing individuals' functioning to an almost able-bodied level, it may occur that these same individuals can't deal with the frustrations they've suddenly been faced [with]. Many people will have unrealistic expectations. We see it in parents, employers, vocational rehabilitation counselors, speech therapists, the physicians here. Many people think that once that person has the appropriate technology, . . . the problem is going to be solved and that person's going to be "normal." It's just not true. (Scherer, 1996a, p. 100)

Like everyone else, people with disabilities vary in how they adjust to and cope with illnesses and physical injuries. The population of clients in a rehabilitation program will reflect a wide range of diversity. There will be pessimists and optimists, passive individuals and those who seem hostile and angry, people with a good social support network and people in social conflict, people who are denying the facts of their disabilities, people who have actively sought out all the information they can about their disabilities, and so forth. To look at the personality of each of these individuals and accurately predict who will adjust well and achieve a high quality of life and who will not is impossible. To think that there is conclusive evidence for predictable emotional and mental patterns in coping and adjustment is to do a tremendous disservice to all people who have disabilities.

Still, a person seen as succumbing to a lifestyle of dependence certainly requires different strategies from the individual who exhibits a spirited determination and drive to overcome obstacles to achievement and independence. To help a person move from withdrawal and hopelessness to adjustment and coping requires attention to physical, social, developmental, and psychological and personal factors.

Within the National Center for Medical Rehabilitation Research (NCMRR) classification of disability into five levels of pathophysiology, impairment, functional limitation, disability, and societal limitation, the diagram in Figure 1 focuses on *disability* and its impact on the *individual* and that person's behavioral adaptation. The center circle depicts AT use or nonuse as one aspect of a person's *quality of life* and *optimal functioning* (other aspects are the development of secondary conditions or returns to the hospital). The primary influences on AT use or nonuse are found in the next circle, which surrounds the center one. These include characteris-

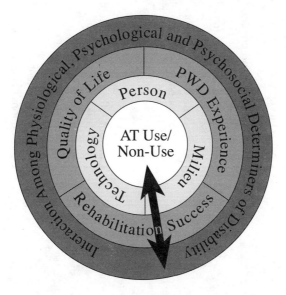

Figure 1.   Factors determining AT use or nonuse by a person with a disability (PWD). (From Scherer, M.J. [1996a]. *Living in the state of stuck: How technology impacts the lives of people with disabilities* [2nd ed., p. 114]. Cambridge, MA: Brookline Books; reprinted by permission.)

tics of the *milieus* or environments in which the assistive device will be used, characteristics of the *person* or user, and characteristics of the *device* itself. Influences in these three areas are listed in Table 1. This is where the person's adjustment and coping strategies as related to AT use become manifest. This is also where decisions regarding discharge destination are made.

The three components of the second circle are most influenced by expectations and definitions of *rehabilitation success* by and for that individual; the person's view of present and future *quality of life*; and the person's current, subjective situation or experiences as a *person with a disability*. These compose the next level of influence and reflect the meaning the person and others have put on the disability and how that frames behavior characteristics of and toward the person. These influences derive from past coping efforts, views of and opportunities offered to the person by therapists, and behavior strategies exhibited and employed by significant others. Although they are partly subjective and culturally determined, they are also determined by more objective and definable influences (i.e., physiological influences, psychological influences, psychosocial in-

Table 1. Assistive technology influences

Attitude	Milieu	Personality	Technology
		Use	
Optimal	Support from family, peers, and employer	Proud to use device	Goal achieved with no pain, fatigue, or stress
	Realistic expectations of family and employer	Motivated	Compatible with and enhances the use of other technologies
	Setting and environment fully supports and rewards use	Cooperative	Is safe, reliable, and easy to use and maintain
		Optimistic	Has the desired transportability
		Good coping skills	No better options currently available
		Patient	
		Self-disciplined	
		Generally positive life experiences	
		Has the skills to use the device	
		Perceives discrepancy between desired and current situation	
Partial or reluctant	Pressure for use from either family, peers, or employer	Embarrassed to use device	Goal not fully achieved or achieved with discomfort and strain
	Assistance often not available	Unmotivated	Requires a lot of set-up
	Setting and environment discourages use or makes use awkward	Impatient and impulsive	Interferes somewhat with the use of other technologies
		Unrealistic expectations	Device is inefficient
		Low self-esteem	Other options to device use exist
		Somewhat intimidated by technology	
		Technology partially or occasionally fits with lifestyle	
		Limitations in skills needed for use	

Nonuse

Avoidance	Lack of support from either family, peers, or employer Unrealistic expectations of others Assistance not available Setting and environment disallows or prevents use	Person does not want device Embarrassed to use device Depressed Unmotivated Uncooperative Withdrawn Intimidated by technology Many changes required in lifestyle Does not have skills for use	*Perceived* lack of goal achievement or too much strain or discomfort in use Requires a lot of set-up Perceived or determined to be incompatible with the use of other technologies Too expensive Long delay for delivery Other options to device use exist
Abandonment	Lack of support from either family, peers, or employer Setting and environment discourages or makes use awkward Requires assistance that is not available	Embarrassed to use device Depressed Low self-esteem Hostile and angry Withdrawn Resistant Poor socialization and coping skills Many changes in lifestyle with device use Lacks skills to use device and training is not available	Goal not achieved and/or discomfort and strain in use Is incompatible with the use of other technologies Has been outgrown Is difficult to use Device is inefficient Repairs and service not timely or affordable Other options to use became available

fluences), which include level of pain, functional status, access to quality care, financial resources, and the like. Influences at the cellular and organ levels occur beyond them.

Although the attitudes of society as a whole and environmental accommodations are crucial (the NCMRR's "societal limitations"), the remainder of this chapter assumes that AT use is reflective of behavioral adaptation and that it is the target outcome. Thus AT nonuse or less-than-optimal use becomes the target for intervention. The effects of characteristics of the milieu, the person, and the technology itself on outcome are discussed as variables deserving clinical and research attention.

IMPORTANCE OF REDUCING
ASSISTIVE TECHNOLOGY NONUSE

Studies of AT nonuse or abandonment, although few in number, have reported consistent overall figures of 30%–50% of all devices recommended; depending on the device, the abandonment figures range from 8% to 75% (Scherer & Galvin, 1994). One of the earliest studies to address the abandonment of recommended technologies was conducted by the Children's Hospital at Stanford (1980) as a follow-up of the use of mobility aids over a 3-year period from 1975 to 1978. The study found that 50% of the devices were being used for an average of 9 hours per day, and 22% of the devices were no longer used. Sixty-nine percent of the study population was under age 18, and the primary reason for nonuse was that the device had been outgrown.

Data from a study of AT device abandonment among a sample of 227 U.S. adults with a variety of disabilities yielded an overall device abandonment rate of 29.3% (Phillips & Zhao, 1993). Most abandoned devices were mobility aids, and most were abandoned either during the first year or after 5 years. The strongest factor influencing abandonment was a change in the needs or priorities of the user (through either improvement or decline in the person's functioning and medical condition or functional changes brought about by personal activities such as returning to work). Other strong influences on abandonment were device performance; the extent to which the consumer was involved in device selection; and whether the device met consumer expectations for effectiveness, reliability, durability, comfort, and ease of use.

Another study surveyed 35 home-based people with hearing impairments over the age of 60 years (mean age = 80.1 years, age range = 60–95 years) regarding the need for and use of AT devices

(Mann, Hurren, & Tomita, 1994). The results of the survey showed that this sample was dissatisfied with 31.9% of their devices. No data were provided regarding the proportion of these devices that were abandoned, so it is not known how many devices were used in spite of dissatisfaction with them.

Although relatively little information is available about technology abandonment, still less is available regarding the numbers of people who must continue to use devices with which they are unhappy because they cannot abandon the devices without more severe consequences. For example, the alternative to using a less-than-perfect wheelchair is reduced options to interact with and within a variety of environments. For individuals, nonuse of a device may lead to decreases in functional abilities, freedom, and independence and increases in expenses. On a service delivery level, device abandonment represents ineffective use of limited funds by federal, state, and local government agencies, insurers, and other providers.

A better understanding of how and why technology users decide to accept or reject a device is critical to improving the costs and general effectiveness of AT interventions (DeRuyter, 1995) and enhancing consumer satisfaction and quality of life (Scherer, 1995, 1996b). Research must examine different categories of assistive technologies and different ages at disability onset, as well as considering disability severity and the psychological predispositions individuals bring to the process of device selection, evaluation, and use.

RELATIONSHIP OF TWO CONSTRUCTS: TREATMENT ADHERENCE AND OPTIMAL TECHNOLOGY USE

The paucity of data on varying degrees of AT use is indicative of the complex interface between a person and a device and ways to assess the quality of that interface. Although much research remains to be done on the match of person and technology and the abandonment of recommended assistive devices, a related area, failure to adhere to treatment recommendations or prescriptions, has been researched fairly well (especially adherence involving medication). The relationship between treatment adherence and AT use is worthy of exploration.

Treatment Adherence

Treatment adherence is the extent to which patients follow recommended courses of treatment such as medication regimens, weight loss, and lifestyle changes in patterns of exercise and alcohol consumption. The term *adherence* in the medical literature frequently includes the patient-controlled concept of compliance. Rates of adherence failure mirror those of AT device abandonment; on average, they are one third to one half, depending on the type of technology, medication, and the like (e.g., Bloom, 1988; Homedes, 1991; Rand & Wise, 1994; Wright, 1993). Adherence failure has been related to treatment characteristics (e.g., the complexity of the recommended treatment, the discomfort and lifestyle changes it represents), patient characteristics (i.e., demographic and psychosocial factors), and characteristics of patient–provider interactions and communication (e.g., Drozda, Allen, Turner, Slusher, & Cain, 1993; Franklin, Kolasa, Griffin, Mayo, & Badenhop, 1995; Mann, 1993). Studies of adherence within particular populations of individuals with disabilities suggest more differential adherence according to age and gender (e.g., Krasnegor, 1992; Lerman & Schwartz, 1993; Morrow, Leirer, & Sheikh, 1988) than according to race or culture (e.g., Piane, 1990). The measurement of adherence is problematic because patient self-reports of adherence are relied on most. Objective measures of adherence (e.g., blood levels of medication) can be intrusive.

Bloom (1988) believed adherence is composed of a psychological readiness for adherence and a belief that the treatment will be effective, factors to modify or enhance readiness, and reinforcement for adhering to the treatment. His description of the major approaches to the improvement of adherence is as follows:

> Three approaches have been explored in attempting to improve adherence rates to medical treatment programs. [1]] . . . the development of patient education programs and the assessment of whether such programs result in improved adherence-related behavior. [2]] . . . changes in the treatment program, including changes in the behavior of the health care practitioner in the hopes that such changes will enhance adherence rates. [3] the use of] . . . behavioral modification approaches with the patient in order to improve adherence rates directly. . . . The greatest number of studies are probably in this category. (Bloom, 1988, p. 321)

Bloom reported that improved patient education efforts have had relatively little impact on adherence, whereas the modification of the patient's behavior through behavioral approaches (manipulating antecedents or consequences) and techniques to improve provider–patient communication have met with considerable success. Modifying aspects of the treatment program—for example, tailoring the timing of medications to existing habitual patterns of the patient—has also been successful with many patients.

Optimal Technology Use

Regardless of the type of technology under consideration, an individual is either a user or a nonuser. As shown in Figure 1 and Table 1, the outcome of the process of matching person and technology may be nonuse, wherein the person avoids an assistive device altogether (e.g., a person will not show up for an evaluation or fitting or will not purchase a recommended device), or complete abandonment of the device after initial use. Alternatively, use may be optimal (e.g., according to recommendation and done willingly) or partial and done reluctantly. (The latter most frequently occurs with people whose device use is optional or with people who will use a device in one environment but not in another.)

An assistive device must be adapted to a person's needs and preferences, and the user of that device must adapt to the realities important to its optimal use. Options in the functions and features of various assistive devices allow differences among individual users to be accommodated. However, as shown in Table 1 under personality influences, people's reactions to assistive technology are highly personal and individual. They emerge from varying needs, abilities, preferences, and past experiences with and exposures to technology. Predispositions to technology use also depend on the outlook and goals a person has for future functioning, expectations of help by others, and financial and environmental support for technology use. Achieving optimal technology use requires a combination of science and engineering with clinical and human services.

Matching an individual with the most appropriate AT device at the right time is multifaceted and complex, as is optimizing treatment adherence. Table 2 compares the major influences on treatment adherence with the major influences affecting optimal assistive technology device use and lists some strategies for enhancing optimal use, which are expanded on in the following discussion.

CONSIDERATIONS FOR ENHANCING THE PERSON–TECHNOLOGY MATCH FOR OPTIMAL TECHNOLOGY USE

Although it is generally presumed that there is a linear relationship between AT use and quality of life, nonuse of a recommended technology does not preclude the achievement of a high quality of life. Just as the lack of use of an inadequate assistive device cannot be considered a failure, neither can less than 100% use. Part-time use may be all that is required for energy conservation, having access to

Table 2.   Some strategies for enhancing AT device use consistent with a treat-
ment-adherence model for a user with low motivation for use and with a history
of poor decision-making skills

Influences on adherence	Influences on AT use	Enhancement of optimal AT use
Patient–provider interactions	Milieu characteristics	Have technology-using peers as role models
		Improve the user's comprehension of information regarding the technology and its use
		Have more tailored and convenient training for the user and significant others in the environments of use
		Ensure that environments of use are reinforcing of use
		Assist rehabilitation engineers in working collaboratively with the user
Patient characteristics	Person characteristics	Ensure that the user participates in all aspects of device selection and evaluation
		Assess the person's knowledge of and comfort with assistive technology
Treatment characteristics	Technology characteristics	Select according to what is already used
		Tailor to the person's preferences and lifestyle

particular places, and so forth. When a device is used appropriately,
then, *part-time use* can be considered *optimal* use.

Determine Current and Desirable
Milieu/Environmental Influences on Use

The environments in which the person uses an assistive device will
either support or deter use. As shown in Table 1, relevant features
of the milieu include the degree of social and economic support for
technology use as well as the existence of physically accessible
community features. In addition, factors such as environmental accommodations, available resources (e.g., private insurance for specialized treatment, availability of personal assistance), and special
opportunities (e.g., placement in a rehabilitation center with
knowledgeable providers and appropriate equipment) are important
influences on AT use.

The availability of training for use of the equipment is crucial.
The AT device that worked so well in the rehabilitation facility often does not work out in the home or in the workplace. The power

wheelchair is tearing up the carpet, or the cane is never in the same place as the need for it. The failure of assistive devices to fit well with the person's environments is a major reason for their being abandoned. Another common reason for abandonment is that AT use is forced on the individual as a condition of being discharged, and the device immediately becomes a focal point for resentment.

The perspectives and expectations of others in the environments of use can be influential, especially if the assistive device inconveniences others. In this fast-paced world, it is often easier (and less emotionally painful) for family members to just jump in and do it for the person than to patiently step aside and watch the individual struggle to accomplish a task independently. Therefore, other people in the environment can nullify the individual's use of AT.

Assessing Milieu Influences   On-site trials of equipment that involve everyone affected by the assistive device have proved to be cost-effective in the long term because obstacles to optimal technology use are identified before nonuse habits can form. When trials are videotaped, the entire rehabilitation team can then participate in identifying solutions to potential obstacles to optimal technology use.

Know the Person

When a person in the process of being matched with an assistive device is involved in selecting the equipment and is encouraged to exercise choice regarding the equipment's features, the likelihood of the most appropriate device being identified is enhanced, as is the probability of its being optimally used. However, many consumers may see only limited alternatives for themselves because they have not been exposed to sufficient options to make informed choices and express informed preferences. Individuals who have not yet come to terms with their disabilities and who may be depressed cannot be expected to exercise good judgment regarding AT selection. In addition, depression may mask capabilities and capacities that would obviate the need for an assistive device. Alternatively, premature introduction of AT may assume capacities and coping skills that in fact must develop over time, which may result in the person feeling confused and overwhelmed. Individuals who have developed a recent severe disability as a result of trauma first need to be helped to understand their changed circumstances. As one person with a C4 spinal cord injury said to me, "In rehab, they handle your broken neck, but the broken neck isn't the problem. The paralysis is the problem. They don't confront the paralysis." Before an assistive device will be optimally used, a person must both need it and want it. If an assistive device enhances the individual's functioning, self-esteem, self-efficacy, and overall quality of life, it will be used.

Assessing Characteristics and Preferences of the Person Proper timing is of the essence. So is privacy. It is best to ask individuals about preferences, needs, and capabilities when their significant others are not present. Significant others want to be helpful and should be involved, but let them know that they will have opportunities to express their preferences at another time.

Find the Best Technology

An assistive device is abandoned when it is perceived as not being worth the effort required to set it up and operate it, is never there when needed, and is costly or inconvenient to maintain. Selecting the most appropriate device with all the right features is a complex process. An AT device must have enough features to be useful and expandable, but not so many that the user becomes overwhelmed. Overload is a concern when an individual already uses or is being matched with more than one device. Multiple-equipment use can bring on overload of many types—electrical circuitry, cognitive stress, and an unwillingness to tolerate further use of AT devices.

For the most part, and for a variety of reasons, people with disabilities have been socialized to minimize their disabilities. Equipment that makes an individual stand out in a crowd yet eclipses the person using it has a high likelihood of being abandoned. Abandonment is also a probable outcome if the individual feels *disenfranchised* when using the equipment and can get by without it.

Increasingly, however, many people with disabilities view assistive devices as desirable markers of a need for accommodation by making one's disability visible enough not to have to defend the need for accommodations. In the context of such legislative backing as the Americans with Disabilities Act (ADA) of 1990 (PL 101-336), when the existence of a disability is addressed up front, the disability *is* minimized and the person can get on with being just that—a person.

Assessing Features of and Comparing Technologies   It has become increasingly difficult to keep up to date with new assistive devices and improvements in existing ones. For this reason, the Technology-Related Assistance for Individuals with Disabilities Act (PL 100-407) was passed in 1988 to help establish state assistive technology centers. A major responsibility of these centers is to provide information about assistive devices and advice on ways to obtain them. Equipment loan and trial programs, user and peer networks, and equipment-funding assistance exist in many states. The lead agency in a given state can be located by contacting the RESNA

Technical Assistance Project (1700 North Moore Street, Suite 1540, Arlington, Virgina 22209-1903; telephone [703] 524-6686 [(703) 524-6639 TTY/TDD]). For information about particular assistive devices, an excellent resource is Co-Net through the TRACE Center (University of Wisconsin–Madison, S-151 Waisman Center, 1500 Highland Avenue, Madison, Wisconsin 53705; telephone [608] 262-6966 [(608) 263-5408 TTY/TDD]).

EVALUATING AND DOCUMENTING THE NEED FOR AND OUTCOMES OF ASSISTIVE TECHNOLOGY USE

Every match of person and technology requires careful consideration. Although some assistive devices are meant to be used only for a short time, premature AT abandonment is costly in terms of both dollars and outcome achievement, regardless of whether the abandoned equipment is low or high tech. Equipment also becomes wasteful when it does not enhance the person's quality of life— even if it is used. Professionals working with assistive devices need to demonstrate that what they do makes a difference in the lives of people with disabilities. Insurance companies and other payers are increasingly asking for documentation showing the effectiveness of all AT services—also known as *quality assurance*. A major part of quality assurance is being able to assess and document outcomes of an intervention.

When evaluating an individual for an assistive device, evaluation forms should be available that will guide professionals in considering those factors influencing an individual's predisposition to the use of AT and to document that such consideration was done (e.g., the Assistive Technology Device Predisposition Assessment[1] [Scherer, 1994]).

Definition of *Outcomes*

Outcomes are the result of an intervention. Examples of outcomes are employability, performance of activities of daily living, and con-

---

[1]The Assistive Technology Device Predisposition Assessment (ATDPA) in Scherer (1994) was developed from a study that looked at differences between AT device users and nonusers. It inquires into individuals' subjective satisfaction with current functioning in many areas and where they want to gain the most improvement. The consumer version has two forms: 1) consumer questions on temperament, psychosocial resources, and views of disability; and 2) technology questions on views of and expectations for a particular assistive device. Companion professional forms are similarly constructed. The ATDPA has adequate content and criterion-related validity and interrater reliability.

sumer satisfaction or subjective well-being. The latter encompasses the person's sense of comfort, happiness, and satisfaction with such specific areas of functioning as work, social relationships, and finances. *Outcomes assessment* has been defined as "what rehabilitation services *ought* to achieve for the persons receiving them . . . and *how* those achievements can be identified and measured" (Fuhrer, 1987, p. 1, emphasis added). In their *1995 Standards Manual and Interpretive Guidelines for Behavioral Health*, CARF . . . The Rehabilitation Accreditation Commission discussed outcome-based evaluation and the need for organizations to "demonstrate that systems have been established to measure outcomes including effectiveness, efficiency, and satisfaction of the persons served" (CARF, 1995, p. 6).

Measuring Outcomes

Outcomes measures are used to demonstrate that particular goals established for a consumer have been identified and then achieved. One outcomes measure is the difference over time between capability and performance (i.e., effectiveness). That is the reason why many functional assessment measures (with their focus on, e.g., self-care, ambulation) are being viewed as means of demonstrating outcome achievement. Without the use of functional assessment measures, the determination of rehabilitation effectiveness can be affected by incongruence in views held by consumers and therapists regarding disability, rehabilitation success, and other aspects. For example, professionals tend to define *independence* in terms of physical functioning, whereas consumers more often equate independence with social and psychological freedoms. Outcomes vary among individuals, and one must obtain the consumer's perspectives of the most desired outcomes as well as the perspectives of secondary consumers (e.g., family members, caregivers), payers, vendors, and employers. Once the goals of the intervention are specified, a time line for goal achievement must be established.

For many people, the ultimate in outcome achievement is a subjective sense of well-being and comfort when in the community. Quality of life has come to mean global happiness and satisfaction as well as satisfaction with specific areas of life functioning such as work, social relationships, and housing. A person's view of his or her quality of life is influenced by such psychological factors as mood and outlook, physical factors (e.g., pain), and his or her perceptions of a broad array of external factors, including available social support, money, and transportation. Furthermore, all of these factors are interrelated: Pain influences mood, which in turn influences perceived resources and needs.

When looking at outcome achievement from a quality-of-life perspective, one means of assessing a person's quality of life is to have the individual report behavioral adaptation at various points in time, prioritize his or her desired outcomes, and then rate over time his or her progress in achieving them. This is the system used in the Assistive Technology Device Predisposition Assessment. In this way, outcomes are measured in terms of changes in, for example, the person's satisfaction in being able to get to a desired location, whether by walking or by some other means, rather than just in terms of the functional capability to do so. Functional capability, however, is an essential means to satisfaction and quality-of-life achievement.

CONCLUSIONS

Quality-of-life enhancement is the ultimate outcome for most people working in AT service delivery, who want to help individuals become more capable, more independent, and able to exercise more choice and take advantage of a wide range of opportunities. Although attention necessarily has been focused on the engineering and production of quality assistive devices, it is now time to attend to the match of these devices with the people they are designed to assist. People with disabilities have preferences, personalities, varying life histories, and networks of support that must be taken into account. Also, these elements may change over relatively short spans of time.

Jim, discussed at the beginning of this chapter, had worked with the insurance company for 13 years when he told me that they had downgraded his job from accountant to clerk. He had lost his private office and was sharing a room with two other people. He reported feeling isolated and believed his supervisors were angry with him "for pushing the ADA issues and equal opportunities." Jim has returned to rehabilitation on an outpatient basis and is in the process of forming an evolved identity as a person with a disability—one in which AT device use is viewed more positively.

People's life situations are influenced by their responses to a disability, not by the disability itself. Jim's example of the need for a psychological readiness for technology use illustrates why the *person* always must come first in rehabilitation—not the *disability* and not the assistive technology or other intervention.

REFERENCES

Americans with Disabilities Act (ADA) of 1990, PL 101-336, 42 U.S.C. §§ 12101 et seq.

Bloom, B.L. (1988). *Health psychology: A psychosocial perspective*. Englewood Cliffs, NJ: Prentice Hall.

CARF . . . The Rehabilitation Accreditation Commission. (1995). *1995 Standards manual and interpretive guidelines for behavioral health*. Tucson, AZ: Author.

Children's Hospital at Stanford. (1980). *Team effectiveness: A retrospective study*. Palo Alto, CA: Rehabilitation Engineering Center. (NARIC Document No. 03850)

DeRuyter, F. (1995). Evaluating outcomes in assistive technology: Do we understand the commitment? *Assistive Technology, 7*(1), 3–8.

Drozda, D.J., Allen, S.R., Turner, A.M., Slusher, J.A., & Cain, G.C. (1993). Adherence behaviors in research protocols: Comparison of two interventions. *Diabetes Education, 19*(5), 393–395.

Franklin, T.L., Kolasa, K.M., Griffin, K., Mayo, C., & Badenhop, D.T. (1995). Adherence to very-low-fat diet by a group of cardiac rehabilitation patients in the rural southeastern United States. *Archives of Family Medicine, 4*(6), 551–554.

Fuhrer, M.J. (Ed.). (1987). *Rehabilitation outcomes: Analysis and measurement*. Baltimore: Paul H. Brookes Publishing Co.

Homedes, N. (1991). Do we know how to influence patients' behavior? Tips to improve patients' adherence. *Family Practice, 8*(4), 412–423.

Krasnegor, N.A. (1992). *Development aspects of health compliance behavior*. Hillsdale, NJ: Lawrence Erlbaum Associates.

Lerman, C., & Schwartz, M. (1993). Adherence and psychological adjustment among women at high risk for breast cancer. *Breast Cancer Research and Treatment, 28*(2), 145–155.

Mann, N. (1993). *Improving adherence behavior with treatment regimens*. Geneva, Switzerland: World Health Organization.

Mann, W.C., Hurren, D., & Tomita, M.R. (1994). Assistive device needs of home-based elderly persons with hearing impairments. *Technology and Disability, 3*(1), 47–61.

Morrow, D., Leirer, V., & Sheikh, J. (1988). Adherence and medication instructions: Review and recommendations. *Journal of the American Geriatrics Society, 36*(12), 1147–1160.

Phillips, B., & Zhao, H. (1993). Predictors of assistive technology abandonment. *Assistive Technology, 5*, 36–45.

Piane, G. (1990). A comparison of the effect of a hypertension education program among black and white participants. *Journal of Health Care for the Poor and Underserved, 1*(2), 243–253.

Rand, C.S., & Wise, R.A. (1994). Measuring adherence to asthma medication regimens. *American Journal of Respiratory Critical Care Medicine, 149*(2), S69–S76.

Scherer, M.J. (1994). *Matching Person and Technology (MPT) Model and accompanying assessment instruments*. Rochester, NY: Author.

Scherer, M.J. (1995). Comments on DeRuyter's "Evaluating outcomes in assistive technology." *Assistive Technology, 7*(11), 11–12.

Scherer, M.J. (1996a). *Living in the state of stuck: How technology impacts the lives of people with disabilities* (2nd ed.). Cambridge, MA: Brookline Books.

Scherer, M.J. (1996b). Outcomes of assistive technology use on quality of life. *Disability and Rehabilitation, 18,* 439–448.

Scherer, M.J., & Galvin, J.C. (1994). Matching people with technology. *Rehab Management, 7*(2), 128–130.

Technology-Related Assistance for Individuals with Disabilities Act of 1988, PL 100-407, 29 U.S.C. §§ 2201 *et seq.*

Wright, E.C. (1993). Non-compliance—or how many aunts has Matilda? *Lancet, 342,* 909–913.

CHAPTER 8

From Hospital to Home

Individual Variations in Experience with Assistive Devices Among Older Adults

Laura N. Gitlin

Research evidence from large-scale national representative surveys suggests an increase in assistive device use and a decline in dependence on personal assistance by older adults who have a disability and live in the community (LaPlante, Hendershot, & Moss, 1992; Macken, 1986; Manton, Corder, & Stallard, 1993; Norburn et al., 1995). Other studies of older adults with functional limitations who are community dwellers (Mann, Hurren, Karuza, & Bentley, 1993; Zimmer & Chappell, 1994), discharged from rehabilitation (Gitlin, Schemm, Landsberg, & Burgh, 1996; Gitlin, Schemm, & Shmuely, 1997), or receiving home care (Bynum & Rogers, 1987) provide further evidence that assistive devices are consistently used as a self-care strategy.

Although it is evident that older adults use AT devices to cope with functional limitations, much less is known about the personal experiences of users. Specifically, we know very little about the experiences of older adults who initially confront the need for assistive devices late in life as a result of a first-time disabling condition.

Most older adults who develop a disability late in life are initially introduced to and instructed in the use of assistive devices in a hospital setting. In rehabilitation, an older patient may receive instruction in the use of as many as 21 different devices for ambulation, dressing, grooming, bathing, feeding, or seating (Gitlin et al., 1996; Schemm & Gitlin, in press). Upon returning home, the individual must incorporate these devices into daily routines and physical environments, often without receiving further instruction and supportive services.

This chapter examines the use of assistive devices by older adults as they confront different functional consequences and life situations in the transition from hospital to home. Case material is presented for three older adults with different impairments who were first-time users of assistive devices. The cases include an 81-year-old widowed African American man with an orthopedic impairment who was issued 10 devices for home use, a 62-year-old divorced African American man with a stroke who was issued 17 devices for home use, and an 81-year-old married Caucasian man with a double below-knee amputation who was issued 6 devices for home use.

The case material draws on personal interviews conducted in the hospital and at home and on home observations of functional status and daily activity needs by a health professional. The use of case material that is derived from multiple perspectives provides an opportunity to examine in depth and qualitatively the issues that present as older adults adapt to new functional limitations using assistive devices (Stake, 1995; Yin, 1989). These cases were purposely selected from a larger study of 250 older rehabilitation clients for their instrumental value in illuminating key issues concerning the fit between hospital-prescribed devices and actual needs upon return home and the factors that may contribute to continued effective device use.

BACKGROUND AND SIGNIFICANCE

Most research on assistive devices has been cross-sectional, with a focus on describing utilization patterns and reasons for nonuse (for reviews, see Gitlin, 1995, in press). A cross-sectional and unidimensional perspective, however, decontextualizes personal experiences and the underlying issues that present to older adults as they master tool use. In contrast, a prospective comparison of multiple cases over time provides an opportunity to explore specific life worlds and differences and similarities in device use and needs. This approach provides a basis for understanding the initial or early stage of device use, as represented in the return home from the hospital.

Furthermore, as a whole, assistive device research has lacked a social science perspective and a conceptual framework from which to examine utilization patterns and experiences (Gitlin, in press; Luborsky, 1993; Strain, Chappell, & Penning, 1993). Unfortunately, this has limited the advancement of research in this area. Although there is not a unified theory of assistive device use, two theoretical constructs are used here to explore the multiple issues involved in becoming a device user: a biopsychosocial framework and the sociological construct of career as a device user.

Biopsychosocial Framework

First, a biopsychosocial framework offers a starting point from which to examine the interplay of functional, psychological, and social conditions that contribute to device use at home. The emerging research on the personal experiences with devices suggests that individuals may need to adapt physically, socially, and psychologically to become successful device users (Frank, 1994). Some studies have shown that there are both physical and psychosocial consequences to using certain types of devices. Mobility aids in particular present a number of personal difficulties for older adults, such as physical discomfort, an inability to propel oneself, or an inability to use the aid within the physical environment of the home (Mann, Hurren, Charvat, & Tomita, 1996). Some mobility-aid users report feeling embarrassed and stigmatized when using aids in public. In a study of adults with severe visual impairments and blindness, it was found that mobility aids (e.g., guide dogs, white canes) provided important opportunities for social engagement, work, and travel while also posing physical challenges and personal feelings of being socially ostracized (Gitlin, Mount, Lucas, Weirich, & Gamberg, 1997; Mount, Gitlin, & Howard, 1997). Similarly, in a study of stroke patients' initial perceptions of devices issued in the hospital, mobility aids elicited concerns about social acceptance and personal identity, although they were also viewed as providing an opportunity for independence (Gitlin, Luborsky, & Schemm, 1997). Other studies on individuals with postpoliomyelitis syndrome and spinal cord injury suggest that, even when it saves lives, the use of equipment can have dramatic consequences for a user's sense of identity and social integration (Locker, Kaufert, & Kirk, 1987; Luborsky, 1993). Thus, changes in biological processes and their impact on self-care practices may be mediated by psychological and social processes.

Career as a Device User

The second theoretical perspective is that offered by the sociological construct of career. The notion of career provides a useful framework for understanding the structural path in assuming the role of an assistive device user and the different transitions and patterns of experiences that emerge. The construct of career has been used to understand the structure of caregiving as it unfolds over time (Aneshensel, Pearlin, Mullan, Zarit, & Whitlatch, 1995; Pearlin, 1992; Pearlin & Aneshensel, 1994). Applied to the context of disability, career is a compelling construct. It emphasizes that device use may extend over many years and may involve transitions marked by new device needs as a consequence of an individual's experiences, functional change, and environmental demands.

It would appear that the path of the career of a user begins in the hospital, where devices are initially prescribed and instruction by trained health professionals occurs. It is in the hospital setting that an older adult usually first acquires the role of an assistive device user. In this initial phase of role acquisition, older adults may begin to accumulate personal, social, and physical experiences using devices that inform early appraisals and influence subsequent use at home.

The first career transition may occur from hospital to home (Bull, 1992; Magilvy & Lakomy, 1991). This transition may pose special challenges in that the user must take knowledge learned in the hospital, adapt it to a different context (that of the home and community), and assume a modified pattern of daily life. Who does what for themselves and how has important clinical and health policy implications (Kart & Engler, 1994). The case material presented here provides insight into the early career stage of self-care with AT devices and the role of biopsychosocial factors in shaping device use. It is of special interest to both the research and clinical communities.

METHOD

The three cases presented were selected from data collected as part of a larger project that examined long-term AT device use by older rehabilitation clients. Participants in the larger study were recruited over a 20-month period from two freestanding rehabilitation hospitals in the Philadelphia area (Magee Rehabilitation Hospital and Chestnut Hill Hospital). Study participants included individuals who were 55 years of age or older and who had been hospitalized with a primary diagnosis of either a cerebrovascular accident (CVA), orthopedic impairment, or lower-limb amputation. Furthermore, participants had to be cognitively intact, able to attend to a 1-hour personal interview, and discharged to their own homes with one or more assistive devices for use in that environment. In the study, individuals were interviewed in the hospital prior to discharge and then monthly at home for 6 months. In addition, individuals were invited to participate in an experimental program that involved assistive device training by an occupational therapist at home following hospital discharge. The program involved up to six home visits, the purpose of which was to examine whether hospital-issued assistive devices were appropriate for the physical dimensions of the home and for carrying out the personal activity choices of individuals. AT device training involved reinforcement or refinement of ways of using issued devices to perform valued activities, recommendation of and instruction in use of new devices or environmental adaptations if necessary, or both. Occupational therapy visits occurred over 6 months, the scheduling of which depended on the specific needs of study participants.

The information presented on these cases is based on open-ended questions and a number of measures that were collected in personal interviews at the hospital and home and during occupational therapy home visits. These measures assessed assistive device use, functional status, and psychosocial well-being. Appraisals of devices were ascertained through interviews using the Reinforcement Motivation Survey (Bruno, 1993), and new device needs were identified through clinical assessment by the occupational therapist. Functional status was assessed in the hospital and home by occupational therapists using the Functional Independence Measure (FIM; State University of New York at Buffalo, 1993). Well-being was assessed using standard measures, including Bradburn's Positive and Negative Affect Balance Scale (Bradburn, 1969) and the Philadelphia Geriatric Center Morale Scale (Lawton, 1975). The cases discussed here are those of individuals who were available for the hospital interview, participated in at least two home interviews, and were involved in the experimental home AT device training program.

CASES

Case 1: Mr. X

In the Hospital   Mr. X, an 81-year-old African American, was hospitalized for a hip fracture resulting from a fall. He had five other previous conditions: arthritis, diabetes, high blood pressure, a heart condition, and visual problems. At the time of his hip fracture, he was a retired widower who lived alone in his daughter's home. His daughter had passed away 8 months prior to his fall.

While in rehabilitation, Mr. X was issued 10 assistive devices (Table 1). Prior to his hip fracture, Mr. X had never needed or used an assistive device. In the hospital, Mr. X presented with high posi-

Table 1. Assistive devices issued in rehabilitation for home use

Case	Mobility	Dressing	Bathing	Feeding	Seating	Grooming
Mr. X (10 devices)	Walker Walker bag Walker basket	Reacher Dressing stick Shoehorn	Commode Long-handled sponge Shower hose	Cup holder	—	—
Mr. Y (17 devices)	Wheelchair Quad-cane Wheelchair bag	Laces Shoehorn Reacher	Tub chair Commode Flexible shower hose Long-handled sponge	Cup holder Rocker knife Dycem	Backboard Arm rest Seat rest	Denture brush
Mr. Z (6 devices)	Wheelchair Walker	Reacher	Commode Tub chair	—	—	Inspection mirror

tive affect and morale. In general, he viewed his issued devices positively. However, he stated that the devices did not facilitate the things he wanted to do, nor did he believe that the devices made him independent. He also noted that it took too long to use some of the devices.

At Home   Once home, a number of factors reflecting biopsychosocial issues placed Mr. X at increasing risk of functional decline. These factors can be summarized as his limited social network, mourning of the loss of his daughter, fear of falling, poor sleep, physical stiffness, and decreased energy. His functional status, as shown in Figure 1, declined in the transition from hospital to home. By his third month at home, Mr. X used only two devices (a 20% device use rate)—a cane that he had received in an outpatient visit and a commode. He did not value his other devices as tools to enable him to accomplish his personal activity goals (see Table 2). His goals represented a primary concern for performing basic activities of daily living. These goals were modified and became more specified from hospital to home as Mr. X confronted new personal and environmental challenges.

New Needs   As shown in Table 3, once Mr. X was home, a number of new device needs and functional issues emerged. Although Mr. X had a hospital bed on the first floor, he preferred to sleep in his own bed on the second floor. However, he had difficulty ascending and descending his stairs, which were steep; getting into and out of his own bed, which was low and lacked adequate support; and bathing and grooming in the second-floor bathroom, which was narrow. The shower hose provided in rehabilitation did not fit Mr. X's spigots. He was frustrated by his inability to achieve

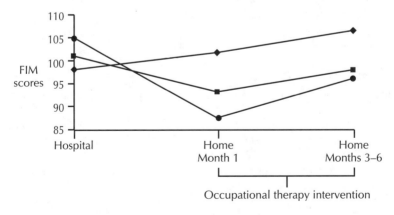

Figure 1.   Functional Independence Measure (FIM) scores for Mr. X, Mr. Y, and Mr. Z in the hospital and at home. (—■—, Mr. X; —◆—, Mr. Y; —●—, Mr. Z.)

Table 2.   Personal activity goals in order of importance in the hospital and the home

Case	Hospital	Home
Mr. X	• Bathing • Dressing • Stairs	• Ascend or descend stairs • Self-care • Get legs on or off bed • Meal preparation
Mr. Y	• Shopping • Housework • Cooking	• Laundry • Shopping • Ambulate outside apartment • Participate in social activities
Mr. Z	• Walking • Driving	• Walking • Transfers • Ascend or descend stairs

his personal self-care goals, which reflected, in part, an attempt to normalize his daily life.

Six new device recommendations and adaptations were made by the occupational therapist at home in response to Mr. X's per-

Table 3.   Overview of device training and new device needs identified at home

Case	Activities used in instruction	Number of devices in which instruction was provided	New device needs or adaptations
Mr. X	• Stair climbing • Bed transfers • Tub chair transfers • Exercise for stiffness	3	• Energy conservation • Shoes • Leg lift • Hand-held shower spray • Grab bar • Raise height of tub chair
Mr. Y	• Wheelchair transfers • Tub chair transfers • Wheelchair safety • Dressing • Meal preparation	12	• Velcro garment fasteners • Doorknob adapter
Mr. Z	• Bathing • Mobility • Stair climbing	6	• Rearrangement of bathroom • Ramp • Stair glide

sonal concerns and difficulties. These included instruction in energy conservation, recommendation of different shoes to ascend stairs safely, provision and instruction in the use of a leg lift and rope to transfer out of bed, adjustment in the height of a tub chair purchased by Mr. X, and recommendation of grab bars and a hand-held shower hose. Mr. X mastered each recommended adaptation and used all of them successfully.

Case 2: Mr. Y

In the Hospital Mr. Y, a retired 62-year-old African American man, was in rehabilitation for a CVA (stroke). The CVA affected the right side of his body, leaving his right upper extremity flaccid. He also experienced mild memory impairment. Previous diagnoses included a history of high blood pressure and a heart condition. Mr. Y was divorced and lived alone in a fourth-floor apartment. He had five children, three daughters and two sons, all of whom provided emotional and physical support.

Mr. Y was a first-time user of assistive devices following his stroke. As shown in Table 1, he was issued and instructed in the use of a total of 17 devices while in rehabilitation. Approximately 4 hours were spent in training to use these devices over 21 days in the hospital. One of his daughters was present during hospital instruction in the use of the shower hose, tub chair, and commode.

Prior to discharge, Mr. Y demonstrated, for the most part, a positive affect. Nevertheless, he also expressed feeling a little lonely and remote from people and stated that he was bored a lot and restless. He stated that he had a lot to be sad about and felt somewhat helpless in coping with his disability. In the hospital, Mr. Y had a positive attitude toward his issued AT devices. He believed that they enabled him to be independent and to do the things that were important to him. Although he considered his disability an inconvenience, he did not feel embarrassed by the need to use assistive devices and maintained high morale. However, he grappled with a sense of personal loss and a change in his personal and social identity as a consequence of the stroke.

At Home During the first few months following hospital discharge, one daughter, who lived close by, stopped in daily to check on Mr. Y to assist him as needed, and another daughter stayed with Mr. Y in the evenings. At home, Mr. Y used 14 (an 82% device use risk) of his 17 assistive devices. Mr. Y had placed each device in such a manner in his apartment that it could be effectively used and incorporated into his daily routine of bathing, dressing, and meal preparation. He purposely chose not to use three devices—his shoe-horn, long-handled sponge, and reacher—because he either preferred to use an alternative approach or did not know how to use the device effectively enough to accomplish an activity.

Mr. Y had a strong and supportive social network. Also, at home and over time, he improved in functional ability (Figure 1). Nevertheless, he expressed a number of concerns that placed him at risk for decline and reflected biopsychosocial issues. These included increasing fatigue, social isolation, depression, and loneliness (see Table 4). His fatigue became an increasing concern because it affected his use of the wheelchair, which he greatly valued as an aid for ambulation. By his third month at home, he found the use of his wheelchair tiring and painful, perhaps a preclinical sign of underlying impairment or physiological change.

New Needs   Although Mr. Y successfully used 14 of his devices at home, additional training was required to reinforce safe and appropriate use. Also, new device needs were identified to enable Mr. Y to accomplish his personal activity goals (see Table 2). His personal goals represented a primary concern for performing instrumental activities and engaging in leisure and social pursuits. First, as Mr. Y accommodated to his home environment, he expressed feeling more alone and isolated. He was unable to successfully leave his own apartment and floor because of decreased strength and an inability to negotiate cumbersome and heavy doors throughout the apartment building. To overcome this barrier, he was shown how to use a non–plastic-coated string for opening doors. This enabled him to resume participation in social activities within the apartment complex. Second, Mr. Y had forgotten how to exit from his wheelchair safely. He needed instruction in locating and

Table 4.   Emerging biopsychosocial risk factors for functional decline at home

Case	Physical function	Psychological	Social
Mr. X	Poor sleep Stiffness Decreased energy	Fear of falling	Death of daughter Restricted social network
Mr. Y	Increased fatigue with wheelchair Inability to dress self	Depression Loneliness	Increased social isolation
Mr. Z	Physical discomfort with aids Declining health	Depression	Increased social isolation Poor health of spouse Death of son

operating the button for the footrest. Involvement of one of his daughters in wheelchair training helped to reinforce safe practice. Third, Mr. Y was shown how to use the reacher to pick up his mail and other objects off the floor and engage in games with his grandchild, activities that were of meaning and importance to him.

Finally, a new area of concern was dressing independently. After the first 3 months at home, Mr. Y's daughter could no longer continue to assist her father in morning routines. Undergarments and clothing with Velcro fasteners were introduced and accepted by Mr. Y as a potential solution (see Table 3).

Case 3: Mr. Z

In the Hospital The third case was that of Mr. Z, an 81-year-old Caucasian who had worked as a truck driver and retired to his own home. He had had both legs amputated below the knees. In addition, Mr. Z had had other major previous health conditions, including stroke, arthritis, diabetes, and a heart condition. In the hospital, he had been issued six devices (Table 1). He had never used an assistive device prior to hospitalization. During his stay in rehabilitation, his wife had also been admitted to a hospital for a heart condition and their son had died.

In the hospital, Mr. Z was initially enthusiastic about the equipment he had received. He expressed feeling depressed and alone because his health had significantly declined and he had experienced significant losses.

At Home During his first few months at home, Mr. Z used three issued devices (a 50% device use rate) with consistency—his wheelchair, walker, and reacher. His commode, tub chair, and inspection mirror were kept on the second floor and thus were not used until he was able to ascend the stairs.

Upon his return home, his level of function dramatically declined (Figure 1). Mr. Z had to contend with significant losses that included the death of his son, his double amputation, dramatic change in function, and the poor health of his wife. With time, he expressed fatigue, awkwardness, and pain in using his wheelchair. This, combined with his increased social isolation and feelings of sadness and depression, placed Mr. Z at increasing risk for functional decline (Table 4).

New Needs Three critical equipment needs were identified (see Table 3). First, Mr. Z was confined to the first floor of his home because he was unable to ascend or descend stairs. His wife had to continually retrieve clothing and other care items as required by Mr. Z throughout the day. This was a significant burden because of the heart condition that put her health at increasing risk. Also, Mr. Z slept on the first floor but preferred to sleep upstairs with his wife. As a temporary solution, Mr. Z was shown a bumping technique to enable him to ascend and descend stairs. He was then referred to a state-funded program that eventually provided him with a stair glide. Second, Mr. Z was unable to get into and out of his house. This became a critical problem because of his need to attend doctors' appointments. A ramp and chairlift were needed for the front of the house and were also eventually obtained through the state-funded program. Third, Mr. Z had difficulty grooming and bathing, which required rearranging the bathroom and reinforcing proper use of the issued tub chair.

VARIATION IN EXPERIENCES

These cases suggest the stages of a career as an AT device user and the interrelated factors that may influence the path that the user takes. Figure 2 graphically shows a hypothetical model of these stages and factors. As shown in Figure 2, in the hospital, the rehabilitation client can be characterized as a novice AT device user. As a novice user, the client is introduced to the need and use of assistive devices and has opportunities to practice use within the hospital setting. At this initial stage, four factors may influence early device acceptance. These factors are personal acceptance of functional loss and the need for an AT device, the quality and scope of instruction in device use (e.g., inclusion of other family members), initial appraisal of the device as useful, and projection of one's self-care needs at home. If, during hospital instruction, the patient perceives assistive devices as unnecessary and not useful to fulfill personal self-care goals, then the potential for nonuse at home may be high. If, however, AT devices are perceived as essential to accomplish projected personal self-care goals and needs, and if instruction in use is appropriate, then continued use is perhaps highly probable. During the first 6 months at home, the rehabilitation client can be characterized as an early AT user. This stage is characterized by personal uncertainty and the need to accommodate a change in physical capabilities, especially in light of the client's returning to an unchanged physical environment. Factors that may influence this stage of adjustment to assistive device use include the emergence of new device needs, biopsychosocial issues that place an individual at continued risk of functional decline, the actual fit of hospital-issued devices within the home environment, and personal goals and preferred self-care practices. Since case material was not available after this stage of early use, one can only speculate as to the nature of the

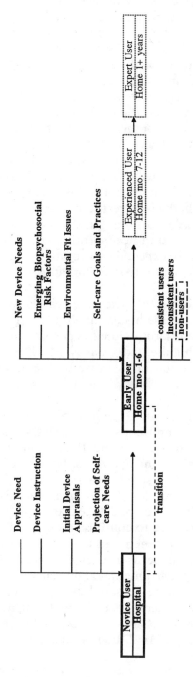

Figure 2.   Theoretical career path of first-time AT device users and factors influencing each stage.

career path following the first 6 months at home. During the next 6 months at home, the client would perhaps be characterized as an experienced AT device user who accommodated to functional change and felt comfortable and safe using issued devices. By the second year of use, the client would perhaps become an expert AT user who possessed the necessary knowledge to acquire and use new devices as new functional issues emerged and adjustments to the physical environment were required.

Obviously, each stage needs further careful articulation and empirical support. However, the cases presented here demonstrate the different constellation of factors that influence the novice and early stages of assistive device use. In the case of Mr. X, his early career as an AT user was characterized by inconsistency. This inconsistency was due primarily to a poor fit of issued devices with his own personal goals, functional needs, and environmental setup. While hospitalized, he had expressed concern about using issued devices, perhaps an early warning sign that he was at risk of rejecting their use at home and in need of other strategies. As other research has shown, early expectations regarding one's course of recovery may predict actual outcome (Borkan & Quirk, 1992; Gitlin et al., 1996).

Mr. X did initiate use of other devices. For example, he had purchased a tub seat to ease his bathing routine. In this case, however, the importance of professional expertise and its interaction with lay practice is highlighted. That is, Mr. X was able to safely and effectively use the apparatus only after the occupational therapist had evaluated its fit, adjusted the height, and provided hands-on training.

In contrast to Mr. X, Mr. Y can be characterized as beginning a career as a successful and consistent assistive device user. He adapted a wide range of self-care practices in an attempt to maintain control over basic living activities. He viewed AT devices as helping him to perform personal activity choices; the devices were integral to his well-being. Mr. Y had organized his apartment in such a way as to enable effective device use and, even over time, he remained highly motivated to continue their use. Even within this context, however, Mr. Y benefited from professional assistance to address new self-care concerns as they emerged at home, particularly those concerning instrumental and leisure needs.

Mr. Z's overwhelming personal and functional losses were compounded by environmental barriers that heightened his inability to begin to use issued assistive devices and normalize daily activity patterns. Although Mr. Z did not reject the use of devices, he needed other environmental adjustments to improve his quality of life. As in the case of Mr. X, hospital-issued assistive devices only partially fit his needs, and thus his career as an AT user began with uncertainty and inconsistency.

Although Mr. X, Mr. Y, and Mr. Z cannot be characterized as nonusers, they each were highly purposeful and selective in their assistive device choices, for several reasons. Personal goals (Table 2) for self-care changed from hospital to home as these three older adults adapted to and became integrated into a pattern of daily life. Each person had a different set of personal goals during rehabilitation that reflected an understanding of his or her physical condition and projections regarding what would be required to function competently in the home environment. Once home, individuals expressed greater specificity in their activity choices and personal goals, which influenced AT device use. Additionally, as function either improved or was accommodated and new self-care needs developed, challenges emerged for which either issued devices were used or other modifications were required. New activity limitations in each case reflected the interaction of physical change, home environmental conditions, and the level of social support available. Attempts to use AT devices to offset new concerns were, in part, thwarted by a poor fit with the environment or lack of appropriate devices.

As shown in Table 3, each case suggests that a combination of physical, psychological, and social factors may place older adults at risk of increasing frailty and in need of additional assistive device training following hospitalization. For example, Mr. Y and Mr. Z both reported that they were experiencing increasing fatigue using their mobility aids. Fatigue placed them at risk for increasing depression and social isolation. Some of these factors were subtle and discernible only by using a combination of self-report and observational measures.

In summary, these cases highlight the complexity of beginning a career as an assistive device user and the situational factors that must be navigated in transferring self-care techniques learned in the hospital to the home environment. Each case demonstrates a different set of biopsychosocial needs, environmental fit issues, self-care goals and practices, and device needs that shifted over time. Clearly, the passage from hospital to home was a critical turning point in the career path, with important implications for service delivery. These cases suggest the need for additional AT device training in the early stage of device use to ease the transition from hospital to home. The individualized, client-driven home training intervention used in this study appeared to be effective in addressing the context-specific functional needs of these three older adults. As shown in Figure 1, functional scores in each case improved from Month 1 to Month 6 at home, suggesting that occupational therapy sessions were beneficial.

CONCLUSIONS

Although older adults constitute a large proportion of individuals who use mobility aids and other equipment, little is known about how this group of users adapt to these tools. This chapter has described the transition from hospital to home for three older adults with different impairments and life circumstances as a basis for proposing a theoretical framework for understanding AT device use and its path for first-time users. These three cases provide insight on some of the intrapsychic, functional, and physical changes or biopsychosocial hurdles that may characterize the early stage of an AT device user's career.

Several implications for health policy and research can be derived from these cases. First, each case demonstrated that assistive device needs changed from hospital to home and over time. Many of these needs could have been identified by a home assessment while the patient was hospitalized. For example, Mr. Z's need for a ramp and interior stair glide as well as Mr. X's need for different transfer techniques and bathroom equipment could easily have been determined by going to the home. As others have shown, a home evaluation conducted while an older adult is hospitalized may be cost-effective (Ramsdell, Swart, Jackson, & Renvall, 1989). It would provide an understanding of the specific context in which AT devices would be used. A home assessment would also enable therapists to provide individualized recommendations. Nevertheless, other needs could not have been identified during hospitalization, and these cases suggest the importance of periodic reevaluation, particularly in the first 6 months at home. For example, Mr. Y's increasing social isolation and depression emerged as he mastered his functional limitations in his immediate environment and was then ready to explore other life options.

Second, in each case, function, as measured by the FIM, improved with time. This may have been due, in part, to the additional AT device training provided by the occupational therapist. Certainly, this trend is encouraging and suggests that the intervention warrants systematic testing with a larger cohort of rehabilitation clients. However, although there were improvements in functional scores, many self-care needs were identified that placed these individuals at risk of falling and of poor mental and physical health. These cases suggest that the use of an independence–dependence continuum to support the need for home care service may not adequately address the complex concerns of older adults with first-time disabilities.

Finally, with regard to research, the cases suggest specific factors that may influence AT device use and reasons for nonuse that should be examined in future research. Reasons for use and nonuse appear in these cases to be more complex than those previously discussed in the literature (Gitlin, 1995). Clearly, these individuals were highly selective in using AT devices, and a combination of conditions supported their decision making and effective use of devices. Figure 2 displays a hypothetical representation of the early stages of the career of device users. Its trajectory warrants careful consideration and mapping with a larger cohort of older adults who confront disability late in life.

REFERENCES

Aneshensel, C.S., Pearlin, L.I., Mullan, J.T., Zarit, S.H., & Whitlatch, C.J. (1995). *Profiles in caregiving: The unexpected career.* San Diego, CA: Academic Press.

Borkan, J.M., & Quirk, M. (1992). Expectations and outcomes after hip fracture among the elderly. *International Journal of Aging and Human Development, 34*(4), 339–350.

Bradburn, N.M. (1969). *The structure of psychological well-being.* Chicago: Aldine.

Bruno, R.L. (1993). *The Reinforcement Motivation Survey.* Hackensack, NJ: Harvest Press.

Bull, M.J. (1992). Managing the transition from hospital to home. *Qualitative Health Research, 2*(1), 27–41.

Bynum, H., & Rogers, J.C. (1987). The use and effectiveness of assistive devices possessed by patients seen in home care. *Occupational Therapy Journal of Research, 3,* 181–191.

Frank, G. (1994). The personal meaning of self-care occupations. In C. Christiansen (Ed.), *Ways of living: Self-care strategies for special needs.* (pp. 27–49). Rockville, MD: American Occupational Therapy Association.

Gitlin, L.N. (1995). Why older people accept or reject assistive technology. *Generations, 19*(1), 41–46.

Gitlin, L.N. (in press). The role of social science research in understanding technology use among older adults. In M. Ory & G. DeFriese (Ed.), *Self-care in later life.* New York: Springer.

Gitlin, L.N., Luborsky, M., & Schemm, R.L. (1997). *Emerging concerns of assistive device use by older stroke patients in rehabilitation.* Manuscript submitted for publication.

Gitlin, L.N., Mount, J., Lucas, W., Weirich, L.C., & Gamberg, L. (1997). The physical costs and the benefits of travel aids for persons who are visually impaired. *Journal of Visual Impairment and Blindness, 91*(4), 347–359.

Gitlin, L.N., Schemm, R.L., Landsberg, L., & Burgh, D.Y. (1996). Factors predicting assistive device use in the home by older persons following rehabilitation. *Journal of Aging and Health, 8*(4), 554–575.

Gitlin, L.N., Schemm, R.L., & Shmuely, Y. (1997). *Predicting home use of mobility aids by older adults following rehabilitation.* Manuscript submitted for publication.

Kart, C.S., & Engler, C.A. (1994). Predisposition to self-health care: Who does what for themselves and why? *Journal of Gerontology: Social Sciences, 49*(6), 5301–5308.

LaPlante, M.P., Hendershot, G.E., & Moss, A.J. (1992). *Assistive technology devices and home accessibility features: Prevalence, payment, need and trends* (Advance data from vital and health statistics; No. 217). Hyattsville, MD: National Center for Health Statistics.

Lawton, M.P. (1975). Philadelphia Geriatric Center Morale Scale: A revision. *Journal of Gerontology, 30*(1), 85–89.

Locker, D., Kaufert, J., & Kirk, B. (1987). The impact of life support technology upon psychosocial adaptation to the late effect of poliomyelitis. *Birth Defects, 23*(4), 157–171.

Luborsky, M.R. (1993). Sociocultural factors shaping technology usage: Fulfilling the promise. *Technology and Disability, 2*(1), 71–78.

Macken, C.L. (1986). A profile of functionally impaired elderly persons living in the community. *Health Care Financing Review, 7*(4), 33–49.

Magilvy, J.K., & Lakomy, J.M. (1991). Transitions of older adults to home care. *Home Health Care Services Quarterly, 12*(4), 59–69.

Mann, W.C., Hurren, D., Charvat, B., & Tomita, M. (1996). Problems with wheelchairs experienced by frail elders. *Technology and Disability, 5*, 81–91.

Mann, W.C., Hurren, D., Karuza, J., & Bentley, D.W. (1993). Comparison of assistive device use and needs of home-based older persons with different impairments. *American Journal of Occupational Therapy, 47*(11), 980–987.

Manton, K.G., Corder, L., & Stallard, E. (1993). Changes in the use of personal assistance and special equipment from 1982 to 1989: Results from the 1982 and 1989 NLTCS. *Gerontologist, 33*(2), 168–176.

Mount, J., Gitlin, L.N., & Howard, P. (1997). Musculoskeletal consequences of travel aid use among visually impaired adults: Directions for future research and training. *Technology and Disability, 6*(3), 159–167.

Norburn, J.E., Bernard, S.L., Konrad, T.R., Woomert, A., DeFriese, G.H., Kalsbeek, W.D., Koch, G.G., & Ory, M.G. (1995). Self-care and assistance from others in coping with functional status limitations among a national sample of older adults. *Journal of Gerontology, 50B*, S101–S109.

Pearlin, L.I. (1992). The careers of caregivers. *Gerontologist, 32*(5), 647.

Pearlin, L.I., & Aneshensel, C.S. (1994). Caregiving: The unexpected career. *Social Justice Research, 7*(4), 373–390.

Ramsdell, J.W., Swart, J.A., Jackson, J.E., & Renvall, M. (1989). The yield of a home visit in the assessment of geriatric patients. *Journal of the American Geriatrics Society, 37*(1), 17–24.

Schemm, R.L., & Gitlin, L.N. (in press). Teaching bathing and dressing assistive device use to patients in rehabilitation. *American Journal of Occupational Therapy.*

Stake, R.E. (1995). *The art of case study research.* Beverly Hills: Sage Publications.

State University of New York at Buffalo. (1993). *Guide for the Uniform Data Set for Medical Rehabilitation (Adult FIM), version 4.0.* Buffalo, NY: Author.

Strain, L.A., Chappell, N.L., & Penning, M.J. (1993). The need for social science research on technology and aging. *Technology and Disability, 2*(1), 56–64.

Yin, R.K. (1989). *Case study research: Design and methods.* Beverly Hills: Sage Publications.

Zimmer, Z., & Chappell, N.L. (1994). Mobility restriction and the use of devices among seniors. *Journal of Aging and Health, 6*(2), 185–208.

CHAPTER 9

Achieving Effectiveness with a Client-Centered Approach

A Person–Environment Interaction

Carolyn M. Baum

If "opportunity is the distance between what is and what could be" (Crimmins, 1995, p. 129), then assistive technology (AT) provides the opportunity for people with physical disabilities who have things to do and places to go. Functional limitations and environmental barriers create obstacles to the accomplishment of objectives; AT, appropriately applied, can remove those obstacles. This chapter raises some issues that must be addressed by professionals as they apply AT and evaluate its effectiveness.

Disability exists only when an individual has an inability or limitation "in performing socially defined activities and roles expected of individuals within a social and physical environment" (Pope & Tarlov, 1991, p. 7). Yet disability affects every individual, community, and family in the United States. It has become more than a medical issue because it has financial, social, public health, and moral aspects (Pope & Tarlov, 1991). It is not feasible to think that disability can be eliminated; but it can be minimized, and the process of minimizing disability requires health professionals to move beyond the medical model, which focuses on cure and management of disease and in which the key relationship is between the patient and his or her physician (Jesion & Rudin, 1983). Overcoming disability requires health care professionals to additionally embrace the social model, which focuses on the psychosocial as well as medical needs of individuals and encourages people to be as autonomous as possible by providing opportunities for choice in decisions and activities (Smith & Eggleson, 1989).

The social model requires clinicians to partner with *clients*, not *patients*, in planning and decision making that will eventually lead to the accomplishment of goals that are important to the person who must live with the consequences of functional limitations that cannot be remediated with traditional medical interventions. This approach is coming to be known as *client-centered care*. Although this approach began to emerge in the 1960s, it was not implemented and tested until the 1990s. The client-centered philosophy is designed to create a caring, dignified, and empowering environment in which clients direct their own care (Matheis-Kraft, George, Olinger, & York, 1990).

Clinicians and researchers at the Neurodevelopmental Clinical Research Unit and McMaster University (Law & Baptiste, 1995) laid out key concepts of client-centered care. This framework can be used in applying AT to the resolution of disability. There are three basic assumptions that professionals using client-centered care must adopt:

1. Clients and their families know themselves best.
2. Clients and their families are different and unique.
3. Optimal client functioning occurs within a supportive family and community context.

The McMaster group (Law & Baptiste, 1995) challenged clinicians to focus on clients' expectations in planning care. Clients expect to lead the decision-making process. They want to use their own resources; define their priorities for intervention; receive timely, individualized services; and be supported in the level of participation they choose. In addition, they expect to be treated with dignity throughout the therapy process.

The client-centered approach requires professionals to alter their behaviors from those traditionally employed in the medical model. Professionals must encourage client partnership in decision making and enable clients to identify their needs and build on their strengths. The approach must be flexible and individualized. The provider of services must respect the client's values, goals, and priorities without judging what is right and wrong. In addition, the clinician must encourage the client to use natural community supports (Law & Baptiste, 1995) rather than become dependent on the medical establishment.

Any new approach requires an evaluation of its effectiveness. Does a client-centered approach make a difference? Research indicates that respectful and supportive services yield improved client satisfaction. In addition, the partnership approach yields better client participation and improved functional outcomes (Dunst, Trivette, Boyd, & Brookfield, 1994; Dunst, Trivette, Davis, & Cornwall, 1988; Greenfield, Kaplan, & Ware, 1985; Moxley-Haegert & Serbin, 1983; Stein & Jessop, 1991).

Perhaps a case study is in order.

> Mrs. Doe is an older adult who has a history of stroke. She lives alone in a congregate housing unit. When a team of clinicians visited her, it was noted that she had been hospitalized three times in the past year. Each time, she had had rehabilitation services and had been given equipment to support her independence at home. Now her tiny dining room was filled with two manual wheelchairs, one electric wheelchair, two walkers, three quad canes, and two commodes. When asked how she got around, she told clinicians that her nephew got her the cart and that she likes it because it carries what she needs and does not make her look different from anyone else. She directed the clinician to the shopping cart in the corner of the living room.

In our haste to help people with disabilities, we may be spending unnecessary financial resources and creating unnecessary stress for families and the people we are trying to serve. How do we create opportunities if the technology that we apply is not focused on the needs, goals, and activities of those to be served? It is time for a new approach.

CLIENT-CENTERED MODEL OF CARE

The National Center for Medical Rehabilitation Research (NCMRR) has proposed a client-centered model that can guide the application of assistive technology. This model (Baum & Law, 1997) (Figure 1) evolved from work that was initially developed as part of the *International Classification of Impairments, Disabilities, and Handicaps*, which was sponsored by the World Health Organization (1980), modified by Nagi (1991), and further developed by the Institute of Medicine and reported in *Disability in America* (Pope & Tarlov, 1991). The uniqueness of the NCMRR model is the addition of a fifth level that allows for consideration of societal limitations associated with barriers to performance by people with disabilities. This fifth level is very important when considering AT. The other

Societal Limitation	Disability	Functional Limitation	Impairment	Pathophysiology
Restriction attributable to social policy or barriers (structural or attitudinal) that limit fulfillment of roles or deny access to services or opportunities	Inability or limitation in performing socially defined activities and roles within a social and physical environment as a result of internal or external factors and their interplay	Restriction or lack of ability to perform an action or activity in the manner or range considered normal that results from impairment	Loss and/or abnormality of mental, emotional, physiological, or anatomical structure or function, including secondary losses and pain	Interruption of or interference with normal physiological and developmental processes or structures
Performance of Roles by Person in Societal Context	Task Performance of Person in Physical and Social Context	Performance of Action or Activity	Organs and Organ Systems	Cells and Tissues
Roles: • Worker • Student • Friend • Parent • Home maintenance • Spouse/Partner Barriers/Issues: • Recreation • Attitudes, customs, beliefs, norms • Accessibility • Inclusion • Accommodation • Quality of life	Task Performance: • Basic self-care • Instrumental tasks • Worker tasks • Leisure activities • Education Context: • Physical environment • Social environment, including family • Cognitive environment	• Initiate, organize, sequence, judge, attend, select • Sit, roll, lift, stoop, squat, stand, climb, ambulate • Reach, pinch, grip, grasp, hold, release • Relate, interact, cope, manage, control, adapt • Read, write, learn, understand	• Cognitive processing • Sensory processing • Perception • Motor • Memory • Physiological function • Psychological function • Pain	• Neurological deficit • Physiological deficit • Immunological deficit

Figure 1. National Center for Medical Rehabilitation Research (NCMRR) client-centered model. (From Baum, C.M., & Law, M. [1997]. Occupational therapy practice: Focusing on occupational performance. *American Journal of Occupational Therapy, 51*[4], 286. Copyright © 1997 by the American Occupational Therapy Association, Inc. Reprinted with permission.)

four levels are very similar to those proposed by the Institute of Medicine.

Most applications of technology to date have been focused at the functional limitation level to support an action or activity. To support a client-centered approach, it is important to focus simultaneously on three levels: functional limitation, disability, and societal limitation. Functional analyses focus on the degree or level of capabilities of organs or organ systems. At the disability level, issues of performance are assessed by integrated actions of the person. Performance of people with disabilities must be put in social and environmental contexts for evaluation of the societal factors that limit levels of participation by people with disabilities in work, relationships, interests, and goals.

CLIENT-CENTERED APPROACH
TO EFFECTIVE ASSISTIVE TECHNOLOGY

Rehabilitation professionals traditionally take measurements to make sure that a piece of equipment is going to fit the individual. To ensure that the equipment is going to enable an individual to be able to accomplish his or her goals, it is necessary to determine what those goals are, how a person will need to use the equipment, and in what environments the equipment will be used. For an individual who has experienced life to the fullest and now, because of a disabling condition, needs AT, it may be possible to get this information from an interview. For a person who has never been motivated to explore his or her boundaries, it is necessary to help him or her envision what might be possible with the assistance of technology. A client-centered planning tool (Figure 2) is offered as a guide for interviewers to explore what a person does or wants to be able to do, so that the individual's activities and interests are considered in designing or selecting AT devices.

A client-centered approach to selecting and fitting assistive devices seems so logical that it might go unsaid. However, periodically, events can remind us of the need to keep the approach on the front burner. A colleague tells of an acquaintance who was fitted for a new electric wheelchair. A functional limitation approach was employed, and the team chose a chair to match his physical capacity. Unfortunately, a difficult series of problems emerged. When the chair arrived, the acquaintance found that the chair was larger than his previous chair, was too big to use in his small apartment, did not fit in his van, and was not compatible with his station at work. Had he not kept his original chair, he would have been socially and

Client-Centered Planning Tool: Person Performance Profile

| | Level of performance | | | | |
Roles and activities	Do	Do with equipment	Choose not to do	Purchase service	Want to do but cannot do
Self-management					
Transfers					
Dressing					
Eating					
Hygiene					
Bladder management					
Bowel management					
Home management					
Shopping (e.g., grocery, personal)					
Cooking/Food preparation					
Light cleaning/Laundry					
Heavy cleaning/Trash removal					
Yard work/Gardening					
Household maintenance					
Driving/Transportation					
Car maintenance/Repair					
Care for a pet					
Manage finances (e.g., bills, investments, insurance forms)					
Talk on telephone					
Home safety					
Family/Spousal					
Parenting					
Partner					
Sexuality					
Reproductive					
Work/School					
Transportation					
Perform essential functions					
Volunteer work					

(continued)

Figure 2.   Client-Centered Planning Tool: Person Performance Profile. (Copyright © 1995 by Carolyn M. Baum; reprinted by permission.)

Figure 2. *(continued)*

Level of performance

Roles and activities	Do	Do with equipment	Choose not to do	Purchase service	Want to do but cannot do
Leisure activities/Play					
Spectator sport (e.g., football, baseball, racing)					
Team sports (e.g., baseball, soccer, football)					
Individual sport (e.g., swimming, bowling, golf, fishing, tennis, hunting)					
Hobby (e.g., woodworking, photography, collecting items)					
Fitness (e.g., walking, running, exercise, hiking, bicycling)					
Camping/Boating/Sailing					
Sewing/Mending/Crafts					
Computer					
Table games/Puzzles					
Musical instrument (e.g., piano, violin)					
Reading books/ magazines					
Writing (e.g., letter writing, keeping a journal)					
Theater/Plays/Concerts/ Movies					
Television/Music					
Rest					
Social activities					
Travel					
Parties/Picnics					
Family/friend gatherings					
Church					
Clubs					

economically compromised. The lesson that was learned was very costly. How often does this happen? We certainly saw a previous example with Mrs. Doe. Regardless of whether the device is a low-tech bathroom item, an expensive wheelchair, or an artificial limb, unless we create partnerships with our clients and obtain environmental data, we stand to compromise the independence of those we are trying to help. When we design programs that distribute assistive devices, it is critical that we design the programs in such a way that families, employers, and others involved with the person needing assistance are a part of the process, if only to receive information.

A major problem remains—that of excess disability. Excess disability occurs when a person is not able to perform at the level of his or her capacity. The Americans with Disabilities Act (ADA) of 1990 (PL 101-336) provides the legal support for people who are capable of working. This support will be possible only when employers understand the value and capabilities of people who, with the assistance of technology, can perform meaningful work. As business people understand human capacity and how AT can work, more resources will be available for technological applications because the benefit of technology to business will be visible.

SOCIAL POLICY AND TECHNOLOGY-SUPPORTED INDEPENDENCE

As we begin to approach assistive technology from a broader perspective, we will see an emerging role for health professionals in the social policy arena. Rehabilitation professionals must partner with consumers to point out environmental and attitudinal barriers that exist in society. The sole focus on technology as a medical intervention makes it appear that AT only adds more cost to overburdened health programs. Perhaps if AT were viewed at the disability and societal limitation level, it would be more obvious that the application of technology overcomes barriers by supporting independence and self-reliance and provides opportunity for self-sufficiency. I know of a director of a vocational program in southwestern Missouri who introduces each client who completes vocational rehabilitation and is placed in a job as a new taxpayer to the local and national congressional representatives. Is community independence not the ultimate purpose of AT?

One way to make assistive technology more visible and more acceptable for reimbursement would be to establish Assistive Technology Advisory Committees with the participation of insurers, legislators, researchers, clinicians, vocational rehabilitation specialists, administrators, business leaders, and consumers. An advisory committee could facilitate broader understanding and propose strategies to evaluate the effectiveness of a given technology.

Rehabilitation has traditionally measured progress at the impairment and functional limitation level. Only in the 1990s have standardized assessments at the disability level been developed, and these have focused primarily on basic self-care. This hardly captures the full potential of AT to support independence. The application of assistive technology requires an expanded approach because the desired outcomes have more to do with satisfaction, community reintegration, and quality of life. Perhaps medical outcome assessments being used for the general population, such as the MOS 36-Item Short-Form Health Survey (SF-36) (Ware & Sherbourne, 1992), the Sickness Impact Profile (Bergner, Bobbitt, Carter, & Gilson, 1981), and the Reintegration to Normal Living Index (Wood-Dauphinee et al., 1988) can be used with technology included as a control variable.

CONCLUSIONS

The use of assistive technology is a very individual experience for the person with a disability. We should try to look at the differences in activities and interests of individuals. Then we can begin to consider different types of assistive technologies to recommend for them to use. Perhaps the first stage of developing methods to measure the effectiveness of AT as applied to life experiences should employ qualitative research methods to explore the role that AT does or does not play in the independence of those users who are satisfied with it and those who are not. Some questions that must be asked in this process include the following: How does an individual arrive at the decision to accept or reject AT? How long does it take to integrate a new piece of equipment into everyday life? Do individuals have ideas for other assistive devices or modifications of the devices they have that would make them more effective? Qualitative studies have often preceded quantitative work to get an accurate description of the issues and to develop categories that will eventually yield standardized assessments. The absence of such instruments will eventually compromise the gains that will be achieved when efficacy can be demonstrated.

AT is more than a tool for rehabilitation professionals to employ. It offers opportunities that will minimize disability for thousands, if not millions, of Americans. The application of AT must be approached as a partnership with the person with a disability, who is the only one who knows what it is he or she wants to do. A client-centered approach that includes an exploration of the potential activities in a person's life and of the individual's environment should be integrated with functional and impairment measures to create the best fit for technology to support the individual's goals and health.

REFERENCES

Americans with Disabilities Act (ADA) of 1990, PL 101-336, 42 U.S.C. §§ 12101 *et seq.*

Baum, C.M., & Law, M. (1997). Occupational therapy practice: Focusing on occupational performance. *American Journal of Occupational Therapy, 51*(4), 277–288.

Bergner, M., Bobbitt, R., Carter, W., & Gilson, B. (1981). The Sickness Impact Profile: Development and final revision of a health status measure. *Medical Care, 19,* 955–962.

Crimmins, J.C. (1995). *The American promise: Adventures in grassroots democracy.* San Francisco: KQED Books.

Dunst, D.J., Trivette, C.M., Boyd, K., & Brookfield, J. (1994). Help-giving practices and the self-efficacy appraisals of parents. In C.J. Dunst, C.M. Trivette, & A.G. Deal (Eds.), *Supporting and strengthening families: Methods, strategies, and practices* (Vol. 1, pp. 212–220). Cambridge, MA: Brookline Books.

Dunst, D.J., Trivette, C.M., Davis, M., & Cornwall, J. (1988). Enabling and empowering families of children with health impairments. *Children's Health Care, 17,* 71–81.

Greenfield, S., Kaplan, S., & Ware, J.E. (1985). Expanding patient involvement in care: Effects on patient outcomes. *Annals of Internal Medicine, 102,* 520–528.

Jesion, M., & Rudin, S. (1983, Summer). Evaluation of the social model of long-term care. *Health Management Forum,* 64–80.

Law, M., & Baptiste, S. (1995). Client-centered practice: What does it mean and does it make a difference? *Canadian Journal of Occupational Therapy, 62,* 250–257.

Matheis-Kraft, C., George, S., Olinger, M.J., & York, L. (1990). Patient-driven health care works! *Nursing Management, 21,* 124–128.

Moxley-Haegert, L., & Serbin, L.A. (1983). Developmental education for parents of delayed infants: Effects on parental motivation and children's development. *Child Development, 54,* 1324–1331.

Nagi, S.Z. (1991). Disability concepts revisited: Implications for prevention. In A.M. Pope & A.R. Tarlov (Eds.), *Disability in America: Toward a national agenda for prevention* (pp. 309–327). Washington, DC: National Academy Press.

Pope, A.M., & Tarlov, A.R. (Eds.). (1991). *Disability in America: Toward a national agenda for prevention.* Washington, DC: National Academy Press.

Smith, V., & Eggleson, R. (1989, Summer). Long-term care: The medical versus the social model. *Public Welfare, 26–29.*

Stein, R.E.K., & Jessop, D.J. (1991). Long-term mental health effects of a pediatric home care program. *Pediatrics, 88,* 490–496.

Ware, J.E., & Sherbourne, C.D. (1992). The MOS 36-Item Short-Form Health Survey (SF-36): I. Conceptual framework and item selection. *Medical Care, 30,* 473–483.

Wood-Dauphinee, S.L., Opzoomer, A., Williams, J.I., Marchand, J.I., Marchand, B., & Spitzer, W.O. (1988). Assessment of global function: The Reintegration to Normal Living Index. *Archives of Physical Medicine and Rehabilitation, 69*(8), 583–590.

World Health Organization. (1980). *International classification of impairments, disabilities, and handicaps.* Geneva: Author.

SELECTING, DESIGNING, AND DEVELOPING ASSISTIVE TECHNOLOGY FOR USE BY PEOPLE WITH DISABILITIES

CHAPTER 10

Incorporating Human Needs into Assistive Technology Design

Rory A. Cooper

It is not enough to teach man a specialty. Through it he may become a kind of useful machine but not a harmoniously developed personality. It is essential that the student acquire an understanding of and a lively feeling for values. He must acquire a vivid sense of the beautiful and of the morally good. Otherwise he—with his specialized knowledge—more closely resembles a well trained dog than a harmoniously developed person. He must learn to understand the motives of human beings, their illusions, and their sufferings in order to acquire a proper relationship to individual fellowmen and to the community.

Albert Einstein (1952)

The lives of many people with disabilities can be improved through the careful and considerate application of engineering principles to the design, manufacture, and application of assistive (also called adaptive) technology (AT) that improves human functions. *Rehabilitation engineering* can be defined as the application of engineering principles to the design, development, and assessment of AT and techniques (Cooper, 1995). Assistive technologies are devices and techniques that are used to optimize human function through enhancing residual capacities (e.g., orthotic splints), replacing missing structures (e.g., prosthetic limbs), substituting structures (e.g., wheelchairs), providing alternate means of function, and minimizing environmental barriers (e.g., universal design of buildings) by promoting access and egress.

EXTENT AND NATURE OF THE PROBLEMS ADDRESSED BY REHABILITATION ENGINEERING AND ASSISTIVE TECHNOLOGY

The number of individuals with disabilities living in the United States is estimated by several government agencies to range from 20 million to more than 49 million (U.S. Bureau of the Census, 1990). The wide range of estimates of the number of people with disabilities stems from the manner in which *disability* is defined. *Disability* may be defined on the basis of limitations in functional ability, quality of life, or employment. Findings from a 1989 study of demographic data on disability in the United States (National Institute on Disability and Rehabilitation Research, 1989) estimated that there are 13.5 million people with disabilities between the ages of 16 and 64 who are not in institutions. Of these, 13.3 million people were considered to have disabilities that interfere with their capacity to work, with 7.25 million having a severe disability in this regard. Only 20% of the 13.3 million people with disabilities interfering with their capacity to work are employed full time. Of this group, 26% have incomes below the poverty level. (*Note:* These figures might be contrasted with the Harris Poll findings discussed under "Cost Factors" on page 160.)

No simple direct relationship exists between those individuals variously defined as having a disability and those individuals who use AT to improve function. In part, this is a result of inadequate surveys of AT use, lack of information available to potential consumers of AT, insufficient funds for purchase of assistive devices by consumers who might use them, and poorly designed devices that are discarded. To estimate the number of people with disabilities who use AT is a difficult task. One approach is to sum the number of products considered to be assistive devices that have been manufactured or purchased. However, this task is somewhat like collecting the parts of a very large puzzle and placing them together to get a look at the whole picture. No such compilation is available, and many parts of the puzzle are missing.

Pope and Tarlov (1991) estimated that 6.5% of the gross national product of the United States is consumed by the total direct cost of disability (including lost productivity both by individuals with disabilities and by members of their families). The portion of these funds used to purchase and maintain assistive devices has not been determined for the total population of people with disabilities. However, Berkowitz, Harvey, Greene, and Wilson (1992) addressed the issue for two physically disabling conditions: paralysis and multiple sclerosis. These studies estimated the annual costs of AT, home modifications, and AT provider services to be about $14,000 per year on an ongoing basis for people with spinal cord injuries. The lifetime costs for paraplegia resulting from spinal cord injury are estimated to be about $800,000, whereas the costs for quadriplegia resulting from spinal cord injury exceed $1 million. These estimates include the cost of home modifications, wheelchairs, adaptation to cars and vans, and medical care. Although the populations surveyed in these reports do not mirror the general population of people with disabilities, the finding that payments for AT come from a variety of sources, including government programs, private insurance, and personal savings, probably reflects the general principle that people with disabilities must use multiple resources to afford AT. For these two groups of people with physical disabilities, the cost of assistive technology is a significant portion of their annual expenditures.

PROBLEMS AND SOME SOLUTIONS ASSOCIATED WITH ACQUISITION AND USE OF ASSISTIVE TECHNOLOGY

The cost of assistive technology is significant to individuals with disabilities and to society, yet people with disabilities purchase and use AT. Probably many more could benefit from AT if they could afford it. Increasing the number of people with disabilities who are employed could provide a market demand for assistive technology. Recognizing that, through the use of AT, individuals with disabilities can become less dependent on others for care and more likely to be employed, in 1986 and 1992 Congress amended the Rehabilitation Act of 1973 (PL 93-112) to include assistive technology as a part of vocational rehabilitation plans (Rehabilitation Act Amendments of 1986 [PL 99-506]; Rehabilitation Act Amendments of 1992 [PL 102-569]). The Technology-Related Assistance for Individuals with Disabilities Act of 1988 (PL 100-407) provided resources for funding state and regional centers to inform people with disabilities of available AT. Unfortunately, neither of these acts made adequate provision for initial and replacement purchases of work-related assistive devices or for maintenance of such equipment.

In most instances (a notable exception being the work of Hotchkiss [1993] in developing countries), the design, development, manufacture, and application of AT require skilled professionals. The Rehabilitation Act of 1973 and the Technology-Related Assistance for Individuals with Disabilities Act of 1988 mandate that professionals trained in rehabilitation technology should be available for people with disabilities as they search for devices that will improve their lives. The former U.S. Office of Technology Assistance estimated that one third of assistive devices purchased for use by people with disabilities are discarded within 1 month of purchase (Berkowitz, 1987). The reasons for discarding recently purchased devices are not well understood but probably include that the devices provide little or no improvement in function, break easily, are difficult to learn to use, are unreliable, are grossly stigmatizing, or do not fit into the individual's home or work environment. To optimize the benefits of AT for people with disabilities, trained engineers, technologists, therapists, and counselors are needed to guide and make recommendations regarding development and application of assistive devices. In addition, employers hiring people with disabilities need guidance in purchasing and configuring devices for work-related tasks. Finally, third-party payers may benefit from knowledge provided by a cohort of trained personnel who make recommendations on AT that will be used and not discarded. The lack of clear data on what will be used is often a source of conflict between providers and consumers of AT.

Although the field of rehabilitation engineering and the vocations specializing in the application of assistive technology require specialized training, the level and content of training programs do not have the solid foundation familiar to other disciplines. Rehabilitation engineers, occupational therapists, rehabilitation physicians, prosthetists, orthotists, and Vocational Rehabilitation counselors gain knowledge of AT, human function, and the rehabilitation process through multidisciplinary academic coursework. They acquire skills in designing, building, testing, modifying, prescribing, and ordering AT as they progress through clinical internships. In the process of this training, they learn to empower the consumer and involve other team members in the decision-making process; evaluate the fit of specific assistive devices to the needs of individual consumers; develop an acute awareness of the consumer's environment in which the devices must perform; and provide answers to unique problems that can be solved with technology intervention.

These professionals employ a systematic approach to applying their knowledge of human capacities and AT in developing solutions to difficulties faced by people with disabilities. The key to problem resolution is making provision for the person with the disability to function optimally in a variety of settings and activities. For example, these professionals may use a controlled, clinical setting to begin analyzing and solving problems associated with seating and positioning of individuals who use mobility devices (e.g., manual and powered wheelchairs). However, these solutions must be tested and modified as the consumer uses the mobility device while driving an adapted van, using a computer, or moving through work and home sites. Thus, problem resolution associated with the use of AT is not limited to assessment of optimal performance in a single setting for simple tasks. Other examples of problems faced by people with disabilities successfully addressed by those trained in skillful application of AT include but are not limited to the following:

- Computer hardware and software that allows access and use of standard programs
- Work, home, and recreational site modifications that provide access to use of these facilities
- Augmentative communication technologies that give access to learning and using alternative languages for people with limited capacities for producing or hearing spoken language
- Adaptive driving equipment for individuals with auditory, cognitive, and mobility impairments
- Sensory aids to improve vision or hearing impairments
- Independent living implements to reduce reliance on care providers
- Recreational accoutrements that make possible participation in individual and team sports; in exploration of nature by trail, water, or air; and in discovery of literature, music, and the visual arts

A CONTEXTUAL MODEL FOR
ASSISTIVE TECHNOLOGY DESIGN AND DELIVERY

All too often technology has been developed devoid of meaningful consumer input, or consumer input has been severely limited. This common circumstance has resulted in a common aggravating cycle for consumers:

1. The consumer is provided an assistive device for use and evaluation based on some clinical or personal selection process. This is often done with all parties having only limited information about the device.

2. The consumer uses the assistive device and determines its inadequacies for his or her needs. The device often undergoes moderately successful modification or alteration.
3. The consumer continues to use the assistive device, although not completely satisfied, until the device is obsolete or the consumer abandons it.
4. The consumer selects another assistive device that meets some of the needs unmet by the previous device but has shortcomings of its own.

To avoid this costly, destructive, and unproductive cycle, professionals who develop AT and assist people with disabilities in the selection process need a model to guide their deliberations. A valuable heuristic contrivance to use when developing AT is to visualize a person with an impairment doing something somewhere. In other words, there is a person, a task, and an environment (i.e., a human, an activity, a context). Understanding how these components interact can be aided by a human engineering perspective. Initially, the engineer may conduct separate analyses of the person's capacities and the characteristics of existing or developing AT. Eventually, the engineer should work with a team that includes the consumer to develop simultaneous solutions for use of different types of AT for enhancing optimal change of function in a variety of settings (Bailey, 1989).

Some of the problems in fitting assistive devices to individual differences of users can be avoided by working with consumers early in the design process and having them follow the development of the device through its production. The advent of new computer software and manufacturing processes may be used to produce a new generation of AT. Ideally, a computer model of a given assistive device designed to the individual's unique characteristics would be made. Then, simulated trials of a variety of alterations to this model would be conducted for the purpose of assessing which best fit the individual's capabilities for use. These variations would be tested for rate of acquisition of product use and ultimate change in performance of the functions targeted for improvement. Construction of inexpensive component-part prototypes for initial tests of function hold promise for reducing costs; improving performance; and breaking the cycle of purchase, trial, and discard of assistive technology. Using this approach to production of AT should result in devices that better meet the functional needs of the consumer.

However, some problems may never be solved by changing the manufacturing process. The specific needs of some people with disabilities require customized, unique products that can be produced only by rehabilitation engineers working directly with the consumer in his or her environments. This approach is probably best for the integration of several assistive devices to meet the multiple needs of consumers in complex and distinctly different settings. In these cases, input from the AT user is not purely for setting functional and aesthetic goals. Information about user characteristics of the assistive device that are required to optimize the performance of the person with the device can be obtained only during its use. The anthropometry, cognitive abilities, and motivation of the consumer are factors that may be best revealed under actual use conditions. Changes based on findings from these interactions must be considered for modifying the device to optimize its use.

Personal Factors

Variability of human characteristics is a fundamental principle of genetics. With the possible exception of identical twins, no two human beings are the same. People vary in age, gender, size, weight, shape, eye color, skin color, cognitive abilities, emotional stability, aesthetic preferences, and every other category that has been subjected to scientific analysis. When designing AT, all of these characteristics must be determined (Pirkl, 1994). These factors may affect the appearance, size, and strength requirements of the AT device.

Type and severity of impairment influence the design of assistive technology (see Figure 1). For example, the rehabilitation engineer must consider whether the person has proprioceptive perception. The engineer must be aware of the existence and degree of spasticity. The degree of impairment alters the relationship between the assistive device and the user. The engineer needs to plan for these differences in designing the device.

The independence level and the attitude of the person toward assistive technology will alter the use of AT devices. Some people are not receptive to technology and must therefore be approached differently from others. People with similar impairments achieve different levels of independence because each individual is motivated by a unique set of life goals. Achieving these goals may require different types of AT for people with similar impairments. The successful rehabilitation engineer needs to be an astute observer, a good listener, and amenable to change based on individual differences in consumers.

People are motivated to differing degrees to use AT. Learning how to use an assistive device may require a significant time commitment for setup, fitting, modifying, and training. The greater the

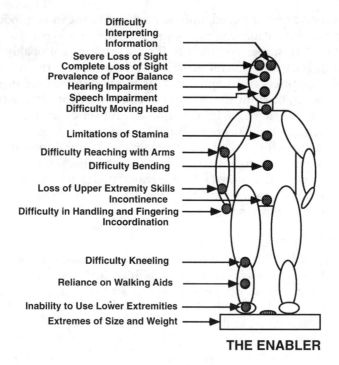

Difficulty
Interpreting
Information
Severe Loss of Sight
Complete Loss of Sight
Prevalence of Poor Balance
Hearing Impairment
Speech Impairment
Difficulty Moving Head

Limitations of Stamina

Difficulty Reaching with Arms
Difficulty Bending

Loss of Upper Extremity Skills
Incontinence
Difficulty in Handling and Fingering
Incoordination

Difficulty Kneeling

Reliance on Walking Aids

Inability to Use Lower Extremities
Extremes of Size and Weight

THE ENABLER

Figure 1.   "The Enabler," a simple model used to visualize impairments that must be considered in rehabilitation engineering design.

time demands for user mastery of the device, the greater the returns should be. The user must define the goals for AT use and understand the time commitment he or she must allocate to learning how to use the device. Rehabilitation engineers have the responsibility to clearly define the limitations of the equipment. An assistive device that requires major time commitments to learn to use often meets with opposition from consumers who refuse to take the necessary time to learn how to use it. If the goals of the device user do not match the potential of the technology, the imposition placed on the user can have long-term negative effects.

Task Factors

It must be remembered that, with assistive technology, there is always someone doing something somewhere. Doing something is the task. AT has no intrinsic value. When a consumer has completed tasks to his or her satisfaction, then assistive devices are useful. For an assistive device to be successful, it must incorporate information about the user and the tasks that he or she intends to use it to complete. The desired tasks are a major factor that determines the design. The person for whom the AT device is designed will influence the design by specifying the type and nature of tasks he or she wishes to perform with the device. The rehabilitation engineer then considers the nature of the tasks for which the device will be used. Possible abuses of the equipment or use for unintended purposes by the consumer are important considerations in designing a device. For example, devices designed to enhance the ability of an individual with a hearing impairment to communicate by telephone, watch television, or participate in meetings require different design criteria. Prosthetics designed for walking, running, and lifting may require significantly different components to enhance mobility.

Some tasks are performed many times each day (e.g., talking, listening, eating, typing, moving), whereas others may occur only once or twice during the day (e.g., eliminating, getting out of bed, driving to work). The repetitive nature of the tasks performed may require special design considerations to provide the AT user with a device that can withstand constant high demand for performance enhancement. These features may have to be a compromise of maximal performance possibilities with designs that emphasize average task demands. The features include the force, fit, and appearance of the device.

If a single device is used to perform multiple tasks made possible by modification of equipment, then the frequency of use for each task is an important consideration when designing reliable and durable assistive devices. For example, many power wheelchairs have programmable maximal speed; maximal forward, reverse, and yaw acceleration; and filter parameters. Some of these features are adjusted infrequently to make different task performance possible. The engineer must decide whether these features should be adjustable from an input on the wheelchair or from an external device.

Environmental Factors

Assistive technology is used in particular contexts. The environment in which the activity takes place may determine, to a large extent, the type of the design used to make an AT device. Equipment designed for indoor use will differ from that designed for outdoor use. Combined indoor and outdoor use may require different specifications from those for either indoor or outdoor use. Proper engineering requires consideration of a variety of physical conditions in settings where the device will or may be used. Physical conditions may include dust, fluids, moisture, shock, humidity, vibration, heat, cold, and a number of other hazards. Although designing devices to meet every foreseeable hazard is not possible, understanding the general tolerance levels of the equipment to different environmental conditions is important in constructing reliable, safe, and useful AT devices.

Engineering Design Considerations

Assistive technology requires engineering design as well as human performance design. With consideration for the needs of the consumer, classical engineering design criteria for production of high-quality equipment can be used to guide the development of practical AT.

Cost Factors

Function and cost are often the dominant design criteria used for production of assistive devices. Rehabilitation engineers must evaluate the effectiveness of a device based on a cost–benefit ratio over the life of the product. However, determining the useful life of an assistive device requires looking beyond profit. Consideration must be given to the rate of development of improved technology to meet the needs of the consumer because new equipment that better meets consumer needs will shorten the life of existing devices.

When considered as a group, people with disabilities have a very low average income level. A Harris Poll conducted in 1986 found that approximately 80% of people with disabilities were unemployed (Berkowitz et al., 1992). This low level of income and high level of unemployment result in most AT devices being purchased by third-party providers (e.g., Medicare, Medicaid, Social Security, veteran benefits, charitable organizations, private health insurance). Third-party providers make funding decisions based on meeting the consumer's minimal needs, not based on normal market forces such as comfort, convenience, or productivity. The result is selection of the least costly assistive device that meets a generic description of an average user's needs. This practice may be responsible in part for the high rate of AT device return or storage after little use. Thus, this apparently economical system may not be the most cost-effective approach for the consumer, third-party payer, or society. However, it is the system in place.

Expensive technology must be justified based on longer product life, greater improvement in function for the consumer, or both. Cost amortized over the life of the product is one method of justifying higher cost devices. For example, if a high-quality electric wheelchair with a 10-year life-use and features that reduce costly hospital care for skin sores and episodes of dysreflexia can be purchased for $24,000, it may have a lower net cost than a less expensive wheelchair (e.g., $10,000) that has a short life-use and no features to reduce secondary complications. When third-party payers begin to analyze their total lifetime costs for insuring people with disabilities, instead of obsessing on the cost of single items independently of how they fit into the total cost–benefit analysis, then the quality of AT may improve.

A second justification for the purchase of complex AT is that it provides a method for accomplishing a task that is not possible with any other equipment (e.g., communication devices for individuals who have severe hearing and visual impairments). The reasonable accommodation requirements for employers described in both Section 504 of the Rehabilitation Act of 1973 as amended and the Americans with Disabilities Act of 1990 (PL 101-336) may stimulate employers to purchase high-quality AT for employees with disabilities.

Under the current economic conditions and social policies that influence the purchase of AT, three basic paths are open to the rehabilitation engineer interested in working on developing new assistive devices. One approach is to invent sophisticated devices that perform important tasks other systems cannot perform. Unfortunately, developing advanced technology is expensive and may be difficult to justify. A second approach is to make devices that last longer than those made by competitors. The caveat here is that the rapid rate of development of improved products may result in the durable product becoming obsolete prior to the end of its useable life. The most frequent path taken by rehabilitation engineers is to modify inexpensively manufactured products to better meet the unique functional needs of the consumer. The low price of the equipment promotes selection by third-party payers, but payment for adapting these products for actual use by the consumer is rarely covered.

QUALITY ISSUES IN ASSISTIVE TECHNOLOGY DESIGN

Thus, the economic realities involved in development and purchase of AT challenge the rehabilitation engineer to provide quality equipment for a low cost that meets the needs of consumers. Engineers define the quality of assistive devices in terms of function, durability, reliability, and robustness. Three important additional features of AT play an important role in an engineer's concept of quality products—simplicity of the manufacturing process, ease of repair of equipment, and interactive control of "smart" AT.

Function has been discussed previously but in this context means a high-quality assistive device that allows the consumer to perform tasks for which the device was designed. In some cases, emphasis may be placed on high-quality AT that enhances a single but essential function allowing the consumer to survive (e.g., phrenic nerve stimulator, self-operated lifts for transfer to and from bed). Other examples of high-quality engineering may be directed at AT that provides the user with the flexibility to perform a variety of tasks (e.g., six-degrees-of-freedom artificial ankles, computer on-line trail guides to numerous national parks).

Durability defines a product's resistance to wear, fatigue, and other forms of damage or decay. The International Standards Organization develops standards related to durability for assistive technology. Simulating the use of AT under harsh environmental conditions is a common test of durability. Assistive devices should provide maximal durability without limiting function or exceeding cost.

Reliability is a measure of the amount of time the product functions properly over its lifetime or the percentage of time the product functions properly over a given interval. Because people use their assistive devices to achieve a goal, reliability is related to the percentage of time the person is not able to reach that goal because of the failure of the device. Nearly 100% reliability is desired. Within the budget provided for device development, product reliability must rank very high on the list of desirable product features. In some cases, the reliability of the product is so important that the product will not be marketed unless reliability approaches 100% (e.g., artifical organs, portable oxygen sources, implantable pumps).

Robustness determines the degree to which a system is able to function when components vary in tolerance or fail. Robustness can refer to the degree of variability in the environment that a system can tolerate. Robustness is important from a manufacturing perspective because robust designs permit normal operation with some variation in component tolerances. Robustness is important to the consumer because robust designs will function properly longer as components wear, deteriorate, or, in some cases, fail. Robust designs also permit systems to operate acceptably in environments for which they may not have been intended.

Manufacturing approaches for the production of AT are highly variable, depending to a large extent on the quantity, quality, and specificity of the device. If a rehabilitation engineer is planning to make a single device for a specific consumer, then the availability of resources for its fabrication is of primary concern. Components that must be custom ordered or that come from a single supplier (sole source) may cause undue hardship on the user if they delay initial delivery and subsequent repair of the assistive device. To avoid these problems, rehabilitation engineers making one-of-a-kind devices should use high-quality parts that are both reliable and widely available.

When the assistive device is to be manufactured in quantity, the rehabilitation engineer must consider the appropriate manufacturing methods for making the device. Nearly all mass-manufactured AT requires some degree of customization. Manufacturing plans must incorporate this in initial product design, manufacturing process design, and postmanufacturing modification plans. Special considerations of the needs of consumer populations must be made even for AT that is manufactured in relatively large quantities. For example, operation of many assistive devices requires power flowing from a source external to the user (i.e., battery or power distribution network). The use of these devices will be limited by the cost, availability, reliability, duration, weight, and other characteristics of the power source. Generally, designing products for minimal power consumption improves the quality of AT because minimal power consumption will lead to less heat being generated, longer periods of operation, and lower cost. Lightweight, long-acting battery power allows production of an assistive device that is portable, enabling the consumer to use the device in a variety of locations.

The *repair* of assistive devices is inevitable. The mark of high-quality AT is that it can be easily repaired at a reasonable cost. These two desirable aspects are heavily influenced by the design of the device. However, designing AT to maximize these features may conflict with designs that target improving reliability. These conflicts require making trade-offs that may reduce overall product quality. One solution to this dilemma is to design AT that can be assembled from several components or modules. This approach allows repairs to be made in one or more components relatively quickly and easily. When a part no longer functions reliably, the module containing the defective part can be sent to the factory or service center for repair. While the module is being repaired, the customer can use the device with a loaned replacement module. This strategy allows customers to have reliable assistive devices, gives the service provider an option for repair without replacement, and provides the manufacturer with a device that has a longer operating life. Modular construction of AT lowers the cost, allows for rapid repair, and provides the option of modification without replacement. This new approach gives product designers more freedom to develop high-quality, moderately customized, affordable products. In addition, service centers and field sites do not have to invest in expensive test equipment.

The *interactions* of people with disabilities and their assistive devices can range from totally person controlled to autonomous functioning by the device. When people use AT to perform work, function and control often are shared. Many devices are purely passive and convert the input of the user into another form of motion or energy. An orthotic hand splint that converts the power of wrist extension to a functional grip illustrates this type of function and control relationship. One approach to increasing shared control of AT is to design devices that operate differently in one or more modes. The user controls the mode of operation by his or her action. For example, leg braces may be locked into position by the user when he or she is performing an activity that requires standing for long periods of time. In some cases, the device may set boundary conditions for operation in the different modes. Speed settings on electric wheelchairs may be changed by the user, but the range of speed, power, turn rate, and other motion parameters are fixed by preset characteristics of a limited number of modes.

Developments in miniaturization of components, computer program control of operations, and new materials are allowing rehabilitation engineers to build new types of AT that have varying degrees of intelligence. In designing this new generation of AT, rehabilitation engineers must decide which segments of performance are to be controlled by the device, which components can operate with shared input, and which elements must be controlled exclusively by the user. For shared control, the engineer must build in decision rules for device or human control under varying task demands in a variety of settings. In some cases, control of devices may change as the device "learns" the consumer's desired actions. When the device has acquired the user's preferred response patterns, then some portions of the operation may be relinquished to the device or the device may provide cues (suggestions) for optimal operation to the user. For example, operation of an electric wheelchair by an individual with upper limb spasticity may improve as the module controlling direction "learns" to average the variable input from the user. Control of the movement of the wheelchair by the module would be relinquished when the user decided to change direction.

APPLYING TOTAL QUALITY MANAGEMENT PRINCIPLES TO REHABILITATION ENGINEERING

Rehabilitation engineers work in teams with other disciplines, service providers, and consumers for the purpose of developing new assistive devices that are used by consumers in a safe and productive manner. Very often, however, the level of satisfaction with and use of AT by consumers is less than satisfactory. Clearly, a replicable method for involving all parties in a shared problem-solving approach must be developed that maximizes the expertise of each team member and meets the needs of consumers for AT.

One promising approach is to apply the principles of total quality management (TQM) to the development of AT. The principles of TQM were formulated in the 1950s by Deming (1982) and have been applied by Japanese industry to produce high-quality products. TQM is a process and atmosphere that promotes quality products from a consumer's perspective and that engages the skills of qualified experts. It is accomplished by treating people as intelligent colleagues who strive to do a good job (Crosby, 1988). TQM provides a framework for achieving high-quality rehabilitation engineering services, device designs, and AT products. TQM tools can assist rehabilitation teams in developing optimal solutions for challenges faced by people with disabilities through promotion of optimal interaction between consumers and rehabilitation professionals.

The "Plan-Do-Check-Act" cycle (Deming, 1982) is used to describe how productivity and quality can be maximized while maintaining a healthy working environment. This cycle is the core of TQM. The Plan-Do-Check-Act cycle as applied to rehabilitation engineering service is illustrated in Figure 2. The cycle emphasizes a team approach.

The Plan portion of the cycle for production of useful AT entails rehabilitation professionals and consumers working together to articulate problems, define goals, and describe solutions. The notion is that this planning team is likely to address all of the critical issues required to develop optimal solutions to problems encountered by consumers as they use AT to perform tasks of their daily activities. The basic concept is that members of the team have a variety of experiences and perspectives that no single person can bring to problem resolution.

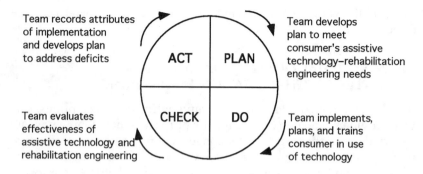

Figure 2.   Example of Deming's (1982) "Plan-Do-Check-Act" cycle applied to reha-bilitation engineering service delivery. Definitions for each portion of the cycle can be used to describe research, design, or developmental tasks.

During the Do portion of the cycle, rehabilitation professionals and consumers design, modify, or purchase an assistive device considered to be appropriate for meeting the consumer's goals. Following selection of the device, the consumer receives training in its use and care. This training is an essential component of AT service delivery. This is evidenced by the fact that numerous good products designed by rehabilitation engineers working in laboratories by themselves have been rejected by therapists, consumers, or both on the basis of inadequate training in device use. To realize the benefits of a specific device, the consumer and the therapist must take the time to learn how to perform activities with it. The rehabilitation engineer must take responsibility for making clear to the consumer or therapist the advances in task perfomance that can be attributed to use of the new device.

The amount of time devoted to learning to use complex AT may prove to have a large payoff for the consumer in terms of speed or ease of task completion or both. For example, if a consumer is presented with two power wheelchairs, one with simple controls and one with complex controls, he or she must plan for an extended period of training during the Do phase of TQM if the complex controls are to have a chance of being used. In this example, the simple operation of one type of foot-controlled electric wheelchair requires the use of four switches. The consumer can learn to perform simple driving maneuvers within a very short time (usually within a few hours). However, simple switch control makes it difficult to maneuver in close quarters (e.g., offices, small rooms, rooms with much furniture). An electric wheelchair that operates through the use of a proportional foot control (foot joystick) and several switches requires many more hours of training for proficient use. Complex learning is involved in acquiring skills needed for common driving maneuvers. However, for those who can learn to use a foot-operated joystick control, the reward is greater control over the wheelchair. This additional control allows safe access and passage through many more physical environments than the wheelchair controlled by switches alone.

The first step in the Check portion of the TQM cycle is a quantitative and qualitative evaluation of the effectiveness of the consumer's current means of functioning with existing AT. Comparisons are made of performance with the existing equipment and with the new assistive device developed during the Plan and Do cycles. Training techniques used to improve abilities of consumers to perform tasks with the new device are reviewed and suggestions for improvements are made. Qualitative analyses of differences in user satisfaction with the current and proposed methods for enhancing task performance are made. Quantitative data on performance with old and new AT are collected to provide for statistical analyses of performance on separate components of complex tasks.

The Act part of the TQM cycle is used to record the contributions of differing elements of the process (i.e., evaluation, design, selection, training, task performance). Positive and negative aspects of the process are assessed. The team then develops a plan to address the limitations. Training can have a tremendous influence on the Act part of the cycle. What is learned during training will affect decisions about modifying the assistive device, the method of rehabilitation intervention, or both. Without incorporating an Act component into the quality control cycle, consumers are apt to be dissatisfied or to abandon the equipment, even if they took part in developing it.

Economic constraints can interfere with the optimal use of TQM. Use of the TQM cycle assumes that the process of providing rehabilitation engineering and assistive technology services is iterative. Comparison of different types of AT to solve performance goals of the consumer requires that several devices be available for testing. However, third-party providers are often skeptical when asked to pay for several assistive devices for evaluation purposes. One solution to this problem is to rent assistive devices until a satisfactory solution is obtained. Another possibility is to conduct assessment at sites where there is a large selection of assistive devices and broad rehabilitation engineering capabilities. In these types of settings, a number of iterations of the Plan-Do-Check-Act cycle may be made prior to purchase.

METHODS USED FOR SELECTION OF AND PROBLEM DETECTION IN THE OPERATION OF ASSISTIVE DEVICES

When using the Plan-Do-Check-Act cycle is not practical for selection of AT, several other options are available to rehabilitation teams. Identifying device components that contribute to a problem in the use of AT can be a difficult task. One approach is to use a diagram in the form of the skeleton of a fish (fishbone) as a visual aid in problem analysis. The horizontal arrow of the fishbone points to the problem. A series of major components leading to the problem are depicted as ribs of the fishbone flowing into the primary axis from above and below the shaft of the arrow. Subcomponents of the problem flow into the major components. This type of diagram provides a tool for focusing the rehabilitation team on problems associated with development and use of AT. However, the fishbone diagram does not incorporate the important interactions between various components that may contribute to problems fundamental to the process of matching consumer needs with appropriate AT.

Another frequently used method for analyzing problems with the process of AT selection is the use of flowcharts. The process is illustrated as a sequence of activities beginning at the top and ending at the bottom of a chart. Several steps may be directly connected, whereas others incorporate feedback loops. Typically, arrows are used to illustrate the direction of information flow. Different line types are used to discriminate between forward and feedback paths. Tasks are placed in rectangular boxes. Decisions are placed in diamond shapes. These flowcharts are useful for illustrating interactions between components and for identifying feedback loops. They can be used to show weaknesses in the process flow, feedback loops, or interactions of components. Once problem areas are identified and their interactions with other factors are understood, solutions can be developed.

Although the use of fishbone diagrams and flowcharts is widespread in the assessment of AT, the lack of input by consumers using several types of assistive devices in comparative performance trials limits these approaches to assessment of single devices. If the problem could be resolved by means of an entirely different type of device, these approaches would miss the recommended solution. If the device selected does not meet the consumer's needs even after a thorough fishbone diagram and flowchart analysis, then the device is likely to be abandoned. The outcome may be a very dissatisfied consumer or a costly additional set of fishbone and flowchart analyses of a series of different types of AT.

CONCLUSIONS

Each person has a finite set of abilities and resources that can be used to address their life goals. People with physical impairments often bring different, lesser, or fewer physical abilities to perform some tasks. When task demands exceed the capacity of a person with disabilities to complete the task, then changes must be made in the task, the environment, or the person. For rehabilitation professionals, the challenge is to design, develop, and produce assistive devices that enable people with disabilities to improve their capacities to meet the task demands of activities in which they choose to engage within a variety of different environments in which the skills are needed. Successful solutions to performance problems presented by people with disabilities will be best developed by using a team approach that has significant consumer involvement. Fundamental engineering principles of quality control must be incorporated into the design and production of AT. A form of TQM should be adopted to ensure that the best type of AT is produced for and used by people with disabilities. Training the consumer in the optimal use of a device is essential to long-term satisfaction with the product. When these basic tenets are followed, the chances of people with disabilities using AT to improve their quality of life will be maximized.

> There is as much difference between us and ourselves as between us and others.

> Michel de Montaigne (in Pirkl, 1994, p. 1)

REFERENCES

Americans with Disabilities Act (ADA) of 1990, PL 101-336, 42 U.S.C. §§ 12101 et seq.

Bailey, R.W. (1989). *Human performance engineering* (2nd ed.). Englewood Cliffs, NJ: Prentice Hall.

Berkowitz, M. (Ed.). (1987). *Disability policy*. New York: Cambridge University Press.

Berkowitz, M., Harvey, C., Greene, C.G., & Wilson, S.E. (1992). *The economic consequences of traumatic spinal cord injury*. New York: Demos Publishing.

Cooper, R.A. (1995). *Rehabilitation engineering applied to mobility and manipulation.* Bristol, England: Institute of Physics Publishers.

Crosby, P.B. (1988). *The eternally successful organization: The art of corporate wellness.* New York: McGraw-Hill.

Deming, W.E. (1982). *Out of the crisis.* Cambridge, MA: Productivity Press.

Einstein, A. (1952, October 5). *New York Times.*

Hotchkiss, R.D. (1993, July/August). Ground swell on wheels. *The Sciences,* 14–19.

National Institute on Disability and Rehabilitation Research. (1989). *Chartbook on disability in the U.S.* (Contract HN88011001). Washington, DC: U.S. Department of Education.

Pirkl, J.J. (1994). *Transgenerational design: Products for an aging population.* New York: Van Nostrand Reinhold.

Pope, A.M., & Tarlov, A.R. (Eds.). (1991). *Disability in America: Toward a national agenda for prevention.* Washington, DC: National Academy Press.

Rehabilitation Act of 1973, PL 93-112, 29 U.S.C. §§ 701 *et seq.*

Rehabilitation Act Amendments of 1986, PL 99-506, 29 U.S.C. §§ 701 *et seq.*

Rehabilitation Act Amendments of 1992, PL 102-569, 29 U.S.C. §§ 701 *et seq.*

Technology-Related Assistance for Individuals with Disabilities Act of 1988, PL 100-407, 29 U.S.C. §§ 2201 *et seq.*

U.S. Bureau of the Census. (1990). *1990 decennial census.* Washington, DC: U.S. Government Printing Office.

CHAPTER 11

Engineering for
People with Disabilities

Kenton R. Kaufman

The engineering design process involves the application of both science and technology to obtain a product that serves a valuable purpose. People with disabilities may benefit greatly from engineering designs aimed at improving their abilities to fulfill their functional requirements and needs for independence. Engineering design involves developing a methodology to proceed from concept to final product while knowing which technological resources to use, as well as considering economics, timeliness, reliability, safety, and practicality during the design process. Good engineering design must encompass all of these issues to create products that benefit humanity and improve the quality of life. This chapter describes the application of engineering design for people with disabilities.

THE DESIGN PROCESS

Engineering design is a creative process that devises or develops something new or arranges existing things in a new way. Engineering design is a continuous process whereby scientific and technological information are used to innovate a system, device, or process that will benefit society in some way (Hill, 1970). Engineering design is both a science and an art. The science of engineering

This chapter was supported in part by National Center for Medical Rehabilitation Research Grants RO1 HD30150 and RO1 HD31476. Appreciation is also expressed to Jill Jordano for her careful assistance with manuscript preparation.

design can be learned through the systematic application of problem-solving techniques and experience. The art of engineering design must be practiced to become proficient. Good design needs both analysis and synthesis. The analysis is learned through formal training. It involves separation of the overall product into constituent parts that are individually designed to meet the overall goals of the system. However, analysis should not be confused with design. A device may be well analyzed but not well designed. A good design requires synthesis of the constituent elements into an integrated system. The parts of this integrated system must be assembled with imagination and creativity in a unique way. The science and art, as well as the analysis and synthesis, must occur simultaneously in the process of design in order to devise uniquely useful systems, devices, or processes. The design of a device, system, or process can develop in one of two ways; it can be either evolutionary or revolutionary. Evolutionary design presents a slow, low-risk process whereby the product is allowed to develop over time with only slight improvements. The risk of making major mistakes is minimized, but the creative capabilities of the design engineer are used minimally. In contrast, the revolutionary or innovative design represents a paradigm shift in the application of science and art to create a new product. The creative skills and analytical ability of the design engineer are used to their utmost to obtain a design that carries a high risk and high yield.

The methodology of good engineering design parallels the methodology for good science (Hill, 1970). It is important to understand the similarities and differences between these two techniques. Gaining a complete understanding of these two methodologies will ensure appropriate cross-fertilization of engineering design and scientific investigation. This cross-fertilization will promote appropriate research that can be applied to yield enhanced engineering designs for people with disabilities. The components of the scientific method and the design method are similar (Figure 1).

The scientific method uses a body of existing knowledge as the basis for investigation. This knowledge can be in the form of published literature, scientific laws, or research experience. A scientist observes nature with respect to this knowledge base and asks questions regarding his or her observations. The scientist conceives a hypothesis to explain the phenomenon or idea and then devises a research plan to test the hypothesis. Data are collected, and the hypothesis is subjected to logical analysis that either confirms or fails to confirm the idea. The hypothesis and analysis phases are iterative: The analysis may reveal a flaw in the hypothesis, which must

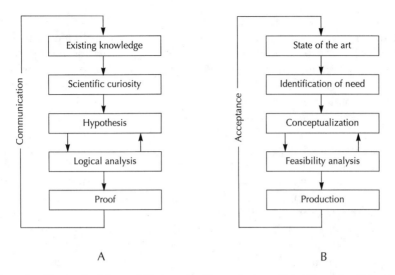

A   B

Figure 1.   The methodology of (A) the scientific method parallels (B) good engineering design.

be altered and then reanalyzed. Once the idea has been tested and confirmed by the scientist, it must be accepted by fellow scientists. The idea is shared with the scientific community in the form of research publications and is subjected to peer review. Once accepted by the scientific community, it becomes part of the existing body of knowledge, which is communicated via oral and written modalities, and the scientific process is repeated.

The design method begins with a body of knowledge that encompasses the state of the art for that particular device, process, or technique. Given the state of the art, a person, company, or society identifies a need that requires fulfillment. A system is conceptualized to satisfy the need that has been identified. The conceptualization may take the form of sketches and task specifications, which control the design process as it moves toward the desired goal of satisfying the identified needs. The feasibility of these specifications is tested against known mathematical and engineering principles as well as economic objectives. Several design concepts are generated that define possible pathways to the stated goal. These concepts are tested against physical laws. This verification with the laws of nature is known as an *engineering design analysis* and forms an iterative loop with conceptualization. After an optimum design has been selected, it is constructed and tested to verify the concept and analysis of the design with regard to performance and durability characteristics. After several cycles of testing, analysis, and redesign, a product emerges that satisfies the previously identified need. This product is then manufactured and distributed through commercial channels. The general public has the opportunity to purchase the product. The consumption records dictate the usefulness and success of the design. Acceptance is defined in terms of sales volume. Acceptance by the public enlarges the state of the art, and the design process begins again.

The scientific method and the design method differ in terms of motivation for the participant. The scientist is motivated by curiosity and is driven by a desire to obtain answers to personal observations, professional acceptance, and recognition among peers. In contrast, the design engineer desires to produce something that is useful to society and will be sold for a profit. The scientist faces uncertainty in terms of funding and peer acceptance. The design engineer faces uncertainty in terms of cost competition and public acceptance of a product that is unique. Both individuals require intellectual curiosity and knowledge to achieve success.

IDENTIFICATION OF NEED FOR ASSISTIVE TECHNOLOGY

People with neurological disorders are among those most often treated by rehabilitation professionals (Bohannon, 1995). These individuals frequently have reductions in skeletal muscle strength. Estimates made in 1994 indicated that there are 1,752,000 people in the United States with partial or complete paralysis of the extremities (U.S. Department of Health and Human Services, 1994). The prevalence of paralysis of the extremities increases with age (Figure 2). These individuals require assistive technology (AT) in the form of a leg brace to maintain erect support during stance and to enhance mobility. It is estimated that 866,000 people use a leg brace (U.S. Department of Commerce, 1994). In addition to people who require a leg brace for ambulation, there are 184,000 individuals who use a foot brace and an additional 184,000 individuals who use an artificial leg or foot (U.S. Department of Commerce, 1994). Thus, 1,234,000 people need some form of AT for the lower extremity (Table 1). It is important to note that, although there is a greater need for assistive technology as age increases (Figure 2), the use of AT actually decreases with age (Figure 3). The prevalence of leg brace use is higher among younger individuals (Figure 3), and the use of an artificial limb is highest among people in the 45- to 64-year age range (Figure 4).

Thus, a need for assistive technology in people with partial or complete paralysis of the lower extremity has clearly been identi-

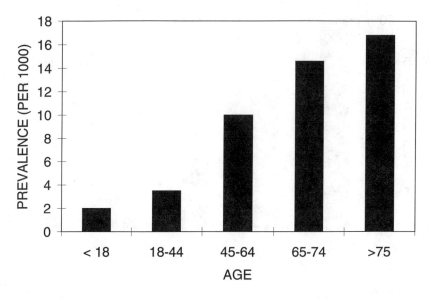

Figure 2.   Prevalence of people in the United States with partial or complete paralysis of the extremities. There is a greater need for assistive technology as age increases. (*Source:* U.S. Department of Health and Human Services [1994].)

fied. Functional needs of individuals are utmost in importance. The following sections discuss how AT can be used to assess and restore function in individuals with paralysis of the lower extremity.

METHODS FOR ASSESSMENT OF MUSCLE STRENGTH

Instrumented and Noninstrumented Methods

Several instrumented and noninstrumented methods exist for measuring the strength of individuals with neuromuscular weakness. Manual muscle testing has been the most common noninstrumented method for measuring muscle strength since it was introduced by

Table 1.   U.S. population requirements for assistive technology for the lower extremity

Device	Population
Leg brace	866,000
Foot brace	184,000
Artificial leg or foot	184,000
Total	1,234,000

Source: U.S. Department of Commerce (1994).

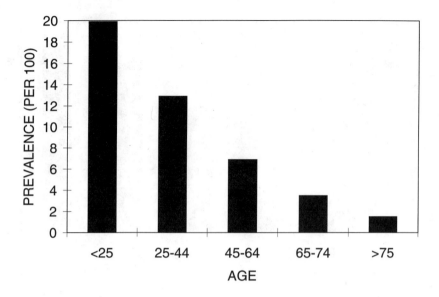

Figure 3.   Prevalence of people in the United States who use a leg brace. The use of a leg brace decreases with age. (*Source:* U.S. Department of Commerce [1994].)

Lovett in 1917. The most often used scoring system for manual muscle testing is the six-level scheme (Table 2). This scoring system ranges from a 5 (normal strength) to 0 (no evidence of contractility). The muscle grade is determined by the ability of the subject to move voluntarily against gravity and to resist a force applied by an examiner (Beasley, 1961; Daniels & Worthingham, 1980; Kendall & McCreary, 1983; Wakim, Gersten, Elkins, & Martin, 1950). Several other noninstrumented methods, which include functional tests and measurements with weights, have also been used. These other noninstrumented methods do not measure muscle strength but rather provide a nonspecific indication of muscle capacity to perform an activity of daily living. The most commonly selected tasks are sit-to-stand (Bohannon, Hull, & Palmeri, 1994; Csuka & McCarty, 1985; Guralnik et al., 1994) and stair climbing (Amundsen & Graves, 1991; Olgiati, Burgunder, & Mumenthaler, 1988). These tests are thought to test lower-extremity muscle strength in a functional capacity because the joint moment required to perform activities such as sit-to-stand and stair ascent and descent is considerable (Andriacchi, Andersson, & Fermier, 1980; Wrentenberg, Lindberg, & Arborelius, 1993). Noninstrumented testing fails to predict the ability to walk because people with muscle weakness can modify muscle action timing to avoid threatening postures and obtain protective alignment during stance (Perry, 1992). Also, they

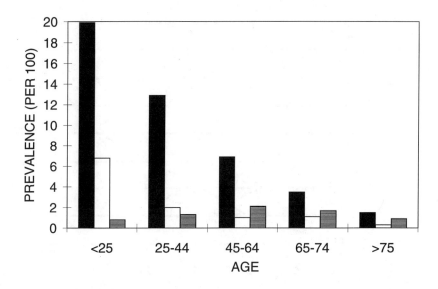

Figure 4.   Prevalence of people in the United States who use some form of assistive technology for the lower extremity. (□, leg; ■, foot; ▤, artificial limb.) (*Source:* U.S. Department of Commerce [1994].)

find subtle ways to advance the limb in swing by postural substitution (Perry, 1992).

Manual muscle tests have limited value in the lower extremity (Figure 5). A normal muscle (Grade 5) ranges in strength between 53% of true nonparalytic normal for the knee and 80% for the ankle. The earliest display of weakness (Grade 4) represents 40% of normal strength (Sharrad, 1953). A Grade 3 muscle is approximately 15% of normal strength. During normal walking, normal muscles function at a 3+ level (Perry, Ireland, Gronley, & Haffer, 1986). This effort, averaging about 25% of normal strength, allows adequate reserves so that fatigue is avoided (Perry, 1992). However, people whose muscles have only fair strength (3+) will have no endurance or reserve, because they must function at a

Table 2.   Scoring system for manual muscle testing

Muscle grades	Description
5—Normal	Complete range of motion against gravity with full resistance
4—Good	Complete range of motion against gravity with some resistance
3—Fair	Complete range of motion against gravity
2—Poor	Complete range of motion with gravity eliminated
1—Trace	Evidence of slight contractility; no joint motion
0—Zero	No evidence of contractility

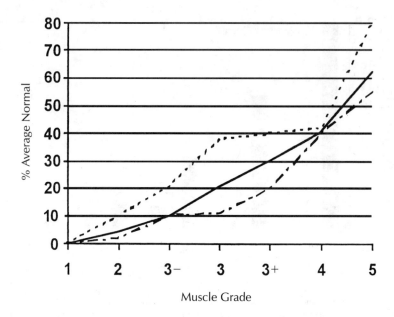

Figure 5.   Relative value (percentage of true normal) of a manual test for the lower-limb muscles. (---, ankle; ———, hip; – - – -, knee.) (*Source:* Beasley [1961].)

100% effort level. Thus, manual strength grading can be misleading. Although strength testing is critical, noninstrumented muscle testing has serious limitations.

Instrumented strength testing is a more accurate indication of actual strength status and is needed to define true capability. Instrumented methods include hand-held dynamometers (Bohannon, 1988, 1990; Wickholm & Bohannon, 1991), load cells (Fowler & Gardner, 1967), hand-grip dynamometers (Sunderland, Tinson, & Bradley, 1989), and isokinetic dynamometers (Armstrong et al., 1983; Tripp & Harris, 1991). Instrumented measurement has been shown to be more sensitive to differences in muscle strength than noninstrumented manual measurement (Aitkens et al., 1989; Beasley, 1956; Bohannon, 1986; Schwartz, Cohen, Herbison, & Shah, 1992). Hand-held dynamometers are held by the examiner, who then applies force to the person being tested. The examiner must be strong enough to withstand the forces generated by the person; otherwise, the measurement tests the examiner's strength rather than the strength of the patient. Load cells are fixed in position and measure only isometric strength. Hand-grip dynamometers measure only hand-grip strength and, thus, are limited in terms of applications. The most common strength testing device is an isokinetic dynamometer, the popularity of which may be attributed to the ease with which it provides information. Isokinetic testing, however, can provide generalizations only about muscle function. It cannot be used to determine the function of an individual muscle. Also, the location of the peak joint moment does not necessarily correspond to the position of maximum muscular output for a muscle (Lieber & Boakes, 1988). In general, instrumented methods are better than noninstrumented methods for providing information about muscular strength. However, these methods fail to provide detailed information about individual muscles. Electromyography is customarily used to provide quantification of individual muscle function.

Electromyography

Electromyography has been used with motion and force plate data to assess muscle function during gait and has been useful in defining the phasic activity of muscles. Although considerable progress has been made in quantifying electromyographic activity (Bogey, Barnes, & Perry, 1992, 1993), the basic problem remains that an electromyogram (EMG) provides a quantitative measurement of muscle tension only under isometric conditions (Bigland-Ritchie, Kukulka, & Woods, 1980; Dempster & Finerty, 1947; deVries, 1968; Lippold, 1952; Maton & Bouisset, 1977; Messier et al., 1971; Metral & Cassar, 1981; Moritani & deVries, 1978; Woods & Bigland-Ritchie, 1983; Zuniga & Simons, 1969). Inman, Ralston, Saunders, Feinstein, and Wright (1952) first observed changes in myoelectric signal amplitudes that corresponded to variations in muscle load. Since then, much work has been done to determine the degree to which EMG signals and muscle loads are related (Bigland & Lippold, 1954; Bouisset, 1973; Hatze, 1978; Hof & Vandenberg, 1977; Komi, 1973; Milner-Brown & Stein, 1975). However, the EMG signal is a measure of the bioelectric events that occur in conjunction with contraction of muscle fibers. Thus, it is a phenomenon related to the initiation of muscle contraction rather than an effect of the muscle's mechanical action.

Problems occur in dynamic situations when using electromyographic activity as a measure of a muscle's functional capability. The dynamic force produced by a muscle is not proportional to the degree of muscular activity. Other factors may affect the muscle force, such as a change of the muscle length, change of the contraction velocity, the rate and type of muscle contraction, joint position, and muscle fatigue. Several authors agree that the integrated EMG value is not affected by a length change of the muscle at maximal effort (Komi & Buskirk, 1972; Seliger, Dolejs, & Karas, 1980), whereas others report a contrary behavior (Lunnen, Yack, & Le Veau, 1981; Rosentswieg & Hinson, 1972). Barnes (1980) reported a decreasing value for the integrated EMG at maximal effort with increasing contraction velocity. In contrast, Rosentswieg and Hinson (1972) stated that isokinetic contractions elicited significantly greater integrated EMG values than either isotonic or isometric contractions. Others reported that the integrated EMG value at maximal effort is not affected by a change of velocity (Hinson & Rosentswieg, 1973; Komi & Rusko, 1974; Rothstein, De Litto, Sinacore, & Rose, 1983). Muscle force varies with the type of muscle action. The relative strength of eccentric contractions was reported to be equal to that of isometric contractions (Smidt, 1973) or greater by 10%–20% (Vandervoort, Kramer, & Wharram, 1990). Concentric muscle contraction results in approximately 20% less force than isometric contraction (Osternig, 1975; Smidt, 1973). Strength varies nonlinearly with the speed of effort (Osternig, Hamill, Corros, & Lander, 1984). During maximum efforts at any speed, the EMG is relatively constant even though the force differs (Perry, 1992). As a joint moves, both the muscle fiber length and the muscle moment arm change. Whereas the intensity of the EMG remains constant, the strength of the quadriceps declines by 50% when the joint position is changed from 50° to 10° of flexion (Haffajee, Maritz, & Sauntesson, 1972). Estimation of muscle force from the myoelectric signal is limited to nonfatiguing contractions because the myoelectric signal changes with fatigue, which is unrelated to changes in muscle force (Lippold, Redfearn, & Vuco, 1970; Parker, Körner, & Kadefors, 1984). Because the relationship between muscle force and EMG is not known for dynamic conditions, EMG cannot be used to quantify muscle force.

Direct Muscle Force Measurement

In vivo internal muscle forces are difficult to measure directly. Experimental measurements have been performed on cats. The first was done by Walmsley, Hodgson, and Burke (1978), who measured the force of the cat soleus and medial gastrocnemius during standing and walking. This work was extended by other researchers using the same model and a similar protocol (Gregor et al., 1988; Hodgson, 1983; Lovely, Gregor, Roy, & Edgerton, 1990; Whiting, Gregor, Roy, & Edgerton, 1984). Abraham and Loeb (1985) also measured muscle forces in the cat hind limb. Data from direct muscle force measurements in humans are very limited because of the invasive nature of the experiment. Komi (1990) and Komi, Salonen, Jarvinen, and Kokko (1987) performed direct muscle force measurements on the human Achilles tendon. The results of these studies must be regarded cautiously, however, because the measurements obtained were from a group of muscles rather than individual muscles.

Intramuscular Pressure Measurement

It is desirable to find an alternative measurable mechanical parameter related to muscle force that would be less invasive to obtain. The electromyographic signal does not furnish adequate information to assess the tension produced by a muscle, because the tension reflects the sum of both the active contraction and the passive stretch. Measurement of intramuscular pressure (IMP) is a conceivable solution. It is possible to obtain IMP measurements during gait and relate these measurements to the timing and intensity of muscle contraction.

Two types of systems are available for recording IMP. One system is fluid filled and the other system uses a fiberoptic transducer. The fluid-filled systems include the needle manometer (Burch & Sodeman, 1937; Landerer, 1884) and the wick catheter technique (Mubarak, Hargens, Owen, Garetto, & Akeson, 1976; Snashall, Lucas, Guz, & Floyer, 1971). However, pressure recording systems that are fluid filled require infusion to maintain accuracy (Matsen, Mayo, Sheridan, & Krugmire, 1976; Rorabeck, Castle, Hardie, & Logan, 1981; Styf, Crenshaw, & Hargens, 1989). Fluid-filled systems are sensitive to hydrostatic artifacts and may be used only with limited types of movement that do not involve limb position changes relative to the horizontal plane. Thus, this technology would not be adaptable to measurements of IMP during gait. Furthermore, use of fluid-filled systems increases the risk of a collusion at the tip of the catheter. In contrast, a fiberoptic transducer–tipped system is not sensitive to hydrostatic artifact (Crenshaw, Styf, Mubarak, & Hargens, 1990) and has been shown to be effective for measuring IMP during exercise (Crenshaw, Styf, & Hargens, 1992).

IMP has been used to quantify muscle function during dynamic activities (Kaufman & Sutherland, 1995). IMP was measured during passive motion and active contraction of the ankle and was found to be capable of recording the passive stretch component of muscle (Figure 6). The electromyographic activity of the gastrocnemius was silent because the motion was obtained passively. Nevertheless, the IMP curve followed the motion of the ankle. When the gastrocne-

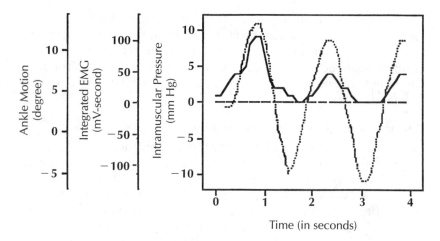

Time (in seconds)

Figure 6.   Intramuscular pressure (IMP) and electromyogram (EMG) activity during *passive motion* of the ankle. The recordings are from the gastrocnemius. The motion was recorded with an electrogoniometer. Ankle dorsiflexion is positive. (· · · ·, motion; – – – –, EMG; ——, IMP.) (From Kaufman, K.R., & Sutherland, D.H. [1995]. Dynamic intramuscular pressure measurement during gait. *Operative Techniques in Sports Medicine, 3*[4], 252; reprinted by permission.)

mius was stretched passively (dorsiflexion), the IMP increased. When the stretch was removed from the gastrocnemius (plantar flexion), the IMP returned to zero. Timing of peak dorsiflexion and peak IMP coincided. During active motion (Figure 7), the IMP was measured during both plantar flexion and dorsiflexion, whereas the EMG was present only during contraction of the gastrocnemius (plantar flexion). Thus, the IMP was able to quantify the contribution of both the passive stretch of muscle and the active contraction of muscle, whereas the electromyographic activity recorded only the active tension of the muscle force.

Measures of IMP and electromyographic activity have also been obtained during gait (Figure 8). The stance portion of the gait cycle starts with the foot strike and continues to toe-off. The swing portion of the gait cycle starts at toe-off and continues to foot strike. Single-limb stance begins at opposite toe-off and ends at opposite foot strike. It can be seen in Figure 8 that IMP increased at the beginning of single-limb stance (opposite toe-off) and peaked at the end of single-limb stance (opposite foot strike). The increase of IMP corresponded with the increase in electromyographic activity of the gastrocnemius. The greatest muscle activity in the plantar flexors was required near the end of single-limb stance to meet the

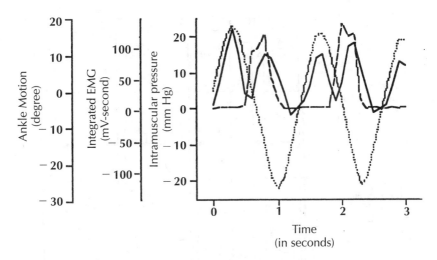

Time
(in seconds)

Figure 7.   Intramuscular pressure (IMP) and electromyogram (EMG) activity during *active motion* of the ankle. The recordings are from the gastrocnemius. The motion was recorded with an electrogoniometer. Ankle dorsiflexion is positive. (· · · ·, motion; – – – -, EMG; ———, IMP.) (From Kaufman, K.R., & Sutherland, D.H. [1995]. Dynamic intramuscular pressure measurement during gait. *Operative Techniques in Sports Medicine, 3*[4], 252; reprinted by permission.)

high extrinsic dorsiflexion moment occurring at the ankle joint (Figure 9B) and to reverse the direction of ankle movement (Figure 9A). However, it should also be noted that the IMP reading continued briefly after cessation of the EMG. Furthermore, it can be noted that there is a lower-level intramuscular pressure recording during the swing phase of gait. The peaks in IMP during gait can be correlated with the peaks of active contraction and passive stretch of the gastrocnemius. During the stance phase of gait, the peak IMP recording corresponds to the time when the ankle moment is at a maximum (opposite foot strike) (Figure 9B). Furthermore, during the swing phase of gait, the peak of IMP corresponds to the point of time when the ankle is at peak dorsiflexion (Figure 9A).

Currently available fiberoptic pressure transducers are too large for optimum comfort (1.35 mm). The Mayo Clinic is conducting research and development efforts in cooperation with Lawrence Livermore National Laboratory to develop a smaller IMP biosensor. This microsensor has an outer diameter of 200 μm, a 75% decrease in size. This will allow the IMP transducer to be inserted with a 25-gauge needle, thereby obviating the need for surgical implantation. Measurement of IMP under dynamic conditions, such as walking or running, has obvious application in research and clinical problems.

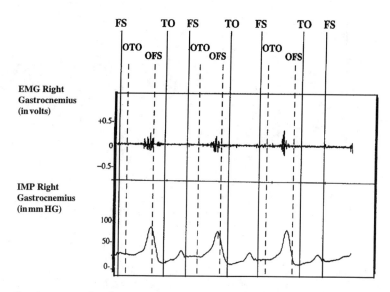

Figure 8.   Raw data for a single subject during gait. Both electromyogram (EMG) activity and intramuscular pressure are being recorded from the gastrocnemius muscle. The stance phase of gait occurs from foot strike (FS) to toe-off (TO). The swing phase of gait occurs from TO to FS. Single-limb stance occurs from opposite toe-off (OTO) to opposite foot strike (OFS). (From Kaufman, K.R., & Sutherland, D.H. [1995]. Dynamic intramuscular pressure measurement during gait. *Operative Techniques in Sports Medicine, 3*[4], 253; reprinted by permission.)

ASSISTIVE TECHNOLOGY METHODS TO RESTORE FUNCTION

Provision of mobility for an individual with neuromuscular disabilities is a complicated problem. Three alternatives are available: surgery, functional electrical stimulation, and orthoses. Regardless of which modality is selected, the goals of locomotion are similar: 1) rotate and coordinate the joints to achieve forward progression, 2) support the body's weight during the stance phase of a locomotion cycle, 3) adjust the limb length by flexing the knee during the swing phase of gait, and 4) further smooth the trajectory of the center of gravity by slightly flexing the knee in mid-stance (Perry, 1967). The overall goal is to obtain forward locomotion in the most energy-efficient way possible.

Surgical techniques for obtaining these stated goals of locomotion are muscle transfers or arthrodesis (fusion) of joints. Although arthrodesis achieves stability during stance, the mobility of the individual is severely limited. These limitations in mobility require compensatory movements to be made in order to obtain foot clearance during swing. These compensations result in increased mus-

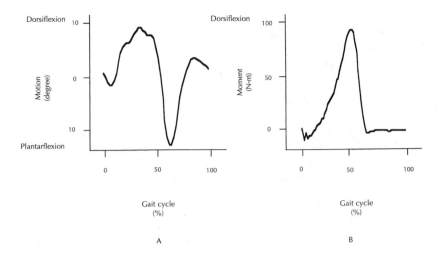

Figure 9.   Ankle motion (A) and moment (B) during gait. The gait cycle is defined as the events that occur between successive footsteps of the same foot. The gait cycle begins with foot strike, continues through stance and swing phases, and ends with foot strike of the same foot.

cular effort and increased vertical displacement of the body's center of mass. The net result is an increase in energy consumption to achieve locomotion. The effect of restricted joint motion on the metabolic cost of walking has been studied. The increase in energy consumption varied with the joint that was immobilized (Mattsson & Broström, 1990; Waters, Barnes, Husserl, Silver, & Liss, 1988; Waters, Campbell, Thomas, Hugos, & Davis, 1982).

Functional electrical stimulation (FES) has also been used to obtain mobility. It has been used by people with paralysis to restore functional movement to the extremities, assist in bladder and bowel evacuation, provide respiratory pacing, and counteract some of the secondary complications of paralysis. FES typically applies low-level electrical current to the neuromuscular system. There are two major classifications of FES—functional and therapeutic. Functional applications provide restoration of movement or function. An example is the use of an FES system by a person with paraplegia for standing. Therapeutic applications are aimed at slowing, halting, or reversing the progress of a disabling condition. A therapeutic application of FES is to strengthen muscles weakened from lack of use. FES is used primarily by people with neuromuscular disorders resulting from spinal cord injury, brain injury, or stroke. An FES system generally consists of a control unit, a stimulator unit, and electrodes. The control unit determines the intensity of the electrical stimulus to be applied to the individual through electrodes. The stimulator unit generates the electrical stimulus. Depending on the application, electrodes are either attached to the skin surface, inserted through the skin, or surgically implanted.

The third alternative for restoration of lower-limb locomotion is accomplished through the use of orthoses. People with partial or complete paralysis of the lower extremity require bracing for stability during stance. These individuals are often prescribed knee-ankle-foot orthoses (KAFOs), also known as long leg braces. KAFOs are used to compensate for severe weakness of the lower-limb muscles. Two types of KAFOs are generally prescribed: eccentric (or free) knee joint or locked (or fixed) knee joint. Eccentric knee orthoses are stable in extension as long as the ground reaction force vector passes anterior to the knee hinge axis. The eccentric hinge orthosis design provides limited stance stability and allows flexion and extension at all times. However, the individual must maintain the force vector anterior to the knee hinge axis during stance for stability. The locked KAFO achieves maximum stability through the use of drop locks. These drop locks keep the knee joint locked at all times. This design allows stance-phase stability but does not allow any swing-phase knee flexibility. Surveys show that the rejection rate for long leg braces ranges from 60% to nearly 100% (Kaplan, Grynbaum, Rusk, Anastasia, & Gassler, 1966; Phillips & Zaho, 1993; Rossman & Spira, 1974). People who require KAFOs typically accept braces for a very short period following injury or disease but soon choose to stay in wheelchairs, presumably because walking with locked knees is so energy-inefficient. Cerny, Waters, Hislop, and Perry (1980) showed that walking with KAFOs is more inefficient than wheelchair propulsion in individuals with paraplegia who are dependent on KAFOs to walk, even those who customarily use the orthoses for locomotion. Walking with KAFOs is much less energy efficient than typical walking, whereas values for wheelchair propulsion approximate values for typical walking. These data suggest that wheelchair propulsion is selected as the primary mode of locomotion because walking with two KAFOs is more taxing. Most of the research and development efforts that are aimed at improving impaired gait have been directed at prosthetic systems. This is because design engineers face fewer technical problems in developing a prosthetic limb replacement as compared with the development of an orthotic brace system. The difficulties of an orthotic device include the added weight and volume of the lower extremity, which limit the size and weight of the orthotic device that can be accommodated. Other than the application of modern plastics to orthotic designs, there have been no real changes in the function of conventional long leg braces for decades (Lehnis, 1993).

A new design for a KAFO has been developed (Irby, 1994; Kaufman et al., 1994; Malcolm, Sutherland, Cooper, & Wyatt, 1980). The system is composed of two major parts: mechanical hardware and an electronic control system. The mechanical hardware portion consists of a polypropylene long leg brace design, a mechanical knee flexion restraint mechanism, and a knee release actuator solenoid. To adapt the electromechanical components to a standard orthosis, the medial-side knee hinge struts are left intact and the lateral hinge is removed. Specially fabricated stainless steel brackets connect the clutch mechanism to the lateral thigh and shank struts. The knee-hinge clutch mechanism is a wrap-spring clutch, which is a special class of overrunning clutch, a mechanism that allows torque to be transmitted from one shaft to another in one direction or rotation but not in the other. A solenoid is used to control the clutch. The electronic control system is composed of digital logic integrated circuits. A combinational logic network monitors input data and produces electrical output commands based on the input states. The inputs to the control circuitry are signals generated by strategically located foot contact sensors. Based on the input, the controller algorithm generates an actuation signal that is sent to the solenoid for release of the electromechanical knee joint mechanism during the swing phase of gait.

Dynamic gait analysis has clearly shown improvements in the knee motion pattern while using this new KAFO (Figure 10). When the brace was tested in the locked configuration to simulate a standard locked KAFO, the knee motion did not change during stance or swing. A significant improvement in swing-phase knee flexion was recorded when the brace was switched from the standard knee-locked configuration to free-knee operation. When the free-knee control algorithm was actuated, the knee maintained a stable, locked configuration during stance, yet the knee swing-phase motion pattern obtained was the motion of typical walking.

The energy consumption while using the new KAFO design was compared with conventional bracing (Kaufman, Irby, Mathewson, Wirta, & Sutherland, 1996). Tests were performed on a treadmill at speeds ranging from 15 to 80 meters per minute. At each treadmill speed, oxygen consumption rate increased in a linear manner for both brace-locked and brace-unlocked conditions (Figure 11). The increase in oxygen consumption rate was significant for both the brace-locked ($r^2 = .96$, $p = .001$) and the brace-unlocked ($r^2 = .96$, $p = .001$) conditions on level ground (0% slope). Similar

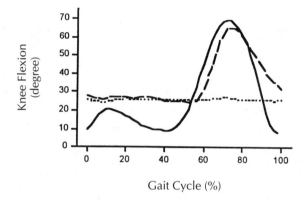

Gait Cycle (%)

Figure 10. Knee motion when walking with stiff-knee gait (i.e., brace locked) and free-knee gait (i.e., brace free). Both bracing conditions provided a locked, stable knee during stance. The brace-locked condition did not allow knee motion during swing, whereas the brace-unlocked condition allowed normal knee swing-phase motion. (——, normal; – – –, brace free; •••, brace locked.) (From Kaufman, K.R., Irby, S.E., Mathewson, J.W., Wirta, R.W., & Sutherland, D.H. [1996]. Energy-efficient knee-ankle-foot orthosis: A case study. *Journal of Prosthetics and Orthotics, 8*[3], 82; reprinted by permission.)

findings were obtained for the 5% slope: The increase in oxygen consumption rate was again significant for the brace-locked $(r^2 = .99, p = .027)$ and brace-unlocked $(r^2 = .98, p = .099)$ conditions. For each slope condition, oxygen consumption rate was always greater for the brace-locked configuration. Comparison of the regression lines at 0% slope revealed that the intercepts were not significantly different $(p > .05)$ but that the slopes of the two lines were not the same $(p < .025)$. Comparison of the regression lines for 5% slope showed that the slopes are parallel $(p < .05)$ but that the lines are not coincident $(p = .07)$. Thus, the brace-unlocked configuration reduced metabolic energy requirements for ambulation. Nevertheless, the energy requirements for the participant were higher than those of individuals without mobility impairments (Figure 11a).

COST

Although costs are relatively easy to determine, the benefits, which encompass social and psychological intangibles such as earning capacity, personal independence, and quality of life, are not easily quantified. Economic data can be quoted but may be too simplistic in nature. Cost–benefit analyses must be undertaken. However, benefits are sometimes economically intangible or must be derived

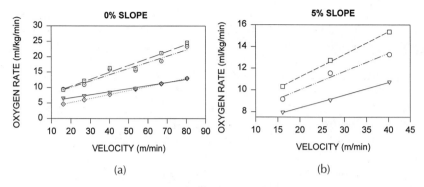

Figure 11.   Oxygen consumption rates. (a) Walking on level ground (0% slope). (▽, normal [Bobbert, 1960]; ◈, normal [Waters, Barnes, Husserl, Silver, & Liss, 1988]; ⊙, unlocked; ⊡, locked.) (b) Walking on a 5% slope. (▽, normal [Bobbert, 1960]; ○, unlocked; □, locked.) Data are presented for stiff-knee gait (i.e., brace locked) and free-knee gait (i.e., brace free). The oxygen consumption rate increased linearly for both conditions. The energy consumption rate increased linearly for both conditions. The energy consumption was significantly less for the brace-free condition. (From Kaufman, K.R., Irby, S.E., Mathewson, J.W., Wirta, R.W., & Sutherland, D.H. [1996]. Energy efficient knee–ankle–foot orthosis: A case study. *Journal of Prosthetics and Orthotics, 8*[3], 82; reprinted by permission.)

from what are typically perceived as noneconomic values. The cost of disability and rehabilitation are strongly related to social structure and a country's level of economic development. Nevertheless, it is difficult to explain a cost differential in a reciprocating gait orthosis (RGO) between two developed countries such as the United States and Australia. It has been documented that an RGO costs $2,270 in Australia (Phillips, Field, Broughton, & Menelaus, 1995). In contrast, the cost of an RGO in the United States is approximately $7,000. It is difficult to understand why there should be a threefold difference in cost for equivalent technology in these two countries. Perhaps at least a portion of it could be explained by the litigious aspects of society in the United States.

The costs of disability can be divided into four areas: 1) personal and domestic costs, 2) service costs, 3) lost surplus production, and 4) other costs to society (Taylor, 1978). The first two categories are the most important. The personal and domestic economic consequences of disability range from loss of earnings suffered by someone unable to work or someone who must accept a low-paying job because of a disability to the effect on family life of having a family member who may not be able to fully perform his or her role. Even disability among children can have significant costs. It has been estimated in France that the average cost for a child with a disability is five times that for a child without a disability (Fourastie, 1977). Service costs are the amount of expenditure for rehabilitation and other care provided to people with physical disabilities. As of 1994, 48.2% of payment for assistive technology came from the family, 34% came from third-party reimbursement, and 17.9% came from a combination of out-of-pocket and third-party reimbursement (U.S. Department of Health and Human Services, 1994). The amount of out-of-pocket expenses increases with age, whereas third-party reimbursement decreases with age (Figure 12). Consideration must be given to the fact that a person with a disability may have lowered economic production capabilities, which may severely limit both access to appropriate AT and that person's potential contribution to society. In the end, the goal should be to add life to years rather than years to life.

SAFETY ISSUES IN ENGINEERING DESIGN

The concept of safety must be discussed because of its complexity and its interaction with risk factors. There is always risk involved in designing products. The issue of how much risk an engineer should allow in designing a product is unresolved. An engineering judgment of product safety is made by calculating the factor of safety. For structural designs, this factor is expressed as Factor of safety = Yield stress/Actual stress. The numerical value is always

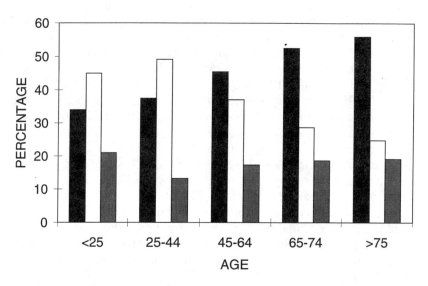

Figure 12.   Source of payment for people using devices or features to assist with impairments. The amount of out-of-pocket expense increases with age, whereas the amount of third-party reimbursement decreases with age. (□, out of pocket; ■, third party; ■, combination.) (*Source:* U.S. Department of Commerce [1994].)

greater than 1 and may range as high as 4 in the worst loaded conditions. In actuality, loads may vary and loading conditions may be encountered that require a large factor of safety. There are not many rules for determining a suitable value for the factor of safety. It is always assumed that engineers will use the latest design tools and techniques and upgrade their technical competence as design practices change over time. Nevertheless, variations and nonuniformity of materials must be considered when determining a reasonable factor of safety.

In general, the term *factor of safety* is meant to include the uncertainties or risks in a design. If the magnitude and direction of various forces are not known, it is difficult to determine a reasonable factor of safety. Factors such as corrosion, lack of lubrication, loading, temperature, and history of use can all affect the life of a component. Knowledge of engineering materials is required when performing engineering design. This knowledge may be obtained from suppliers or from experimental tests of samples. The choice of the factor of safety is related to the amount of time available for engineering and testing. A large factor of safety might be costly if a failure involves only a slight loss of time or inconvenience and might be acceptable. Fatigue testing will raise the cost of a product and may or may not be justified. As stated in the preceding paragraph, there are not many reliable rules for determining the factor of safety. Ultimately, experience accumulated over a long period of time is the best method for choosing the correct factor of safety in engineering design. However, it is certain that if the safety of human life is involved in an engineering design, the factor of safety should definitely have a high value applied to it during the design process.

Although systems should be designed to avoid catastrophic failure, overdesign is wasteful. The reliability of a design should be assessed by using statistical methods to determine the chance of success of the design. Any system will fail under extreme conditions. The reliability of a system can range from 0 (unreliable) to 1 (will never fail). Similarly, values for the factor of safety range from 0 to infinity. Components attached in series will have an overall factor of safety equal to the weakest component in the system. Therefore, the system factor of safety equals the smallest factor of safety of all of the components. For a system with components in parallel, the probability of system failure is a product of the individual components' probabilities of failure. Redundant designs have parallel systems to ensure fail-safe operations. The disadvantage of parallel systems is the added cost for redundancy. In the case where human lives are involved, this system is more costly but may be necessary. Overall, the design goal of minimizing overall cost requires balancing the cost of reliability with repair costs and the consequences of a system failure.

CONCLUSIONS

The goal of the design engineer is to combine creativity, judgment, technical expertise, economic awareness, and analytical abilities to devise a uniquely useful system that serves a valuable purpose for humankind. Rehabilitation engineers provide AT that is helpful to people with disabilities. This chapter has presented an overview of the design process. Specific examples have been given with regard to techniques for assessing paralysis and methods used for restoring function in people with paralysis.

REFERENCES

Abraham, L.D., & Loeb, G.E. (1985). The distal hind limb musculature of the cat (patterns of normal use). *Experimental Brain Research, 58,* 580–593.

Aitkens, S., Lord, J., Bernauer, E., Fowler, W.M., Jr., Lieberman, J.S., & Berck, P. (1989). Relationship of manual muscle testing to objective strength measurements. *Muscle and Nerve, 12,* 173–177.

Amundsen, L.R., & Graves, J.M. (1991). Testing knee extensor muscles of survivors of poliomyelitis. *Journal of Human Muscle Performance, 1,* 25–34.

Andriacchi, T.P., Andersson, G.B.J., & Fermier, R.W. (1980). A study of lower limb mechanics during stair climbing. *Journal of Bone and Joint Surgery, 62A,* 749–757.

Armstrong, L.E., Winant, D.M., Swasey, P.R., Seidle, M.E., Carter, A.L., & Gehlsen, G. (1983). Using isokinetic dynamometry to test ambulatory patients with multiple sclerosis. *Physical Therapy, 63,* 1274–1279.

Barnes, W.S. (1980). The relationship of motor unit activation to isokinetic muscular contraction at different contractile velocities. *Physical Therapy, 16*(9), 1152–1158.

Beasley, W.C. (1956). Influence of method on estimates of normal knee extensor force among normal and post-polio children. *Physical Therapy Review, 36,* 21–41.

Beasley, W.C. (1961). Quantitative muscle testing: Principles and applications to research and clinical services. *Archives of Physical Medicine and Rehabilitation, 42,* 398–425.

Bigland, B., & Lippold, O.C.J. (1954). The relationship between force, velocity, and integrated electrical activity in human muscles. *Journal of Physiology, 123,* 214–224.

Bigland-Ritchie, B., Kukulka, C.G., & Woods, J.J. (1980). Surface e.m.g./ force relation in human muscles of different fibre composition. *Journal of Physiology, 308,* 103–104.

Bobbert, A.C. (1960). Energy expenditure in level and grade walking. *Journal of Applied Physiology, 15*(6), 1015–1021.

Bogey, R.A., Barnes, L.A., & Perry, J. (1992). Computer algorithms to characterize individual subject EMG profiles during gait. *Archives of Physical Medicine and Rehabilitation, 73,* 835–841.

Bogey, R.A., Barnes, L.A., & Perry, J. (1993). A computer algorithm for defining the group electromyographic profile from individual gait profiles. *Archives of Physical Medicine and Rehabilitation, 74,* 286–291.

Bohannon, R.W. (1986). Manual muscle test scores and dynamometer test scores of knee extension strength. *Archives of Physical Medicine and Rehabilitation, 67,* 390–392.

Bohannon, R.W. (1988). Make versus break tests of elbow flexion force using a hand-held dynamometer. *Physical Therapy, 68,* 93–194.

Bohannon, R.W. (1990). Make versus break tests for measuring elbow flexor muscle force with a hand-held dynamometer in patients with stroke. *Physical Therapy Canada, 42,* 247–251.

Bohannon, R.W. (1995). Measurement, nature, and implications of skeletal muscle strength in patients with neurological disorders. *Clinical Biomechanics, 10*(6), 283–292.

Bohannon, R.W., Hull, D., & Palmeri, D. (1994). Muscle strength impairments in gait performance deficits in kidney transplantation candidates. *American Journal of Kidney Disease, 24,* 480–485.

Bouisset, S. (1973). EMG and muscle force in normal muscle activities. In J.E. Desmedt (Ed.), *New developments in EMG and clinical physiology* (pp. 547–583). Basel, Switzerland: Karger.

Burch, G.E., & Sodeman, W.A. (1937). The estimation of the subcutaneous tissue pressure by a direct method. *Journal of Clinical Investigation, 16,* 845–850.

Cerny, K., Waters, R., Hislop, H., & Perry, J. (1980). Walking and wheelchair energetics in persons with paraplegia. *Physical Therapy, 60*(9), 1133–1139.

Crenshaw, A.G., Styf, J.R., & Hargens, A.R. (1992). Intramuscular pressures during exercise: An evaluation of a fiberoptic transducer-tipped catheter system. *European Journal of Applied Physiology, 65,* 178–182.

Crenshaw, A.G., Styf, J.R., Mubarak, S.J., & Hargens, A.R. (1990). A new "transducer tipped" fiber optic catheter for measuring intramuscular pressures. *Journal of Orthopaedic Research, 8,* 464–468.

Csuka, M., & McCarty, D.J. (1985). Simple method for measurement of lower extremity muscle strength. *American Journal of Medicine, 78,* 77–81.

Daniels, L., & Worthingham, C. (1980). *Muscle testing technique of manual examination* (4th ed.). Philadelphia: W.B. Saunders.

Dempster, W.T., & Finerty, J.C. (1947). Relative activity of wrist moving muscles in static support of the wrist joint: An electromyographic study. *American Journal of Physiology, 150,* 596–606.

deVries, H.A. (1968). "Efficiency of electrical activity" as a physiological measure of the functional state of muscle tissue. *American Journal of Physical Medicine, 47,* 10–22.

Fourastie, J. (1977). *Rehabilitation for the disabled.* New York: United Nations.

Fowler, W.M., & Gardner, G.W. (1967). Quantitative strength measurements in muscular dystrophy. *Archives of Physical Medicine and Rehabilitation, 48,* 629–644.

Gregor, R.J., Roy, R.R., Whiting, W.C., Lovely, R.G., Hodgson, J.A., & Edgerton, V.R. (1988). Force-velocity potentiation in cat soleus muscle during treadmill locomotion. *Journal of Biomechanics, 21,* 721–732.

Guralnik, J.M., Simonsick, E.M., Ferrucci, L., Glynn, R.J., Berkman, L.F., Blazer, D.G., Scherr, P.A., & Wallace, R.B. (1994). A short physical performance battery assessing lower extremity function: Association with self reported disability and prediction of mortality and nursing home admission. *Journal of Gerontology, 49M,* 85–94.

Haffajee, D., Maritz, U., & Sauntesson, G. (1972). Isometric knee extension strength as a function of joint angle, muscle length and motor unit activity. *Acta Orthopaedica Scandinavica, 43,* 138–147.

Hatze, H. (1978). A general myocybernetic control model of skeletal muscle. *Biocybernetics, 28,* 143–157.

Hill, P.H. (1970). *The science of engineering design.* New York: Holt, Rinehart & Winston.

Hinson, M.M., & Rosentswieg, J. (1973). Comparative electromyographic values of isometric, isotonic, and isokinetic contraction. *Research Quarterly, 44*(1), 71–78.

Hodgson, J.A. (1983). The relationship between soleus and gastrocnemius muscle activity in conscious cats: A model for motor unit recruitment. *Journal of Physiology, 337,* 553–562.

Hof, A.L., & Vandenberg, J.W. (1977). Linearity between the weighted sum of the EMG's of the human triceps surae and the total torque. *Journal of Biomechanics, 10,* 529–539.

Inman, V.T., Ralston, H.J., Saunders, J.B., Feinstein, B., & Wright, E.W., Jr. (1952). Relationship of human electromyogram to muscle tension. *Electroencephalography and Clinical Neurophysiology, 4,* 187–194.

Irby, S.E. (1994). *A digital logic controlled electromechanical free-knee brace.* Master's thesis, San Diego State University, San Diego, CA.

Kaplan, L.K., Grynbaum, B.B., Rusk, H.A., Anastasia, T., & Gassler, S. (1966). A reappraisal of braces and other mechanical aids in patients with spinal cord dysfunction: Results of a follow-up study. *Archives of Physical Medicine and Rehabilitation, 47,* 393–405.

Kaufman, K.R., Irby, S.E., Mathewson, J.W., Wirta, R.W., & Sutherland, D.H. (1996). Energy efficient knee-ankle-foot orthosis: A case study. *Journal of Prosthetics and Orthotics, 8*(3), 79–85.

Kaufman, K.R., Irby, S.E., Wirta, R.W., Ussell, D., Mathewson, J.W., & Sutherland, D.H. (1994). Knee–ankle–foot orthosis for free knee gait. In L. Blankevoort & J.G.M. Kooloos (Eds.), *Proceedings of the Second World Congress of Biomechanics* (Vol. I, p. 280). Nijmegen, the Netherlands: Stichting.

Kaufman, K.R., & Sutherland, D.H. (1995). Dynamic intramuscular pressure measurement during gait. *Operative Techniques in Sports Medicine, 3*(4), 250–255.

Kendall, F.P., & McCreary, E.K. (1983). *Muscles: Testing and function* (3rd ed.). Baltimore: Williams & Wilkins.

Komi, P.V. (1973). Relationship between muscle tension, EMG, and velocity of contraction under concentric and eccentric work. In J.E. Desmet (Ed.), *New developments in clinical neurophysiology* (pp. 596–606). Basel, Switzerland: Karger.

Komi, P.V. (1990). Relevance of in vivo force measurements to human biomechanics. *Journal of Biomechanics, 23*(1), 23–34.

Komi, P.V., & Buskirk, E.R. (1972). Effect of eccentric and concentric conditioning on tension and electrical activity of human muscle. *Ergonomics, 15*, 417–434.

Komi, P.V., & Rusko, H. (1974). Quantitative evaluation of mechanical and electrical changes during fatigue loadings of eccentric and concentric work. *Scandinavian Journal of Rehabilitation Medicine, 3*(Suppl.), 121–126.

Komi, P.V., Salonen, M., Jarvinen, M., & Kokko, O. (1987). In vivo registration of Achilles tendon forces in man: II. Methodological development. *International Journal of Sports Medicine, 8*, 3–8.

Landerer, A.S. (1884). *Die Gewebesspannung in ihrem Einfluss auf die ortlich Blut-und-Lymphbewegung [Tissue contraction and its influence on local blood and lymph flow]*. Leipzig, Germany: Vogel.

Lehnis, H.R. (1993). Orthotics: The state of the art. *Journal of Rehabilitation Research and Development, 30*(4), vii–viii.

Lieber, R.L., & Boakes, J.L. (1988). Sarcomere length and joint kinematics during torque production in the frog hindlimb. *American Journal of Physiology, 254*, C759–C768.

Lippold, O., Redfearn, J., & Vuco, J. (1970). Electromyography of fatigue. *Ergonomics, 3*, 121–131.

Lippold, O.C.J. (1952). The relation between integrated action potentials in a human muscle and its isometric tension. *Journal of Physiology, 117*, 492–499.

Lovely, R.J., Gregor, R.J., Roy, R.R., & Edgerton, V.R. (1990). Weight-bearing hind limb stepping in treadmill exercised cats. *Brain Research, 514*, 206–218.

Lovett, R.W. (1917). *The treatment of infantile paralysis* (2nd ed.). Philadelphia: Blakiston's Son & Co.

Lunnen, J.D., Yack, J., & Le Veau, B.F. (1981). Relationship between muscle length, muscle activity, and torque of the hamstrings. *Physical Therapy, 61*(2), 190–195.

Malcolm, L.L., Sutherland, D.H., Cooper, L., & Wyatt, M. (1980). A digital logic-controlled electromechanical orthosis for free-knee gait in muscular dystrophy children. *Orthopaedic Transactions, 5*, 90.

Maton, B., & Bouisset, S. (1977). The distribution of activity among the muscles of a single group during isometric contraction. *European Journal of Applied Physiology, 37*, 101–109.

Matsen, F.A., Mayo, K.A., Sheridan, G.W., & Krugmire, R.B., Jr. (1976). Monitoring of intramuscular pressure. *Surgery, 79*, 702–709.

Mattsson, E., & Broström, L. (1990). The increase in energy cost of walking with an immobilized knee or an unstable ankle. *Scandinavian Journal of Rehabilitation Medicine, 22*, 51–53.

Messier, R.H., Duffy, J., Litchman, H.M., Paslay, P.R., Soechting, J.F., & Stewart, P.A. (1971). The electromyogram as a measure of tension in human biceps and triceps muscles. *International Journal of Mechanical Science, 13*, 585–598.

Metral, S., & Cassar, G. (1981). Relationship between force and integrated EMG activity during voluntary isometric anisotonic contraction. *European Journal of Applied Physiology, 46*, 185–198.

Milner-Brown, H.S., & Stein, R.B. (1975). The relationship between surface electromyogram and muscle force. *Journal of Physiology, 246*, 549–569.

Moritani, T., & deVries, H.A. (1978). Reexamination of the relationship between the surface integrated electromyogram (EMG) and force of isometric contraction. *American Journal of Physical Medicine, 57*, 263–277.

Mubarak, S.J., Hargens, A.R., Owen, C.A., Garetto, L.P., & Akeson, W.H. (1976). The wick catheter technique for measurement of intramuscular pressure: A new research and clinical tool. *Journal of Bone and Joint Surgery, 58A*(7), 1016–1020.

Olgiati, R., Burgunder, J.-M., & Mumenthaler, M. (1988). Increased energy cost of locking in multiple sclerosis: Effect of spasticity, ataxia, and weakness. *Archives of Physical Medicine and Rehabilitation, 69*, 846–849.

Osternig, L.R. (1975). Optimal isokinetic loads in velocities producing muscular power in human subjects. *Archives of Physical Medicine and Rehabilitation, 56*, 152–155.

Osternig, L.R., Hamill, J., Corros, D.M., & Lander, J. (1984). Electromyographic patterns accompanying isokinetic exercise under varying speed and sequencing conditions. *American Journal of Physical Medicine, 65*(6), 289–297.

Parker, P.A., Körner, L., & Kadefors, R. (1984). Estimation of muscle force from intramuscular pressure. *Medical and Biological Engineering and Computing, 22*, 453–457.

Perry, J. (1967). The mechanics of walking: A clinical interpretation. In J. Perry & H.J. Hislop (Eds.), *Principals of lower extremity bracing* (pp. 9–32). Washington, DC: American Physical Therapy Association.

Perry, J. (1992). *Gait analysis: Normal and pathological function* (pp. 381–411). Thorofare, NJ: Slack.

Perry, J., Ireland, M.L., Gronley, J., & Haffer, M.M. (1986). Predictive value of manual muscle testing and gait analysis in normal ankles by dynamic electromyography. *Foot and Ankle, 6*(5), 254–259.

Phillips, B., & Zaho, H. (1993). Predictors of assistive technology abandonment. *Assistive Technology, 5*, 36–45.

Phillips, D.L., Field, R.E., Broughton, N.S., & Menelaus, M.B. (1995). Reciprocating orthoses for children with myelomeningocele: A comparison of two types. *Journal of Bone and Joint Surgery, 77B*(1), 110–113.

Rorabeck, C.H., Castle, G.S.P., Hardie, R., & Logan, J. (1981). Compartmental pressure measurements: An experimental investigation using the slit catheter. *Journal of Trauma, 21*, 446–449.

Rosentswieg, J., & Hinson, M.M. (1972). Comparison of isometric, isotonic, and isokinetic exercises by electromyography. *Archives of Physical Medicine and Rehabilitation, 68*, 249–252.

Rossman, M., & Spira, E. (1974). Paraplegic use of locking braces: A survey. *Archives of Physical Medicine and Rehabilitation, 55*, 310–314.

Rothstein, J.M., De Litto, A., Sinacore, D.R., & Rose, S.J. (1983). Electromyographic, peak torque, and power relationships during isokinetic movement. *Physical Therapy, 63*(6), 926–933.

Schwartz, S., Cohen, M.E., Herbison, G.J., & Shah, A. (1992). Relationship between two measures of upper extremity strength: Manual muscle test. *Archives of Physical Medicine and Rehabilitation, 73*, 1063–1068.

Seliger, V., Dolejs, L., & Karas, V. (1980). A dynamometric comparison of maximum eccentric, concentric, and isometric conditions using EMG and energy expenditure measurements. *European Journal of Applied Physiology, 45*, 235–244.

Sharrad, W.J.N. (1953). Correlations between the changes in the spinal cord and muscular paralysis in poliomyelitis. *Proceedings of the Royal Society of London, 40,* 346.

Smidt, G.L. (1973). Biomechanical analysis of knee flexion and extension. *Journal of Biomechanics, 6,* 79–92.

Snashall, P.D., Lucas, J., Guz, A., & Floyer, M.A. (1971). Measurement of interstitial "fluid" pressure by means of a cotton wick in man and animals: An analysis of the origin of the pressure. *Clinical Science, 41,* 35–53.

Styf, J.R., Crenshaw, A.G., & Hargens, J.R. (1989). Intramuscular pressures during exercise: Comparison of measurements with and without infusion. *Acta Orthopaedica Scandinavica, 60,* 593–596.

Sunderland, A., Tinson, D., & Bradley, L. (1989). Arm function after stroke: An evaluation of grip strength as a measure of recovery and a prognostic indicator. *Journal of Neurology, Neurosurgery and Psychiatry, 752,* 1267–1272.

Taylor, D.G. (1978). The economics of rehabilitation. In R.M. Kenedi, J.P. Paul, & J. Hughes (Eds.), *Disability* (pp. 87–100). Baltimore: University Park Press.

Tripp, E.J., & Harris, S.R. (1991). Test–retest reliability of isokinetic knee extension and flexion torque measurements in persons with spastic hemiparesis. *Physical Therapy, 71,* 390–396.

U.S. Department of Commerce. (1994). Persons using devices and or features to assist with impairments, by age: 1990. In *Statistical abstract of the United States* (Table 217). Washington, DC: Author.

U.S. Department of Health and Human Services. (1994). Number of selected reported chronic conditions, by age: United States, 1993. *Vital and Health Statistics, Series 10: Data from the National Health Survey, 190,* 94.

Vandervoort, A.A., Kramer, J.F., & Wharram, E.R. (1990). Eccentric knee strength of elderly females. *Journal of Gerontology, 45*(4), 125–128.

Wakim, K.G., Gersten, J.W., Elkins, E.C., & Martin, G.M. (1950). Objective recording of muscle strength. *Archives of Physical Medicine and Rehabilitation, 31,* 90–100.

Walmsley, B., Hodgson, J.A., & Burke, R.E. (1978). Forces produced by medial gastrocnemius and soleus muscles during locomotion in freely moving cats. *Journal of Neurology, 41,* 1203–1216.

Waters, R.L., Barnes, G., Husserl, T., Silver, L., & Liss, R. (1988). Comparable energy expenditure after arthrodesis of the hip and ankle. *Journal of Bone and Joint Surgery, 70A,* 1032–1037.

Waters, R.L., Campbell, J., Thomas, L., Hugos, L., & Davis, P. (1982). Energy cost of walking in lower extremity plaster casts. *Journal of Bone and Joint Surgery, 64A,* 896–899.

Whiting, W.C., Gregor, R.J., Roy, R.R., & Edgerton, V.R. (1984). A technique for estimating mechanical work of individual muscles in the cat during treadmill locomotion. *Journal of Biomechanics, 17,* 685–694.

Wickholm, J.B., & Bohannon, R.W. (1991). Hand-held dynamometer measurements: Tester strength makes a difference. *Journal of Orthopaedic Sports Physical Therapy, 13,* 191–198.

Woods, J.J., & Bigland-Ritchie, B. (1983). Linear and non-linear surface EMG/force relationships in human muscles. *American Journal of Physical Medicine, 62*(6), 287–299.

Wrentenberg, P., Lindberg, F., & Arborelius, U.P. (1993). Effects of arm rests and different ways of using them on hip and knee load during rising. *Clinical Biomechanics, 8,* 95–101.

Zuniga, E.N., & Simons, D.G. (1969). Nonlinear relationship between averaged electromyogram potential and muscle tension in normal subjects. *Archives of Physical Medicine and Rehabilitation, 50,* 613–620.

CHAPTER 12

Enhancing Human Movement in the 21st Century

Internal to External Dimension

P. Hunter Peckham

Control of human movements takes place both internally and externally. One must be able to exercise regulation of internal body system functions to retain even a modest level of independence in life. Equally important for a self-directed life is the command of the body as it moves through the external environment. People with movement disabilities rely on technology to provide some measure of control over their lost functional capacities. For those with severe physical disabilities, the quality of life and the degree to which they can live independently are directly related to the assistive technology (AT) that is available to them. Fundamental to the concept of AT is the dimension of use or implementation. The *internal dimension* is defined as technology that directly interfaces with the individual's neuromusculoskeletal system to restore control over a variety of body functions. Internal dimension AT includes neurostimulation of end organs and muscles (i.e., functional neuromuscular stimulation or functional electrical stimulation), surgical reconstruction, and neural control interfaces. Assistive devices that are external to the individual's body are termed *external dimension devices*. They are devices that are in contact with the person's body that are used to augment the individual's ability to perform tasks. Examples of these devices are orthoses (e.g., ankle braces, hand splints), wheelchair interfaces (e.g., sip and puff, toggle, joystick control of electric wheelchairs), and environmental controls (e.g., remote control of van doors, garage doors, and audio equipment). This chapter postulates that

1. Assistive technology can have a major impact on increasing independence and quality of life of people with physical disabilities.
2. Devices that restore the individual's body functions reduce the need for environmental modifications.
3. Internal dimension devices provide more flexibility in the individual's attainment of independence.
4. Neural activation provides an approach to restoring function that is unavailable by other means.

In addition, the premise is set forth that assistive devices that restore internally mediated function *complement* those that modify the environment. Clearly, both approaches are necessary to maximize the independence of individuals with severe paralysis.

NEUROPROSTHESES

The development of a new generation of neuroprostheses has played an important role in efforts to improve the lives of people with disabilities. Neuroprostheses are internally located devices that control body functions through the electrical stimulation of muscles or organs that are dysfunctional as a result of injury or disease. Control over at least five basic life activities (breathing, eating, defecating, urinating, and moving) is lost or substantially reduced following traumatic injury to the spinal cord. Neuroprostheses that restore or improve these functions can dramatically change the lives of people with spinal cord injury (SCI). Implanted neuroprostheses for controlling breathing and urinating have been in clinical use since the mid-1980s (Creasey & van Kerrebroeck, 1996; Creasey et al., 1996). New neuroprostheses for regulating eating have received Food and Drug Administration approval, and those for regulating defecating are presently in clinical trials. One system for improving personal mobility (stepping) uses surface electrodes to deliver stimulation. This device has completed clinical trials. Other mobility-enhancing neuroprostheses that use implanted devices remain in an earlier stage of clinical research. Each of these neuroprostheses has been demonstrated to provide individuals with paralysis the capacity to improve their performance. A worldwide survey conducted by Creasey (see Peckham et al., 1996) revealed that approximately 3,000 implantable neuroprostheses for these previously mentioned functions as well as for other functions have been deployed and are used. Each of these neuroprostheses has had a remarkable impact on the lives of people with severe physical disabilities. The vast majority of these systems are reported to function acceptably for many years with minimal failures and have reached a level of clinical acceptance by practitioners and consumers.

Two examples of internally located assistive devices (neuroprostheses) are provided to give the reader a clear idea of how these somewhat complex devices improve and restore function. One enables the individual with paralyzed upper limbs to open and close his or her hand to provide grasp-and-release functions, and the second provides control of micturition, enabling the individual to control urination upon activation of the urinary system. The first was developed in the MetroHealth Medical Center laboratories in Cleveland, Ohio (Kilgore et al., 1997; Peckham & Keith, 1992), and the second in the laboratories of the Neuroprosthesis Unit of Professor Giles Brindley in London (Brindley, 1990; Brindley, Polkey, Rushton, & Cardozo, 1986).

DESCRIPTION AND IMPLEMENTATION OF TWO NEUROPROSTHESES

Neuroprosthesis for Restoration of Grasp and Release

The neuroprosthesis for restoration of hand function provides both opening and closing of the hand in response to command signals provided by the user. Two hand configurations are provided with the neuroprosthetic grasp. In lateral prehension, the thumb develops force against the side (lateral aspect) of the user's index finger. This key grip is used to grasp small objects. In the second configuration, palmar prehension, the thumb comes into contact with the index and long fingers. This grasp is often called the *three-jaw pinch* and is used to grasp larger objects.

The grasp neuroprosthesis consists of internally implanted and externally worn electrical components. The implanted components are the receiver-stimulator, leads, connectors, and electrodes. The external components are the control sensor, an external control unit (ECU), and a transmitting coil. A detailed description of the system can be found elsewhere (Scott, Peckham, & Keith, 1995). Operation of the neuroprosthetic grasp is as follows. The user wears the control sensor on a part of his or her body that retains voluntary control. Voluntary movements generated by the user's contralateral (i.e., opposite side) shoulder or the ipsilateral (i.e., same side) wrist are sensed by the control sensor and fed to the ECU. Then they are translated into command signals by the ECU and are telemetered to the implanted receiver. The ECU is uniquely tailored to the individual user's capabilities during a training period that establishes stimulation and control levels. The user has a switch that enables him or her to select the type of grasp (key grip or three-jaw pinch) and to lock the hand in position for activities such as eating or writing. The motion of the stimulated hand muscles is coordinated into the desired patterns of movement by voluntary movements of the shoulder, which can be graded proportionally by the command sensor. Thus, a gradual hand movement or a fast hand movement is possible by the rate at which the user changes the command movement (i.e., shoulder movement).

Attaining skilled use of this neuroprosthesis for improved grip is a process that takes place over several months, mostly outside of the hospital. This process includes preoperation muscle strengthening, device implantation, muscle stimulation trials for system programming, user training, and use in home and office settings. An individual who is a candidate for the grasp neuroprothesis generally has atrophied muscles as a result of his or her paralysis. A 4- to 6-week period of stimulation using surface electrodes is used to build muscle strength and fatigue resistance. Often tendon transfers are made to enhance functional movement of the fingers.

Surgical implantation of the device is then performed. Incisions are made over each of the muscles to be implanted, the proper point is selected for each muscle, and the electrode is sutured into place. Leads are then tunneled beneath the skin to an incision on the mid-upper arm. The receiver is placed on the chest wall and the leads are passed subcutaneously to the mid-humeral incision. The leads are joined at the mid-lead connector. The receiver detects command signals generated by the voluntary muscle movements of the shoulder as processed by the ECU. These signals control the stimulation of electrodes that have been attached to the appropriate muscle of the hand and forearm for the purpose of causing finger and thumb (and sometimes wrist) movements. The muscle stimulator has eight channels. Seven are used for creating movement; the eighth is placed near the clavicle to produce an electrocutaneous (i.e., sensory) feedback to the user. As noted, tendon transfers can often augment function by adding wrist or elbow extension through providing more uniform movements and can augment function lost because of weak musculature (Keith et al., 1996).

Electrical stimulation of the finger, thumb, and wrist muscles begins after a healing period that may take 3–6 weeks. The muscles are stimulated to ascertain proper stimulus parameters for flexion and extension. Exercise patterns for these muscles are programmed by therapists in the clinic setting. After adequate strengthening (generally requiring 4–6 weeks), programming and training of grasp for daily activities is begun and lasts for a 3-week period. Data collection on grasp reacquisition was the focus of a multicenter clinical trial. These training procedures and the multicenter clinical trial were initiated in the MetroHealth Medical Center and subsequently transferred to NeuroControl Corporation (Cleveland, Ohio) for distribution.

To understand how effective these grasp neuroprostheses are, one need only consider some of the dimensions in which an individual must have grasp functionality in order to be independent. At home, gripping abilities are critical in self-care involving grooming (e.g., washing, brushing teeth, shaving) and bladder and bowel management (e.g., attaching external urinary catheter, inserting suppositories). The ability to prepare food includes such grasp-dependent actions as removing objects from a refrigerator, cooking foods, and presenting the food on the table for eating. Work tasks (e.g., data and text entry, writing, answering telephones) are enhanced by a neuroprosthetic grasp. Hobbies and recreational activities (e.g., playing cards, board games, and pool; creative painting, sculpting, needlepoint, and music; remote control operation of telephone, television, and audio equipment) are aided by the use of a neuroprosthetic grasp.

Neuroprosthesis for Restoration of Bladder Control

Control of the urinary system is one of the most fundamental needs of an individual who has sustained an SCI. The bladder must provide a means of both storing and voiding urine. These are both lost with an SCI. Retaining urine in the bladder for even relatively short periods dramatically increases the chances of infection and kidney damage. Prior to the advent of powerful antibiotics in the 1980s, urinary tract infections (UTIs) were a leading cause of death for those with SCI. Discharge of urine without adequate means of capturing the fluid results in embarrassment for the individual as well as increased risk for skin breakdown. The current solution to the problem of urine collection and storage is the use of external collection devices. This solution necessitates connection of either an indwelling catheter or an external condom device by a tube to a urine collection bag. These devices are another source of UTIs. Although pharmaceutical treatment has reduced mortality, the frequency of

UTIs in individuals with SCI remains high, resulting in lost work days, high medical costs, and many periods of time filled with pain and depression.

The Brindley-Finetech system (Brindley, 1990; Brindley, Polkey, Rushton, & Cardozo, 1986) is a neuroprosthetic solution to the control of urine storage and release. It was designed to address these problems by providing controlled voiding through electrical stimulation of the bladder. In concept, the overall system resembles the neuroprosthetic grasp system. The Brindley-Finetech system consists of implanted and external components; the implanted components are the receiver, leads, and electrodes, and the external components consist of the ECU and transmitting coil.

In operation, the user places the transmitting coils (there are three joined together, as opposed to one in the neuroprosthetic grasp system) over the receiver and presses a switch on the external controller to begin the stimulation. Stimulation is generated for approximately 3 seconds, during which time the pressure in the bladder builds and the external urinary sphincter contracts, holding urine in the bladder. Upon cessation of the 3-second stimulation, the urinary sphincter relaxes and the increased bladder pressure causes voiding to occur. Repeating this sequence allows almost complete voiding of the bladder. This is critically important because eliminating urine from the bladder decreases the possibility of bladder infections and kidney stones. The Brindley-Finetech system allows the user to be free of a catheter and external collection system.

Operation of the bladder neuroprosthesis requires a surgical procedure for placement of the electrodes and the receiver. This is accomplished by surgical removal of a portion of spinal bones (laminectomy) to gain access to the spinal cord. The electrodes are placed intradurally on the ventral roots, although extradural stimulation has been used. An additional procedure that is often combined with the electrode implantation is transection of the posterior roots to improve bladder capacity and reduce reflex-induced voiding. Surgery is completed in a single procedure. The bladder neuroprothesis is adjusted for the individual's needs during the several days following the operation while the person is in the hospital. When the person leaves the hospital, he or she has control of the bladder.

IMPACT OF NEUROPROSTHESES ON THE USER

Clearly, neuroprostheses can restore functions that are lost following central nervous system injury. In fact, no known alternative approach has been demonstrated that can achieve such dramatic functional restorations for the individual with paralysis. Neuroprostheses enable individuals freedom to achieve their goals without focusing on lost functions. The use of neuroprostheses can lessen the need for attendant care and reduce medical complications that occur secondary to the disability. The individual can improve independent performance in personal hygiene, mobility challenges, work tasks, and recreational activities. Participating in these activities with the greatest amount of independence can be accomplished through the use of neuroprostheses. Attaining independence involves not only the ability to perform each of the individual activities that one desires but also being able to move fluidly from one task to another with minimal assistance. Effective intervention with AT requires the use of a few devices with great versatility in restoring functions. It is in this capacity that neuroprostheses demonstrate their greatest utility. For example, after donning the neuroprosthetic grasp, the individual user gains the ability to perform a wide variety of functions without having to use other assistive aids or ask for assistance from attendants or family members. With the neuroprosthetic grasp, one may independently pick up a telephone, talk privately, and replace the receiver; pick up a pen, write a letter, and place a letter in an envelope; and brush his or her teeth, shave, and dress.

A user satisfaction survey is one of the tools being used to assess the results of the hand neuroprosthesis in the multicenter clinical trial. The data are extremely supportive of the enhancement in function provided to the user by the neuroprosthetic grasp system. The following results were tabulated from 22 people who received the implant and who were surveyed at least 6 months after they had had the system in use outside the rehabilitation facility. Eighteen indicated they would have the system implanted again, two were neutral, and two were negative. Seventeen reported that they benefited from the system, four were neutral, and one was negative. Eighteen reported that the system met their expectations, two were neutral, and two were negative. Nineteen indicated that the system made a positive impact on their life, and three were neutral. Nineteen found the system to be reliable, two were neutral, and one was negative. Twenty were satisfied with their hand function, one was neutral, and one was negative. By nearly similar results, these individuals reported they were more confident in performing activities with their hand with the system on, that they performed activities more "normally," that activities were easier to perform, that they performed more activities, and that the quality of their lives had improved with the hand system. These results suggest the very positive impact that the neuroprosthetic grasp has on the life of a person with upper-extremity paralysis. This neuroprosthesis provides a functional restoration for its users that generally meets their expectations in enabling them to more fully achieve their individual goals.

The impact on the individual who uses a neuroprosthesis is realized across the domains of impairment, functional limitation, disability, and societal limitations. These domains were defined by the National Center for Medical Rehabilitation Research (1993) as the principal domains across which the individual must have restored function. Although the neuroprosthesis does not affect the impairment itself, it provides the individual with the ability to use the remaining neuromuscular system. For users of the hand grasp neuroprosthesis, the result is a reduction in impairment through the ability to grasp and release. This allows the user to develop strength that enables him or her to pick up, hold, manipulate, and use objects. As a result, the individual's functional limitation is reduced. Users' abilities to perform tasks independently increases because they can utilize unmodified objects to accomplish their intended function. This reduces or eliminates their disability. Subsequently, individuals' societal limitations are reduced because they are able to accomplish their own objectives with a reduction in assistance and attendant care.

Similarly, using the urinary control neuroprosthesis allows people with SCI to control bladder voiding. This lessens their dependence on artificial collection systems and reduces the frequency of UTIs. The individual has freedom from concern over accidental voiding and the personal embarrassment associated with such an event. The reduced time spent in inserting indwelling catheters, attaching external catheters, and changing clothing after accidental voiding improves the quality of the lives of people who use urinary control neuroprostheses.

However, there remain many obstacles to overcome in the deployment of neuroprostheses. The time and cost to develop and deploy a neuroprosthesis are considerable. The government regulatory review is extensive (Peckham et al., 1996), approaching that of a new drug from concept to delivery (Young, 1995). The cost of the technology must be balanced by the improvement in function and quality that can be realized. Most important, the neuroprosthesis must achieve acceptance by the consumer (i.e., the person with the disability), the deployer (i.e., the clinician), and the third-party payer. Third-party payment agencies, both private and governmental, must cost-average various rehabilitative options for more than the 1–5 years currently used to establish reimbursement for AT. For example, although a neuroprosthesis for bowel and bladder control may cost $25,000 or more for initial installation and have a modest annual support cost, the reduction in cost of attendant care (ranging from $6,200 to $9,100 annually) would easily be offset if cost accounting were done on a 10-year basis. This type of economic analysis provides a rationale for payment for neuroprostheses as well as a market for the development and purchase of such devices. The problem of transferring the responsibility for rehabilitation from the health industry to a general fund for enabling people with severe physical disabilities to become fully participatory in our society must be addressed. Some portion of AT must surely fall within the purview of making human capital investment for long-term social benefits, both moral and economic.

CONCLUSIONS

Internally implanted assistive technology provides a functionally desirable, cosmetically acceptable, and economically feasible approach to providing control over life functions for individuals with severe disabilities. However, the use of internal AT must not be considered as excluding the need to use external technology. External technology is essential for wheeled mobility and personal transport for people with mobility impairments. Adaptations for a user-friendly environment must not be excluded in consideration of the needs of the individual. Both internal and external AT is needed to restore function to people with disabilities. As clinical successes of neuroprostheses increase, the demand for them from users and clinicians will grow. Although the advantages that the neuroprosthetic approach can offer appear obvious, the approach is in its infancy in the mid-1990s, with truly first-generation devices just reaching clinical implementation in the most advanced treatment centers. The future appears bright for those individuals with severe disabilities who benefit from the advancement provided by neuroprostheses. For development and deployment of neuroprostheses to continue, economic support must be found to allow a broader clinical utilization of these devices for all whose lives could be improved with their use.

REFERENCES

Brindley, G.S. (1990). Treatment of urinary and faecal incontinence by surgically implanted devices. *Ciba Foundation Symposium, 151,* 267–274.

Brindley, G.S., Polkey, C.E., Rushton, D.N., & Cardozo, L. (1986). Sacral anterior root stimulators for bladder control in paraplegia: The first 50 cases. *Journal of Neurology, Neurosurgery, and Psychiatry, 49,* 1104–1114.

Creasey, G.H., Elefteriades, J., DiMarco, A., Talonen, P., Bijak, M., Girsch, W., & Kantor, C. (1996). Electrical stimulation to restore respiration. *Journal of Rehabilitation Research and Development, 33*(2), 123–132.

Creasey, G.H., & van Kerrebroeck, P.E.V. (1996). Neuroprostheses for control of micturition. *Journal of Rehabilitation Research and Development, 33*(2), 188–191.

Keith, M.W., Kilgore, K.L., Peckham, P.H., Wuolle, K.S., Creasey, G., & Lemay, M. (1996). Tendon transfers and functional electrical stimulation for reconstruction of hand function in spinal cord injury. *Journal of Hand Surgery, American Volume, 21,* 89–99.

Kilgore, K.L., Peckham, P.H., Keith, M.W., Thrope, G.B., Wuolle, K.S., Bryden, A.S., & Hart, R.L. (1997). An implanted upper-extremity neuroprosthesis: A five patient review. *Journal of Bone and Joint Surgery, 79A*(4), 533–541.

National Center for Medical Rehabilitation Research. (1993). *Research plan for the National Center for Medical Rehabilitation Research* (NIH Publication No. 93-3509). Bethesda, MD: National Institutes of Health.

Peckham, P.H., & Keith, M.W. (1992). Motor prosthesis for restoration of upper extremity function. In R.M. Stein, P.H. Peckham, & D. Popovic (Eds.), *Neural prosthesis: Replacing motor function after disease or disability* (pp. 162–187). New York: Oxford University Press.

Peckham, P.H., Thrope, G., Woloszko, J., Habasevich, R., Scherer, M., & Kantor, C. (1996). Technology transfer of neuroprosthetic devices. *Journal of Rehabilitation Research and Development, 33,* 173–183.

Scott, T.R., Peckham, P.H., & Keith, M.W. (1995). Upper extremity neuroprostheses utilising functional electrical stimulation. In D.N. Rushton & G.S. Brindley (Eds.), *Neuroprostheses* (pp. 57–75). London: Bailliere Tindall.

Young, W. (1995). Bench-to-bedside lag time: A major problem for SCI. *Paraplegia News, 49*(3), 64–68.

CHAPTER 13

Problem Solving Through Rehabilitation Engineering

Peter W. Axelson

People's lives may be totally out of balance because of an injury or a disease that has resulted in a permanent impairment. This loss of equilibrium may occur because they are required to focus on new methods, techniques, or actions to perform activities that, prior to the impairment, were performed with little effort and no advance preparation. Three dimensions of life can be used to provide a framework for analyzing problems associated with establishing a balance in life after an injury or a disease. Some solutions are found in altering the biology of the person. Others may be discovered within the person's psychological capacity to adjust. Many solutions come from the use of assistive technology (AT) and the modification of the physical environment. The first dimension, experiential, involves areas of daily living, work activities, and leisure and recreational activities. The second dimension addresses the balance among physical, intellectual, and spiritual activities. The third dimension is sociological, which considers the balance between dependence and independence (Axelson, 1983).

The *experiential* dimension involves independent living skills and those assistive devices that enhance the performance of people with disabilities in every part of their daily life activities, including dressing, eating, performing personal hygiene tasks, and moving within their habitat. In the vocational environment, this involves whatever technology is necessary to allow people to continue the kind of work they prefer, whether it is farming or computer-aided design work. The recreational portion of this dimension embodies technology needed to enable people to continue enjoying leisure activities with family and friends.

The second dimension embraces technology that allows the person with a disability a chance to attain *balance among physical, intellectual, and spiritual activities*. After injury, people need to continue exercising and being physical. Even with very high-level spinal cord injuries (SCIs), people still need to be physical to the maximum degree possible. Finding the right balance between physical and intellectual activities involves continuing to use parts of the body and mind that are important to the person with a disability. Designing assistive devices that provide these opportunities is a challenge for rehabilitation engineers. Focusing technology solely on one or the other component of this dimension may not give the individual with a disability an opportunity to regain a sense of personal balance. Everyone's balance points and priorities are different. Some people aspire to be professional athletes who compete in wheelchair races. They need technology that gives them the fastest wheelchairs possible. Others want to continue with their research. They need specific devices that give them access to scientific journals, the capacity to perform laboratory tests, and admittance to the tools of their science. This dimension also includes spiritual activity, however one chooses to define it. For some people, the need might be for an all-terrain vehicle to go for a walk on the beach or through the woods on a trail alone. For others, the need might be a page turner to enable them to reflect on their favorite prose. The importance of providing diversity in AT is that the choice of assistive devices allows people with disabilities to continue their lives in a balanced, meaningful way.

The third dimension, the *sociological dimension*, involves choosing to perform an activity in a dependent, independent, or interdependent manner. People with and without disabilities differ in their preferences for use of AT or assistance from other people to complete tasks. For example, some people with disabilities employ an attendant to perform their personal hygiene, dressing, and cooking tasks. Others are able, with assistive devices (e.g., a robot programmed for cooking meals, remotely controlled urinary sphincters, orthotic hand and wrist braces for dressing), to perform at least some of these personal activities without the assistance of another human being. Reliance on people may and often does result in a very dependent relationship between the provider and recipient. Provision of assistive devices that are safe and reliable allows a person with a disability the choice of the level of interpersonal interactions he or she desires to perform. People with disabilities who are given a choice of assistive devices have the ability to do things with or without others. They can contribute to relationships on a more equal basis if they do not have to rely solely on personal assistance to complete activities. Between independence and dependence lies interdependence. The type and availability of AT sets limits on where a person with a disability falls in the dependence-to-interdependence dimension.

WHAT TO EVALUATE BEFORE DESIGNING

Before designing a device, it is important to evaluate the users' function. At Beneficial Designs, Inc., a Santa Cruz, California, engineering design firm that designs, develops, and tests AT devices, a significant amount of time is spent on research projects to determine the functions required for people to perform a specific activity. Strength, balance, coordination, and cognitive skills that are required are all considered. Methods are then developed to measure these functional skills when a particular device is evaluated by a user. A balance board is employed to evaluate the equilibrium of the user and the effectiveness of an adaptive seating system (Figure 1). The balance board has a rocker underneath it that allows the board to tip left and right. When a user sits on the balance board, a determination can be made about how far the user can angulate to the left and right. When designing seating for a kayak or mono-ski, seating systems are mocked up and the balance board is used to evaluate how well the seating enhances the user's lateral balance.

The development of the Back Support Shaping System (see the "Personal Technology" section in this chapter) included clinical trials involving more than 40 wheelchair users. In this study, participants were fitted and evaluated with the adjustable Back Support

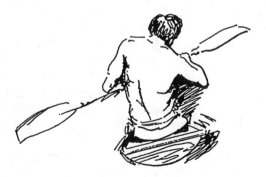

Figure 1.   Balance board.

Shaping System. The appropriate system was selected for each participant based on the height of the back upholstery of the wheelchair, the participant's functional level in terms of balance and stability, and his or her comfort. The exact height of each strap relative to the back of the user was determined based on evaluation of the segmental flexibility of that participant's spine and on his or her feedback regarding comfort. Once the height of the straps was fixed, the amount of tension in the straps was chosen for the initial testing based on comfort and on the optimization of posture (Figure 2).

Seat and back pressures were measured with the Force Sensing Array (Vista Medical) to detect any evidence of increased risk of skin breakdown with the back support system. Participants subsequently underwent mobility testing to determine whether wheelchair propulsion became more efficient with the back support system in place. Each manual wheelchair user propelled him- or herself 3 meters up a standard 1:12 ramp at maximum speed; the time required to propel the 3 meters was recorded. Three trials were conducted without the back support and then with the support. Similarly, each subject propelled the maximum distance possible up the same ramp in one push. Three additional trials were performed without and then with the back support, and the distance traveled each time was recorded. These functional assessment measurements demonstrated that use of the Back Support Shaping System promoted a more upright posture; increased the rigidity of the wheelchair; improved functional posture; and shifted the user's center of gravity forward, resulting in improved propulsion speed and strength (Axelson & Chesney, 1996; Chesney, Hsu, Wright, & Axelson, 1995).

The interests of people with disabilities should be reviewed before designing a product. People have many different preferences regarding what their assistive devices look like and what they hope to achieve with them. Do they want something that is inconspicuous or high profile? Expensive or inexpensive? Recreation oriented or career oriented? Whereas some people may prefer a "stealth black" wheelchair, others may want a pink or yellow one. As far as selecting activities, some preferences involve individual versus group activity, dynamic versus passive activity, and competitive versus noncompetitive sports. Some people are interested in doing things with their family and friends, whereas others want to participate only in sports in which they can be with other athletes with disabilities. For example, playing tennis with the rule modification that permits two bounces allows people who use wheelchairs to be integrated with others on the court. Some people want activities in which they can be completely independent, whereas others are willing to go hiking and be in a dependent situation. There are as many different preferences as there are people, and it is important to consider these when assisting someone in the choice of appropriate technology.

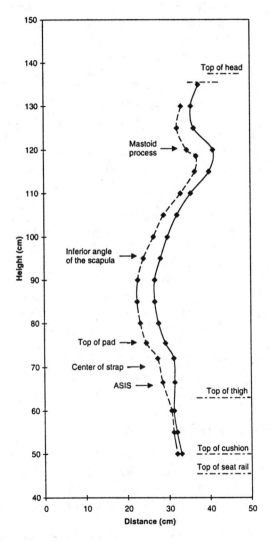

Figure 2.   Spine profile of subject with sling uphol-stery and with Back Support Shaping System. (- -◆- -, with sling upholstery only; —◆—, with Back Support Shaping System.)

DESIGNING FOR ACCESSIBILITY

What is good design? Good design does not necessarily involve a high level of technology. A door knob, for example, is a poor design for people with limited hand function, but switching to a door handle accommodates people with limited function. Going a step further, is the door itself even necessary? Sometimes the environment can be designed to avoid the need for a door at all.

The first thing to do when trying to adapt equipment for people with disabilities is to determine whether a mainstream product exists that will solve the problem being considered. For example, the Bogen Magic Arm was originally designed so that photographers could attach their cameras and lighting systems to various places in their studios. However, it was found to be extremely useful for mounting devices such as cameras, telephones, and remote control devices and for adjusting them in any position relative to a wheelchair user by clamping the other end of the Bogen Magic Arm onto the wheelchair.

If a product or device cannot be used in its originally designed state, it can frequently be modified for use by people with limited function by adding or altering the controls. For example, a shoulder control was designed that allows the fore–aft and up–down movement of the shoulder to control a video game or to operate a computer and perform word processing. A miniature racing yacht (the Mini-12), modified with hand controls so that people without use of their legs can sit inside to sail the boat, is another example in which the control input has been modified. One can modify seating interfaces to make devices usable, especially for people who do not have sensation as a result of SCI. Examples of these modifications include the addition of custom seating to all-terrain wheelchairs, ultralight aircraft, and horse saddles.

THREE KINDS OF TECHNOLOGY

Technology can be categorized into three different types: personal, activity-specific, and environmental. Each represents a different way to approach a problem. One might decide to install an elevator in a building or may prefer to design a ramp to the second floor of the structure. Another way of approaching the problem would be to design a way for wheelchairs to climb stairs. Before the design process begins, a decision must be made to determine the correct way to approach the problem for a given situation. For example, installing a ramp, lift, or elevator provides access for all current and future wheelchair users and others with mobility limitations, but designing the stair-climbing wheelchair assists only individuals who have access to that specific technology.

Personal Technology

Personal technology includes items users wear to assist them in performing in a wide range of activities. Putting on heavy, warm clothing to protect against the cold is an example of personal technology that is used by virtually everyone who lives in a cold climate. Eyeglasses are a personal technology device that assists people with visual impairments in nearly everything they do. Prosthetic arms and legs are examples of personal technologies that enhance a broad scope of actions and activities of users' daily lives. Wheelchairs are another example of a personal technology, one that people with mobility limitations use to accomplish all of their everyday tasks.

In a research project funded by the National Center for Medical Rehabilitation Research, Beneficial Designs developed a Back Support Shaping System for wheelchairs (Chesney, Hsu, Wright, & Axelson, 1995; Zollars & Axelson, 1993; Zollars, Chesney, & Axelson, 1994), another example of a personal technology (Figure 3). Sling upholstery is a cost-effective and creative solution to facilitate seating in a folding wheelchair structure. However, sling upholstery stretches and, even if it is adjustable, facilitates postural positioning only to a limited extent. The user-adjustable Back Support Shaping System consists of postural support pads in combination with tension straps that are fitted behind the back upholstery of wheelchairs

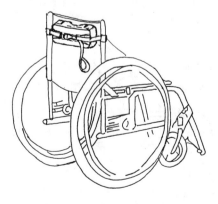

Figure 3.   Back Support Shaping System.

with sling upholstery (Chesney et al., 1995; Zollars & Axelson, 1993; Zollars et al., 1994).

Activity-Specific Technology

Activity-specific technology enables users to enhance their performance or to engage in activities that are impossible without the technology. For example, bicycles are specific technology devices that enable people to travel faster and for longer distances than on foot, motorcycles allow individuals to travel at higher speeds, and cars provide a way to get from Point A to Point B with heavy loads. Hand-powered bicycles (i.e., handcycles) enable people who do not have use of their legs to bike ride with family and friends (Figure 4) (Schwandt, 1983; Schwandt, Leifer, & Axelson, 1987). Many people who were injured during water sports activities want to continue their prior activities. A modified wave ski that a user sits on and propels with a kayak paddle is an example of activity-specific technology that allows people who have mobility impairment to continue participating in surfing. Rowing machines can be modified to enable wheelchair users who tend to overuse the pushing muscles to exercise the opposing (i.e., pulling) muscles. Many different chairs have been designed to provide access to a beach. People with disabilities cannot always get a medical certificate allowing them to fly, so modifying an ultralight aircraft, which does not require a medical certificate to fly, lets them take to the skies.

The cross-country ski is a framelike device that has two typical cross-country skis underneath it that tilt front to rear. One of the newest prototypes currently under development at Beneficial Designs is a dynamic cross-country sit ski. This dynamic orthosis mimics the actions of a person's knees and ankles. Users propel themselves with two poles; when the user reaches forward, a spring

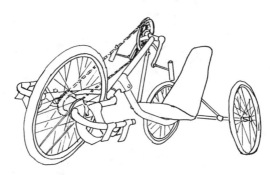

Figure 4.   Handcycle.

loads up, and when the user pushes through, the spring unloads. The ski functions just like a prosthetic foot, mimicking the motion made when someone on a regular pair of skis kicks and glides. This activity-specific technology allows people with disabilities to cross-country ski with family and friends or take part in competitions.

Mono-skis enable people without the use of both legs to ski. The term *mono-ski* may, in fact, be incorrect because the device can have more than one ski. From a technical viewpoint, the equipment could be considered a dynamic skiing orthosis. Many similarities exist between mono-skis and customized leg prostheses. Both must be custom fitted to the remaining functional component of the body. Both use springs, multipivot linkages, and other components to bridge the gap between the body and the ground and hydraulic components to dampen the motion of the body relative to the ground (Axelson, 1988, 1995). In 1985, Beneficial Designs prototyped the first mono-ski in the world with a shock absorber and the ability to go on a chairlift (Figure 5). The motocross shock absorber absorbs bumps and allows speeds of 60–70 miles per hour in downhill and "Super G" (i.e., giant slalom) events. All U.S. Disabled Ski Team members use this kind of technology today in worldwide competition.

Environmental Technology

Environmental technology actually modifies the physical environment itself—a ramp is constructed into a building, or the structure is built at street level so that a ramp is not needed. Generally, these assistive devices are things that do not move from one location to another. Some examples in home environments include a single hot and cold water control, closet rods that can be reached from sitting height, cutting boards that pull out at the height needed, a refrigera-

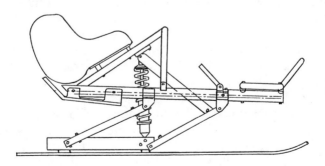

Figure 5.   Mono-ski.

tor with doors that open over a wheelchair user's knees, a table or sink that has the appropriate clearance so a wheelchair user can get underneath and use it, and dish storage space close to the dishwasher. Technology modifications in work environments include mounting a roll of paper that can be pulled out across the wall to use in brainstorming so that it is accessible to people of different heights, designing the layout in all rooms and facilities so that they can be accessed by wheelchairs, applying a presser bar on a sewing machine to provide alternative access to the foot pedal, and positioning power tools so that they are accessible to everyone. Examples in leisure environments include a climbing ladder for exercising the upper body and raised garden beds for wheelchair access. There are many ways to modify the environment—for example, if a person does not have $100,000 for an elevator but does have excellent upper-body strength, one could consider installing a climbing rope for gaining access to the second floor.

COMPUTERIZED MAPPING OF OUTDOOR TRAILS FOR ACCESSIBILITY

The Computerized Mapping of Outdoor Trails for Accessibility research project, conducted by Beneficial Designs and funded by the National Center for Medical Rehabilitation Research, is an example of environmental technology. This project evolved following a 1990 National Council on Disability hearing in Jackson, Wyoming. Several people with disabilities repeatedly expressed that they wanted to have access to the outdoors but did not want to see nature covered with asphalt. The primary obstacle that outdoor environments present to people with disabilities is not lack of access but lack of information. With the right information, outdoor environments can be accessible to everyone. By providing this information, land management agencies will encourage visitation by individuals from a wide range of user groups, including but not limited to those with mobility limitations and visual impairments, older adults, families with small children, experienced and inexperienced hikers, mountain bikers, and equestrians. The trails research project was begun to address this need.

The goal of the trails research project is to provide trail access information about individual recreation trails for users of all abilities by applying universal design principles to the natural environment. The majority of existing trail information is subjective. For example, signage might indicate that a particular trail is "moderately difficult" but provide no information as to how this classification was determined. A moderately difficult trail for some is very difficult for others, depending on each individual's ability and the mobility device used (e.g., wheelchair, stroller, mountain bike). To provide objective information about trails, it is necessary to collect detailed measurements of specific trail characteristics. In the summer of 1992, Beneficial Designs Inc. conducted a pilot study in cooperation with the U.S. Department of the Interior Park Service on three trails in Yellowstone National Park. The study isolated five elements important for providing trail access information: grade, cross-slope, trail width, surface type, and the size and type of obstacles. This project was funded by a grant from the Small Business Innovation Research Program of the National Center for Medical Rehabilitation Research in the National Institute of Child Health and Human Development at the National Institutes of Health.

Project Phases and Research Results

In Phase I of this project, Beneficial Designs developed a trail assessment process. A trail assessment team composed of volunteers measured the trail access elements at regular intervals using simple and inexpensive surveying tools (Chesney & Axelson, 1994; Pasternak, Axelson, Chesney, Wright, & Longmuir, 1996). Using the Universal Trail Assessment Process, teams collected data on several trails in Yellowstone National Park in Wyoming and Gallatin National Forest in Montana (Chesney & Axelson, 1994). Detailed trail guides containing trail access information were created (Axelson, Chesney, Thomas, & Pasternak, 1994; Axelson, Thomas, Chesney, Coveny, & Eve-Anchassi, 1994). The work completed during Phase I demonstrated the feasibility of a system for assessing hiking trails that provides detailed and pertinent information about the characteristics of trails for individuals of all abilities.

In Phase II, the trail guide design was refined, a format for audiotape descriptions with trail guide information for use by people with visual impairments were developed, and comprehensive user evaluations of trail guide materials were performed. An important part of Phase II was the development of a training course and materials for the purposes of training and certifying Universal Trail Assessment Coordinators. Beneficial Designs trained the first group of Universal Trail Assessment Coordinators in April 1995 during two 3-day workshops. Participants included representatives from the National Park Service, the National Forest Service, the Bureau of Reclamation, the Bureau of Land Management, the U.S. Fish and Wildlife Service, and the National Center on Accessibility as well as from other agencies and organizations. Nine additional workshops have been conducted across the United States. Beneficial Designs continues to offer Universal Trail Assessment Coordinator training workshops across the country. Workshop participants learn how to conduct a universal trail assessment and can collect access, mapping, usage, and maintenance information about trails in parks and forests in their regions. Trail data from these assessments can then be incorporated into trail guide products such as trail and trailhead signage (Figure 6) and pocket guides.

The results of this research have been helpful in other ways. The Americans with Disabilities Act (ADA) of 1990 (PL 101-336) accessibility guidelines (U.S. Architectural and Transportation Barriers Compliance Board [ATBCB], 1992) cover only built structures in highly developed areas and routes and ramps leading to these structures. Therefore, the ATBCB created the Recreation Access Advisory Committee to recommend guidelines for outdoor environments. The Outdoor Recreation Area Subcommittee was formed to cover a subset of these outdoor environments, including outdoor recreation access routes and recreation trails. The main goal of this committee was to recommend accessibility guidelines. The committee used the results of the trails research to develop standards to construct new trails and renovate existing ones to provide easy, moderate, difficult, and most difficult degrees of access (Axelson, Chesney, & Pasternak, 1994; Axelson, Chesney, et al., 1994). Building trails that meet each of these levels of access will provide more hiking options for trail users who have differing abilities and interests.

Trail Access Information

Recreational trails are used by many people, including but not limited to hikers, mountain bikers, equestrians, and all-terrain vehicle users. The category of hikers alone includes individuals with a wide range of functional abilities; some use assistive mobility devices. The level of accessibility of a recreational trail can be defined only with respect to the functional abilities and AT needs of a specific individual. For example, a trail that is easy for an experienced hiker may be moderately difficult for a family with a child in a stroller and impossible for a manual wheelchair user with limited upper-body strength. Examination of the needs of different users led to the identification of the five key trail parameters mentioned previously. Objective information about these five parameters will enable all users to determine the level of access and challenge offered by the trail and whether assistance will be required to successfully and safely negotiate the trail.

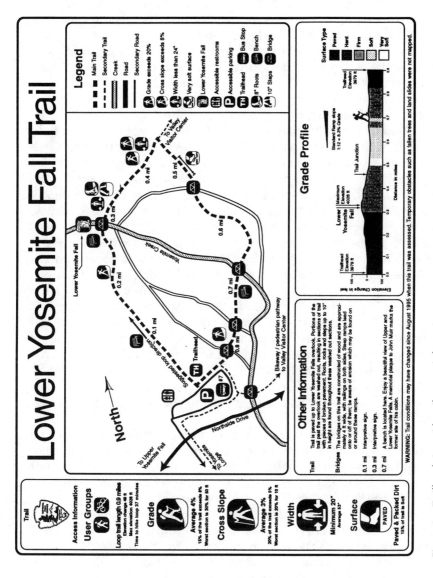

Figure 6. Trailhead sign with trail access information.

The main goal of the Computerized Mapping of Outdoor Trails for Accessibility research project is to make this important access information readily available to recreationalists of all abilities. Nutrition facts can be found on almost all food packaging in a standard format to enable consumers to make informed decisions regarding the food they eat. Similarly, by providing access information about individual hiking trails in a standard format, hikers with or without disabilities will have the opportunity to make informed decisions regarding which trails to hike. The Universal Trail Assessment Process gives land management agencies the tools they need to collect data and create trail access information.

Trail Grade   The effects of grade have a greater impact on individuals who use assistive mobility devices in comparison to weak ambulators. Research conducted by Beneficial Designs and funded by the National Center on Accessibility, a program of Indiana University in cooperation with the National Park Service Office on Accessibility, examined the effects of grade and cross-slope (Chesney, Axelson, & Hamilton, 1996a). An instrumented wheelchair was used to measure the amount of work required to propel a manual wheelchair up various grades. Using this work measurement method for assessing effort to push a wheelchair, it was determined that ramp grades of 14%, 20%, and 24% required approximately 70%, 130%, and 180% more work, respectively, than a standard 8.3% grade (1:12) ramp. The amount of energy required by ambulators is proportionately less than that for wheelchair users. The results of this research showed that the level of difficulty perceived by people negotiating different grades is significantly influenced by level of impairment and the assistive device used. Wheelchair users tended to rate the difficulty of grades higher in comparison to ambulatory individuals.

Trail grade is also critical in terms of the wheelchair user's safety. Wheelchairs, manual and powered, have a certain degree of static and dynamic stability that is dependent on the wheelchair model and setup. The majority of manual wheelchairs, tested according to the wheelchair standards of the American National Standards Institute and the Rehabilitation Engineering Society of North America (ANSI/RESNA Standards Subcommittee on Wheelchairs, 1998), are reportedly stable on grades up to 15.8%–30.6% (9°–17°, respectively), depending on the model. In addition, the ability of the wheelchair rider to compensate for changes in grade by leaning forward or backward in the chair influences how steep a grade the rider will be able to independently negotiate without tipping over backward or forward. Therefore, if wheelchair riders know that a standard 1:12 (8.3%) ramp into a building is at the limit of their abilities, they will be able to compare the average and maximum grade of a specific trail (Figure 7). Then they can determine whether that trail is accessible to them.

Trail Cross-Slope   Similar to grade, cross-slope also has a significant impact on the level of trail access to wheelchair users. In the research study mentioned previously, wheelchair users tended to rate trails with cross-slopes greater than 5% with higher ratings of difficulty than people who were ambulatory (Chesney et al., 1996a). Typically, the potential risk of tipping over sideways in a wheelchair is not as great as tipping over backward or forward. Thus, wheelchair users will use the average and maximum cross-slope values to determine whether they are capable of negotiating the trail (Figure 8).

Trail Width   Objective information about the width of the trail and the locations of the narrowest sections is critical for people who use mobility devices such as strollers, walkers, and wheelchairs. The average manual chair has a wheelbase width of less than 28 inches. If a trail narrows to 26 inches, people in 28-inch wheelchairs know they cannot venture past this point unless they are capable of transferring out of the chair and maneuvering it through this narrow location. If the trail width is disclosed, mobility device users will be able to determine exactly how far they can hike and whether they can reach the destination (Figure 9).

Trail Surface Type   Trail surface type has a great influence on the degree of access for all user groups. Objective test methods and portable devices for the measurement of surface firmness and stability are currently under development (Chesney & Axelson, 1993, 1996; Chesney, Axelson, & Hamilton, 1996b; Chesney, Axelson, & Williams, 1994). Surface firmness primarily affects the amount of energy required to ambulate or propel a wheelchair across that surface. Surface stability mainly influences the amount of energy required to maneuver or turn a wheelchair on the surface. In addition, for people who use crutches or walkers, lack of surface stability

Figure 7.   Grade symbol.

Figure 8.   Cross-slope symbol.

poses a potentially hazardous situation if the device moves while they lean on it for support during walking.

Using a preliminary wheelchair work measurement method, several different surfaces were measured (Chesney et al., 1996b). In comparison to propelling a wheelchair up a standard 1:12 (8.3%) ramp, a trail with the same grade and a decomposed granite surface required 10.6% more work. The results also revealed that level trails with engineered wood fiber surfaces required an average of 25% less work than a standard 1:12 (8.3%) ramp. The development of standardized test methods will enable objective surface firmness and stability measurements to be made. Recreationalists of all abilities can use this information to help make informed decisions about which trails to hike (Figure 10).

Trail Obstacles   Obstacles such as rocks, ruts, and roots can pose a substantial barrier to wheelchair users and strollers, especially if these items occur throughout the trail. Powered wheelchairs have a certain obstacle-climbing ability that is dependent on the model and type of front casters, and the chairs are often limited by the vertical clearance under them. Manual wheelchair users are limited by their own physical strength and maneuverability skills. Information about the types of obstacles found on the trail is also important to people pushing children in strollers, which typically have small wheels that cannot roll easily over larger obstacles. Obstacles can also hinder access to trails by ambulators with poor balance or agility. Therefore, objective information about the type and magnitude of obstacles found on the trail is included in the trail access information.

Figure 9.   Width symbol.

Figure 10.   Surface symbols.

Interactive Computer
Information Trail Guides for Universal Access

In September 1994, Beneficial Designs received funding from the U.S. Department of Education to conduct a research project entitled "Interactive Computer Information Trail Guides for Universal Access." The goal of this project is to provide information about hiking trail accessibility, especially to people with disabilities. Beneficial Designs is developing an interactive, user-friendly, computerized trail guide information system—another example of environmental technology.

The trail guide information system is composed of two main, integrated components: an Interactive Computer Information (ICI) Trail Guide and a Smart Trail Selector program. Both incorporate trail access information useful to people with and without disabilities. The ICI Trail Guide provides information on the degree of access through the use of maps, text, still images, and access data for specific trails. The Smart Trail Selector program allows users to select trails based on easier, moderate, difficult, or most difficult access classifications. This is done by entering specific trail data such as total trail length, elevation, average and maximum grade and cross-slope, minimum trail width, surface type, and magnitude of obstacles. The Smart Trail Selector then determines which trails meet the criteria entered by the user and displays a list of these trails.

In March 1995, Beneficial Designs conducted a pilot study in which individuals of all abilities and ages evaluated both components (ICI Trail Guide and Smart Trail Selector) with respect to their usefulness and effectiveness in providing access information. Questionnaire and interview responses were used to identify each system's strong and weak aspects. In October 1995, Beneficial Designs began to revise and refine the ICI Trail Guide and the Smart Trail Selector program based on the feedback received during the pilot study. A stand-alone trails information kiosk is being designed and developed for use in Yosemite National Park in California (Figure 11). Park visitors will be able to evaluate the kiosk, and their

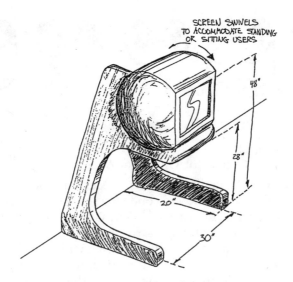

Figure 11.   Trail information kiosk with Interactive Computer Information Trail Guide and Smart Trail Selector.

feedback and use of the system will help to refine the computer programs. A CD-ROM containing the ICI Trail Guide and the Smart Trail Selector program for Yosemite will be created and distributed to reviewers for evaluation.

CONCLUSIONS

When approaching any problem, one should look for products with universal design features that are already accessible or can easily be modified by adapting the control or seating interface. Consider all approaches to the problem: Can a general solution be found that will provide access to everyone, or should a specific assistive device be designed for that individual? Can the device be designed to enhance the person's performance in all situations, or is an activity-specific device needed?

   AT designers should get to know their clients. They must spend time with their clients to determine their greatest needs with regard to establishing or reestablishing balance in their lives. Our efforts must focus on the needs and problems that will have the greatest impact on their life activities. Finally, each individual's function and interest related to the specific tasks he or she is trying to accomplish must be evaluated. Using this approach will help to avert functional limitations or at least to prevent them from becoming disabilities.

REFERENCES

Americans with Disabilities Act (ADA) of 1990, PL 101-336, 42 U.S.C. §§ 12101 et seq.

ANSI/RESNA Standards Subcommittee on Wheelchairs. (1998). *American National Standards for Wheelchairs: Vol. 1. Requirements and test methods for wheelchairs (including scooters)*. New York: American National Standards Institute.

Axelson, P.W. (1983). The humanistic designer: New perspectives. In B.R. Bowman (Ed.), *Proceedings of the Sixth Annual Conference on Rehabilitation Engineering* (pp. 263–266). Bethesda, MD: Rehabilitation Engineering Society of North America.

Axelson, P.W. (1988). Hitting the slopes: Everything you ever wanted to know about mono-skis and mono-skiing. *Sports 'n Spokes, 14*(4), 22–34.

Axelson, P.W. (1995). Snow show. *Sports 'n Spokes, 21*(6), 23–44.

Axelson, P.W., & Chesney, D.A. (1996). Clinical and research methodologies for measuring functional changes in seating systems. In *Proceedings of the 12th International Seating Symposium* (pp. 81–84). Vancouver, British Columbia, Canada: Sunny Hill Health Centre for Children.

Axelson, P.W., Chesney, D., & Pasternak, M. (1994). Research issues relating to making trails accessible: Gradient, cross slope, surfacing, trail classification and mapping. In *Proceedings of the 12th National Trails Symposium: "Connecting our Communities"* (pp. 37–41). Denver, CO: American Trails.

Axelson, P.W., Chesney, D., Thomas, P., & Pasternak, M. (1994). Design specifications for the three levels of accessibility and methods and techniques for measuring trails. In *Proceedings of the 12th National Trails Symposium: "Connecting our Communities"* (pp. 30–36). Denver, CO: American Trails.

Axelson, P.W., Thomas, P.H., Chesney, D.A., Coveny, J.L., & Eve-Anchassi, D. (1994). Trail guides with universal access information. In M. Binion (Ed.), *Proceedings of the RESNA '94 Annual Conference* (pp. 306–308). Arlington, VA: RESNA Press.

Chesney, D., & Axelson, P.W. (1993). A surface accessibility measurement device. In M. Binion (Ed.), *Proceedings of the RESNA '93 Annual Conference* (pp. 341–343). Washington, DC: RESNA Press.

Chesney, D.A., & Axelson, P.W. (1994). Assessment of outdoor environments for accessibility. In M. Binion (Ed.), *Proceedings of the RESNA '94 Annual Conference* (pp. 278–280). Arlington, VA: RESNA Press.

Chesney, D.A., & Axleson, P.W. (1996). Preliminary test method for the determination of surface firmness. *IEEE Transactions on Rehabilitation Engineering, 4*(3), 182–187.

Chesney D.A., Axelson, P.W., & Hamilton, E.J. (1996a). Design specifications for outdoor recreation access routes and recreation trails: A pilot study. In A. Langton (Ed.), *Proceedings of the RESNA '96 Annual Conference* (pp. 444–446). Arlington, VA: RESNA Press.

Chesney D.A., Axelson, P.W., & Hamilton, E.J. (1996b). Draft test method for the measurement of surface accessibility. In A. Langton (Ed.), *Proceedings of the RESNA '96 Annual Conference* (pp. 447–449). Arlington, VA: RESNA Press.

Chesney, D.A., Axelson, P.W., & Williams, J.R. (1994). Surface assessment devices for accessibility. In M. Binion (Ed.), *Proceedings of the RESNA '94 Annual Conference* (pp. 275–277). Arlington, VA: RESNA Press.

Chesney, D.A., Hsu, L., Wright, W., & Axelson, P.W. (1995). Immediate improvements in wheelchair mobility and comfort with use of the adjustable Back Support Shaping System. In A. Langton (Ed.), *Proceedings of the RESNA '95 Annual Conference* (pp. 288–290). Vancouver, British Columbia, Canada: RESNA Press.

Pasternak, M.A., Axelson, P.W., Chesney, D.A., Wright, W.E., & Longmuir, P.E. (1996). The universal trail assessment process. In A. Langton (Ed.), *Proceedings of the RESNA '96 Annual Conference* (pp. 432–434). Arlington, VA: RESNA Press.

Schwandt, D.F. (1983). Para-bike: An arm-powered bicycle. In B.R. Bowman (Ed.), *Proceedings of the Sixth Annual Conference on Rehabilitation Engineering* (pp. 378–380). Bethesda, MD: Rehabilitation Engineering Society of North America.

Schwandt, D.F., Leifer, L., & Axelson, P.W. (1987). Handbike: An arm-powered bicycle. *Journal of Rehabilitation Research and Development, 25*(1), 155.

U.S. Architectural and Transportation Barriers Compliance Board (ATBCB). (1992). *Americans with Disabilities Act (ADA) accessibility guidelines for buildings and facilities, transportation facilities, transportation vehicles.* Washington, DC: Author.

Zollars, J.A., & Axelson, P.W. (1993). The Back Support Shaping System: An alternative for persons using wheelchairs with sling back upholstery. In M. Binion (Ed.), *Proceedings of the RESNA '93 Annual Conference* (pp. 274–276). Las Vegas, NV: RESNA Press.

Zollars, J.A., Chesney, D., & Axelson, P.W. (1994). The design of a Back Support Shaping System: Clinical methodologies for measuring changes in sitting posture with function. In *Proceedings of the 10th International Seating Symposium* (pp. 97–108). Vancouver, British Columbia, Canada: Sunny Hill Health Centre for Children.

CHAPTER 14

The Relationship Between Ability Measures and Assistive Technology Selection, Design, and Use

Stephen Sprigle and Adam Abdelhamied

The assistive technology (AT) field is fairly inconsistent in that the delivery of AT services and devices varies according to geography and service delivery model (i.e., medical, educational, vocational). However, the selection, use, and design of AT share a common thread: the desire to enhance a person's ability, comfort, and function through technical assistance. Therefore, the relationships among ability, function, and assistive technology are quite natural and paramount for all involved.

Because of the varied nature of the AT field, words and phrases adopt multiple definitions. This chapter describes the people and issues involved in assistive technology in the following manner. A *practitioner* or *clinician* refers to a physical therapist, occupational therapist, rehabilitation engineer, or other professional who works with people with disabilities. Professionals trained in assistive technology are referred to as *AT practitioners*. Examples using a particular profession should be considered as such and not suggestive of role delineation. An *assistive device* is any piece of equipment that increases ability or function. It can be a low-tech, high-tech, medical, or mainstream consumer product. An *AT intervention* is any service or assistance that selects an assistive device or improves the use of current assistive technology to meet a person's needs or goals. It might involve better training in device use, alternative strategies of use, or better configuration of the device. An *end user* or *consumer* refers to the person who ultimately uses an assistive device and who may or may not be the customer for the device.

Ability is the quality of being capable of doing something. Ability can be general or task specific. *Physical abilities* refers here to discrete movements such as range of motion (ROM), muscular strength, or levels of sensation. Measurement of physical ability makes no reference to competence or skill. *Functional ability* is task specific and, therefore, includes competence or skill. It is typically a combination of physical abilities that enables a person to perform an action. Measurement of function must be meaningful and practical to the end user (Swanson, 1993). With respect to AT, functional measures are dependent on what the end user experiences when using the device.

The provision and use of AT are very broad topics that can follow different pathways or methodologies. Several related and overlapping topics are covered elsewhere in this book. This discussion concentrates on the process of using physical and functional ability measures to select and design assistive technology. Based on the previous definitions, the provision of AT includes selection and design issues on which both physical and functional measures have an impact. The use of AT is a functional construct that is also related to physical ability determination. This chapter attempts to identify current and future approaches that may improve the selection and design of AT. To illustrate the concepts described in this chapter, examples are provided that are drawn from devices developed to improve functioning in seating, mobility, and augmentative communication.

The process of providing assistive technology to an individual can be loosely divided into eight steps:

1. Identification of need
2. Measurement of physical and functional abilities
3. Description of functional tasks
4. Comparison of abilities to task demands
5. Determination of whether an AT device is indicated
6. Establishment of device criteria and device selection
7. Design of device
8. Evaluation of AT intervention effectiveness

Assistive technology interventions might not include all of these steps, and the order in which these steps are undertaken may vary. For instance, an AT practitioner working with a consumer who uses a simple communication board might skip Step 5 and concentrate on selecting a better system; or the establishment of device criteria might begin in parallel with the identification of need. This process might take a few minutes or several months. These steps are meant as a general guide and are discussed separately.

IDENTIFICATION OF NEED

All AT interventions are reliant on a very good definition of the functional goal or need. The need often involves the desire to perform a task or to improve task performance. Without a clear definition of this goal, interventions are based on incomplete information and are less likely to meet the needs of the consumer. The establishment of functional goals defines the criteria on which to base and evaluate the intervention. A complete definition better ensures that the consumer's needs are reflected and lends itself to being measurable.

This step is arguably both the most important and most difficult in the series, but the technique of identifying consumer needs can be learned easily over time. Payton, Nelson, and Ozer describe a five-question system that forms the basis of consumer participation in planning:

1. What concerns you at this time? (problems)
2. What would you like to see happen? (goals)
3. What has been accomplished in relation to the goals? (outcomes)
4. What may have helped to bring about those results? (methods)
5. What is the plan? (1990, p. 33)

These questions represent a very general intervention model with the goal of involving consumers in their own therapeutic program. Clinicians will add more specific questions as their experience grows. Similarly, consumers will be able to specify needs and goals more clearly with experience. The questions are also general in nature, but the concept of participation can easily be applied to AT interventions.

With regard to an AT intervention, inquiry about problems and goals should address at least three areas:

* The *task* itself: The consumer should describe a functional problem or need (i.e., a need to manage a catheter, a desire to operate several devices at a workstation, a need to get to class on time). Quite often, more than one task will be described.

- The *situation and environment* in which the task is performed: This information begins to describe the context within which the need should be addressed. Is the task done indoors? While alone? Once a day?
- The *criteria for success* or satisfactory performance: Beginning to establish criteria early is as important as defining the goals.

The task might lend itself to measurement (e.g., typing a specific number of words per minute, increased hip ROM to sit erect) or might be difficult to quantify (e.g., decreased pain, more endurance at work). A series of goals can also be described to provide a stepwise progression toward an overall goal. Most functional activities require repetition to maximize performance. Establishing short-term goals might provide a sense of accomplishment and can provide positive feedback to the consumer that can be a source of motivation for using the device (Payton et al., 1990).

Identification of problems and goals is a part of the interview process taught to most clinicians. However, applying this process to an AT intervention requires knowledge about the area of assistive technology in question because the topic is more specific. Knowledge about availablity of assistive devices, their features, and performance trade-offs provides the clinician with better ability to assist consumers in defining functional goals and priorities.

Example 1.   Evaluation forms, consumer profile forms, and AT intervention forms have been developed for certain types of assistive technology. These can be very helpful to clinicians and their consumers by listing important factors that have an impact on need or problem definition. For example, Ragnarsson (1990) listed several factors that should be addressed during the wheelchair prescription process:

1. User's age, size, weight, and so forth
2. User's disability and prognosis
3. User's functional skills and preferences
4. Indoor or outdoor use
5. Portability and accessibility
6. Reliability, durability, and service
7. Cosmetic features
8. Available options
9. Cost

As the list illustrates, factors can become numerous and can even conflict with one another. Establishment of priorities helps resolve conflicting factors. As long as the end user is involved with setting priorities, the selection of a particular device or intervention will be better understood and accepted. The issue of multiple and conflicting factors underscores the complexity of the process and the dependence on the ability of both clinician and consumer.

Certain consumers will have the experience and self-awareness necessary to completely express their goals for selection and use of AT. Some complications will obviously arise when working with certain consumers, such as children or people with cognitive disabilities or communication problems. However, the process can involve others, such as parents, caregivers, or teachers, to assist in this step.

The identification of important factors has been developed for several categories of assistive devices such as wheelchairs, cushions, and augmentative and alternative communication (AAC). Research and development of standards and testing methods is one way that prescription factors can be quantified scientifically. Wheelchair standards will provide documentation about reliability, durability, and service factors. Additional development of objective testing and evaluation protocols is needed to assist clinicians and end users in the formulation of functional goals and the identification of desired device features. For example, wheelchair cushions are made from various materials using different configurations. Clinicians and end users would benefit from research relating clinically important features such as stability and dynamic load distribution to cushion material and design.

MEASUREMENT OF PHYSICAL AND FUNCTIONAL ABILITIES

The processes used to select assistive devices and interventions vary, depending on many factors, but most involve some type of ability measure or assessment. Determination of abilities should be done early in the process of selecting appropriate AT interventions. Many physical and functional abilities—motor, sensory, and cognitive—can be measured. A complete discussion is well beyond the scope of this chapter, so physical abilities, particularly motor abilities, are used as illustrations.

Practitioners in the medical rehabilitation arena are trained to assess physical ability and, ultimately, function, and they commonly base AT decisions on these ability measures. Physical therapists determine a person's upper- and lower-extremity ROM and strength using manual assessment techniques before selecting an ambulation aid (e.g., cane, crutch) most appropriate for a given consumer. An occupational therapist will assess grip strength and fine motor ability before teaching a person to prepare and eat a meal using assistive devices. These discrete abilities are most commonly measured using manual assessment techniques. Manual assessment techniques are certainly the most common means to determine function and will probably remain popular because they are easy to perform and require little or no assessment equipment.

In addition to forming a basis for making AT decisions, clinicians measure physical abilities in order to monitor progress or classify disability. ROM evaluations and manual muscle tests (MMTs) are but two of many discrete measures of performance and are discussed here as examples.

Muscle strength testing determines the capability of muscles to function (Kendall, McCreary, & Provance, 1993). Muscle weakness reduces the capability for movement and stability and, therefore, reduces the abilities of the person. MMTs result in a graded score ranging from 0 to 5. The amount of resistance applied to a muscle group as it acts over a range determines good (5) and normal (4) grades. Movement through a full range against gravity is given a fair (3) grade, and movement with gravity eliminated results in a poor (2) grade. When limb movement is absent, the presence of a muscle contraction distinguishes between trace (1) and no contraction (0) grades. MMT results have been shown to be reliable and valid over the years (Smith, Iddings, Spencer, & Harrington, 1961). Similarly, the measurement of ROM using a goniometer is a simple assessment technique that has proven valid and reliable (Boone et al., 1978; Fish & Wingate, 1987; Gogia, Bratz, Rose, & Norton, 1987; Hamilton & Lachenbruch, 1969). The goniometer is simply aligned with an axis of joint rotation, and the available movement between articulating bones is measured. However, manual assessment does not always provide a quantifiable or objective measure of a person's ability and is subject to errors related to technique, positioning, and muscle substitution.

Providing a means to better quantify these and other discrete measures would benefit the documentation and tracking of outcome measures. Kendall and colleagues (1993) expressed their desire for a simple device better able to distinguish between "good" and normal MMT levels. Many simple devices and techniques are available that can accurately measure range and strength in clinical settings. In addition, commercially available dynamometers (e.g., BTE, Cybex, LIDO) measure and quantify isotonic, isometric, and isokinetic strength and can be configured to determine ROM. However, the fact that a number can be assigned to a discrete physical ability of a person does not mean that it will be useful in the selection of appropriate AT. The usefulness of physical ability measures derives from applying them to function, specifically task performance, device operation, or both.

Functional tasks are measured clinically and most often via observation. For example, pushing a wheelchair up a ramp and donning shoes and socks are common activities of daily living monitored by clinicians. Because the identified need is commonly functional in nature, measuring the consumer's performance in achieving a specific task is an important source of information. The objective is to establish a baseline of performance on which to base intervention decisions and, later, to help judge the intervention. This analysis can be simple or complex and might include both physical and functional measures.

> *Example 2.* When evaluating a person for an AAC device, motor abilities are assessed in a hierarchical structure to determine selection techniques. The appropriate interface method is determined by the quality of movement and control exhibited by the individual who cannot speak. This involves both discrete physical (i.e., ROM, MMT) and functional (i.e., speed, accuracy) measures. The AAC team determines the operating technique of the individual who cannot speak, interface method, area of activation discreteness or key size access, and activation pressure (Kraat & Silver, 1987). The upper extremities are evaluated first. Other interfaces using head or lower extremities are explored next. The interface methods are determined by considering the most appropriate available motor capabilities, including upper extremities, head or mouth stick, head-mounted light pointer, eye gaze, or lower extremities. The area of activation is defined as the largest square area in which the nonspeaking person can successfully manipulate a bodily extremity. The discreteness of this control is determined by measuring the size of the smallest area (key size) that can be consistently selected. The activation pressure is determined by the amount of force deliverable to that key size.

DESCRIPTION OF FUNCTIONAL TASKS

The measurement of ability described in the previous example can be considered specific to the consumer. Functional task description can be considered specific to the task and independent of the person performing the task. In other words, task description is the determination of the abilities required by "some person" to complete the task successfully. It can also identify the "ideal" approach based on performance and safety norms and guidelines, but this information is usually limited to ergonomic applications.

Some studies have defined the amount of motion required to perform certain functional tasks, which an AT practitioner can use as a basis for applying measures of ability. For example, many activities of daily living can be performed within a range of 30°–130° of elbow flexion (Kendall et al., 1993). Clarkson (1989) and Kapandji (1982) discussed movements of the body necessary to perform common functional tasks such as putting on a jacket or tying one's shoes. This information has direct application in assistive technology because clinicians must choose assistive devices or select AT interventions with functional applications in mind. Task description can be rather intuitive and includes a simple biomechanical analysis.

Example 3. Operating a push-button telephone requires adequate physical abilities, including ROM to reach the unit, strength to depress the keypad switches, and grip to hold the receiver. Functional abilities include accuracy in depressing the switches and ability to maintain the receiver in the proper position to listen and speak. However, care must be taken to recognize and identify the alternative approaches people use to perform the same action.

Example 4. Two types of grip, power and precision, can be used to grasp a cup. People choose a certain grip according to the characteristics of the cup (e.g., size, design, weight) or based on habit or other personal reasons. Therefore, task description should not be limited to clinicians' biases of how they would accomplish a task. Rather, it should be a creative process that includes all possible alternatives.

Research has been very helpful in applying biomechanics to functional AT issues. For example, many factors influence manual wheelchair propulsion because people use different strategies to propel their wheelchairs. Research has shown how the biomechanics of propulsion are affected by tire type (Kauzlarich, Thacker, & McLaurin, 1985) and rear wheel position (Hughes, Weimar, Sheth, & Brubaker, 1992). Clinicians can apply this information to improve their consumers' performance by a better propulsion approach or a better wheelchair configuration.

COMPARISON OF ABILITIES TO TASK DEMANDS

Many AT assessments do not result in a new device being provided to the client. In fact, a clinician's first inclination should be to meet the functional goals without additional equipment. The consumer, of course, may identify the desire for a device as a high priority, but this should not be assumed.

At this point, the clinician knows the consumer's needs and goals, has measured certain abilities of the consumer, and has studied the task to be completed. In order to select AT interventions, additional information is necessary: the discrete abilities needed to perform certain functional tasks and the ability needed to use specific assistive devices. Kondraske (1988) offered a useful diagram to illustrate this concept, which has been modified and simplified in Figure 1. This figure describes the relationship between the speed and ROM required to perform a task and the abilities of a given individual. In the top graph, the person's available speed and ROM exceed those required by the task. This person should be able to accomplish the task. However, the bottom graph shows a condition in which a person can exceed the speed requirement but does not have the ROM necessary for the task.

Determining a person's abilities and the abilities required by the task is difficult but important during AT interventions. Equipment matrices, device data sheets, and computerized systems are methods used to help address AT needs. The design of assistive technology builds on this even further by basing a device's capacities on the need to fill the gap between the user's abilities and the abilities necessary to perform a task using a device. Selection or de-

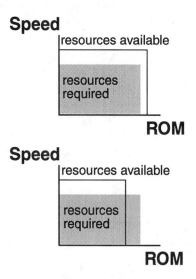

Figure 1.   Comparing available to required task resources. (Adapted from Kondraske [1988].)

sign of appropriate assistive devices requires consideration of three separate interfaces:

- *Human–task interface*: A person might be able to perform all or a portion of the task satisfactorily; this interface is based on the person's functional abilities.
- *Device–task interface*: Any proposed assistive device must interface with the task to supply needed resources.
- *Human–device interface*: The device must be operable by the consumer within the defined situation.

A simple illustration of these interfaces is shown in Figure 2.

Kondraske (1988) described an approach that seeks to define both discrete abilities and the abilities required to perform functional tasks. He suggested that AT interventions and design processes can be made more systematic by 1) identifying, defining, and standardizing a complete array of human performance and task analysis measurements; 2) developing tools to permit easy acquisition of measurement values; and 3) developing a strategy to analyze and characterize assistive devices quantitatively. Kondraske names this systematic approach the Basic Elements of Performance. The factors interact in his plan to provide a useful measure of human performance for device selection. The data derived from this approach are based on available resources that are application independent and are determined through the measurement of discrete abilities that are combined to achieve complex movement. Required resources are identified by task description to determine necessary abilities. These abilities are application dependent and change with the device or the approach to a task.

One complication in Kondraske's (1988) approach is that the definition of *function* affects the required abilities to perform a task. Function can be related to the output or outcome of a task (e.g., Can he shave? Can she enter data into a computer?). These functional goals are much different from those resulting from a def-

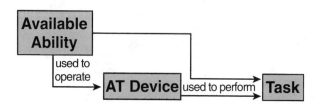

Figure 2.   Interfaces affecting assistive technology interventions.

inition of function relating to the interface or operation or manipulation of a device (e.g., Can he use a razor? Can she type on a keyboard?). Furthermore, because tasks can be performed using alternative approaches, application-dependent required resources become difficult to define. Unfortunately, the principles advocated by Kondraske have not been used systematically by those who select and design AT. These principles and some trade-offs of a systematic approach are discussed in Example 5.

> *Example 5.*   An important aspect of the rehabilitation of people with disabilities is evaluation and training for driving a vehicle. Often, this process involves an evaluation from an occupational therapist or other professional to determine the appropriate equipment necessary to make vehicle controls accessible. A survey of 138 driver evaluators found that over 90% measured upper-extremity ROM, manual strength, and grip strength by using manual evaluation techniques and simple functional tests that were not specifically related to driving (Sprigle, Morris, Nowachek, & Karg, 1995). Very few were able to measure driving-specific abilities, such as steering and brake force. Yet, in a subsequent question, two thirds of the respondents reported being satisfied with their evaluation equipment. Evaluators measure ability in order to determine whether their clients can operate brake, steering, and throttle controls. They informally use physical ability to select an appropriate assistive device, but they do this with incomplete information. The relationship between physical abilities and functional driving abilities is unknown. An improved evaluation would also incorporate the abilities required to operate certain controls. Many different commercial systems incorporate different designs that alter the forces and motions necessary for vehicle operation. An evaluator who knows the available and required abilities can match a consumer to a usable control, thus aiding prescription. One could also use this information to target an exercise program to improve the consumer's function to allow him or her to operate a certain control. This would be very important if a person needed a vacuum-assist hand control because of poor arm strength. The benefits of a simpler mechanical hand control could be realized if the upper-extremity strength improved. Knowing how much strength is needed would facilitate the definition of a strengthening program and provide incentive for the consumer.

DETERMINATION OF WHETHER AN AT DEVICE IS INDICATED

As mentioned previously, not every problem or functional need should be addressed by an assistive device. Not all people with disabilities like to fill their lives with devices or equipment. Practitioners must respect that. The magnitude of the problem or need helps define the amount of effort a person will expend to address the need or overcome the problem. Issues such as cost, frequency of need (i.e., use), and perceived importance all influence a person's definition of *hassle*. In many aspects of our daily lives, we continually judge whether another device or gadget will help us or annoy us by adding clutter to our lives. Assistive technology practitioners probably have a higher gadget tolerance than the consumers with whom they work, simply because they are familiar with technology and use it every day.

A *hassle index* can be defined that simply compares "functional gain" to "hassle to use." Any time AT selection or design is contemplated, the hassle index must be addressed. Factors that affect whether a person will accept or reject a device are the same as those listed previously in this chapter and include setup, storage, transport, complexity, and availability.

> *Example 6.*   Michael is a 30-year-old man with cerebral palsy who uses a powered wheelchair. He does not speak clearly, although those working with him become familiar with his speech. He attends computer training daily for 4 hours on the third floor of a building, which requires Michael to use the elevator. Michael is dropped off by a paratransit and independently drives his powered wheelchair into the building. He waits in front of the elevators for someone to press the "up" button, and, when the elevator arrives and he enters, he asks the person to press the third-floor button. When leaving, he usually asks one of his mentors to press the elevator buttons. Upon learning of this approach, a practitioner approached the engineering department with the request to design a device to allow Michael to depress the elevator buttons.
>
> The engineer's first step involved approaching Michael to get a more complete description of the design specifications. The conversation quickly turned into an explanation of why Michael was not interested in such a device. He offered two reasons:
>
> 1.   Computer training is the only time he uses an elevator alone. Thus, his need for a device would be only twice per day—not enough to warrant carrying a device all day.
> 2.   He does not mind waiting because he prefers to ride the elevator with someone. The elevators do not work well, and, if they ever break down, he would prefer to be stuck with someone who can speak and operate all of the controls well.

ESTABLISHMENT OF DEVICE
CRITERIA AND DEVICE SELECTION

Once the decision is made to use an AT device to meet a consumer's need, the overall goal is to define the characteristics and features of a device that are required to meet those needs. Meeting the consumer's needs can be accomplished by modification of a currently owned device, selection of an available standard device, or design of a new device. Tasks can be completed in many ways. Often, many assistive devices and design solutions exist. However, only a few solutions may be acceptable to the user.

Establishing device specifications and constraints is an extension of the information collected during the identification of need. Often, this information must be expanded because by that time a much better understanding of the consumer and the task has been obtained. Consumer abilities have been determined, the abilities needed to complete the task have been estimated, and the two have been compared. Matching abilities, needs, and desires to device features can be accomplished in many ways, some simple and some complex.

> *Example 7.* The AAC field uses an array of matching tools. The matching process requires a detailed evaluation and characterization of the AAC systems and a systematic method of relating these characteristics to client needs and skills. Some features of an AAC device that have an impact on selection are listed in Table 1. The features that are most limiting are considered first, followed by those that are less restrictive. For example, in an AAC system, the type of symbol system is often the most limiting characteristic. If a consumer requires pictures as symbols, then many devices are eliminated. In contrast, spoken output as a characteristic is not as limiting, because most devices use speech synthesizers (Cook & Hussey, 1995).

Matching systems include both noncomputerized and computerized methods. Noncomputerized methods provide prescription guidance via matrices and poster charts. Examples for AAC include a decision matrix to determine device candidacy (Shane & Bashir, 1980) and a series of three matrices to facilitate decision making and implementation of AAC (Owen & House, 1984). A poster chart with device characteristics listed horizontally and the names of commercial devices listed vertically has also been developed (Kraat & Silver, 1987).

Computerized approaches include the Augmentative Communication Evaluation Systems (ACES) (available from Word+ Inc.)

Table 1.   Augmentative and assistive communication device features

Selection technique	Language	Output	Portability
Interface method	Symbols	Speech	Weight
Key-size access	Storage capacity	Video display	Size
Range of motion	Units	Emergency signals	
Activation pressure	Coding techniques	Control signal	
Selection method	Organization schemes		

and Needs–Features Spreadsheets (NFS; using Lotus 1–2–3) (Good-enough-Trepagnier et al., 1985). ACES consists of software from Word+ and various hardware options from Adaptive Communication Systems. This approach minimizes the amount of time needed to conduct AAC device assessment by guiding the clinician through a consistent evaluation protocol. It produces only a generic prescription of an appropriate device. The NFS employs empirical mathematical formulas to assign a numerical value to each device, based on the number of device features matching a consumer's communication needs. It matches the consumer's capabilities and needs to an appropriate commercial electronic AAC device. The system can explain its results, but its accuracy depends on the expertise of its developer.

Another tool used by AT practitioners to assist in matching the consumer's needs and skills to the appropriate technology is an expert system. Expert systems use a computer program that systematically guides the practitioner through the decision-making process and results in determination of the most suitable device. Expert systems have been developed for AAC (Garrett, Andrews, Olsson, & Seeger, 1990), wheelchair cushions (Ferguson-Pell, 1990), and workstation design (Abdel-Moty & Khalil, 1989).

Several critical issues affecting the use of matching systems can be identified. The output is only as good as the input into the system, and the input, as mentioned previously, is complicated. How are abilities characterized, and how is the problem or need defined? Priorities, trade-offs, and compromises must be defined by the user. The usefulness of the match of tool and function for addressing the individual's needs will separate an academic exercise from a useful clinical tool.

Other limitations can also be identified. The clinician must remember all of the characteristics needed in the device and find a match on the poster chart or computer program. Noncomputerized approaches can be difficult to update without reprinting and redistribution and provide little or no explanation of their results, and their reliability depends on the user's experience. Disadvantages of computerized approaches include the time required to input data, the complexity of the user interface, and their inability to justify their results.

Expert systems or selection matrices have a potential role in the systematic prescription or design of assistive technology and the identification of appropriate AT options to consider. The number of assistive devices on the market complicates the selection process but provides users with increased options. Selection tools that maximize input might be better able to narrow the selection, but at a cost. Is the effort required to collect and enter additional information and the increased complexity of the system worth it? Selection systems should have the dual goals of being time efficient and providing choices. Attempts to identify a particular device or design assume that complete user information and design criteria have been entered. This would be a risky assumption.

Selection tools are beginning to be used to streamline the reimbursement process. Third-party payers can use these tools to determine whether a device is appropriate or necessary. The effectiveness of this approach is still uncertain. The use of selection tools by people who have never seen the users is quite a different process from the use of clinical selection tools by AT practitioners. Tools will have to be developed that reflect the knowledge of the person using them and the information that person is provided.

DESIGN OF DEVICE

Standard equipment design methodology is a multistep approach that generally involves problem definition; identification of design specifications; compilation of design solutions; iterations of prototype fabrication and testing; and, finally, design of the production version of the device. This methodology involves input from many sources, including design, engineering, market analysis, and end user (or customer) input. The design of customized assistive devices usually involves a less structured approach and reduced input. The end users, practitioners, and technical support personnel (e.g., technician, engineer) are often the principal individuals involved. The formality of the design process is dependent on, among other things, the perceived complexity of the device, the available funding for the project, and the time frame. However, AT design involves risks and complications not present in standard equipment design.

Orpwood (1990) provided interesting insights into the problems of assistive technology design by suggesting the differences between standard design methodologies and AT design methodologies. He identified three elements of the problems that usually arise when designing assistive technology: 1) the problems usually involve the device–user interface; 2) the problems are often quite obvious in retrospect but are not at all obvious during the design process; and 3) in order to overcome the problems, the whole device, not just the user interface, must be redesigned. Orpwood then proposed an alternative methodology that separates the user interface aspects of the design from the supporting features of the device. This approach involves the liberal use of prototypes to ultimately determine the appropriate solution and allows the supporting device features to be incorporated into devices for others simply by redesigning the user interface. In other words, the process includes task identification and analysis, design of the interface based on the person's ability, and design of the secondary system to fill in the gap between available and required resources. This concept addresses the interfaces of a person–device–task system and divides the design into two parts. The first question to answer is, can the device be operated using a person's available functional abilities? The next question is, does the device provide the necessary performance to complete the desired (i.e., identified) task? Not all engineers will be able to generate a series of prototypes, but, by following Orpwood's suggestions, an assistive device that is adaptable to the user's abilities will result. This adaptability then provides users with control options that best meet their needs and desires.

EVALUATION OF AT INTERVENTION EFFECTIVENESS

The final step in an AT intervention, regardless of whether a device was provided, is judging the effectiveness of the selected option in meeting the goals of the consumer. A complete discussion of outcome measures and functional outcomes is included elsewhere in this book. Outcomes are mentioned here to underscore the importance of the first step in the series: identification of need.

As mentioned at the beginning of this chapter, the criteria that are to be used to judge effectiveness of an AT intervention must be defined early in the process. Similarly, the means by which to measure the criteria should also be defined early. This information, defined in the "Identification of Need" section, is used in the description of the task, the determination of whether a device is indicated; the identification of design criteria; and, of course, the judgment of AT intervention effectiveness. Without a clear definition, many subsequent steps in the process are adversely affected.

RESEARCH IMPLICATIONS

This chapter has described the process used by practitioners in making recommendations for or against the use of AT for people with disabilities. Each step in the process could be improved by the findings of directed research. The linkages between the steps and the fundamental importance of feedback from consumers remains a largely unexplored area. Several aspects of the AT intervention process could benefit from research.

1. Assessment of consumer needs is largely based on qualitative data from subject reports.
    Recommendation: Develop assessment tools for quantifying consumer needs in relation to the intended use of the AT. For example, studies should address the problem of ordering the consumer's needs in light of the potential for fulfilling his or her goals.
2. Measurement of physical and functional capabilities of the consumer are often conducted in laboratory settings with artificial tasks that may or may not have much to do with the individual's ability to perform the tasks for which the device is being considered as an option.
    Recommendation: Research should be directed to develop means to measure physical and functional abilities that are meaningful during AT interventions. For example, studies should be conducted on how much ROM and strength are needed to drive a car, push a wheelchair, operate switches, and so forth.
3. Functional tasks must be better studied to understand commonalities and differences that could be addressed in designing an AT intervention.
    Recommendation: Studies should be made of how many and what different types of function are required for performance of a task. For example, component analysis of tasks such as activities of daily living and instrumental activities of daily living should be made to provide the practitioner with a guide for the breadth of tasks that might be improved through the use of AT.
4. Comparison of human abilities to the task demands as they relate to potential for improved performance through the use of AT remains an underinvestigated field of study.
    Recommendation: A study should be made of the relation between simple functional measures (e.g., hand strength)

and ability to perform the task (e.g., operate a steering wheel) for a set of tasks required of people with impairments (e.g., spinal cord injury, multiple sclerosis, polio, arthritis) that limit capabilities, for the purpose of discovering commonalities and differences.

5. The determination of the benefit of an assistive device is a complex process that depends on a great number of factors, not the least of which is the ratio of frequency of use to the number of problems involved in having the AT with the consumer at all times.

   Recommendation: The "hassle" value of each assistive device should be considered prior to considering the use of AT. Studies are needed to develop the concept of *hassle* and how it can be measured.

6. Establishing criteria for which devices should be considered and the steps involved in selection of a device could benefit from better testing and evaluation protocols that will help to identify ways to characterize the features of the AT.

   Recommendation: Studies should develop standards for a variety of devices (e.g., personal lifts, driving systems, mobility aids, AAC and computer interface devices) that are based on the methods used in the development of wheelchair standards.

7. Final selection of a device from existing options or the decision to develop a new device rests on knowledge of the defining features and characteristics of available devices that have an impact on their usefulness for the needs of each specific consumer. Although the description previously in this chapter of knowing the features of AAC devices and wheelchairs in the context of the tasks for which they are used illustrated the usefulness of this information in selecting an appropriate device, information about many assistive devices is not available.

   Recommendation: Development of information databases for more devices is desirable.

8. Evaluation of the effectiveness of AT intervention is essential for better utilization of assistive technology as a method for improving the performance of people with disabilities in their daily activities.

   Recommendation: Effectiveness studies that relate interventions to a decrease in secondary complications or to an increase in productivity are needed and should be given a high priority. These studies must emphasize external validity to have clinical impact.

REFERENCES

Abdel-Moty, E., & Khalil, T.M. (1989). Computer-aided design and analysis of the sitting workplace for the disabled. *International Disabilities Studies*, *13*,121–124.

Boone, D.C., Azen, S.P., Lin, C.M., Spence, C., Baron, C., & Lee, L. (1978). Reliability of goniometric measurements. *Physical Therapy*, *58*(11), 1355–1360.

Clarkson, H. (1989). *Musculoskeletal assessment: Joint range of motion and manual muscle strength*. Baltimore: Williams & Wilkins.

Cook, A.M., & Hussey, S.M. (1995). *Assitive technologies: Principles and practice*. St. Louis: C.V. Mosby.

Ferguson-Pell, M.W. (1990, March). Seat cushion selection. *Journal of Rehabilitation Research and Development, Clinical Supplement 2*, 49–73.

Fish, D.R., & Wingate, L. (1987). Sources of goniometric error at the elbow. *Physical Therapy*, *65*, 1666–1670.

Garrett, R., Andrews, P., Olsson, C., & Seeger, B. (1990). Development of a computer-based expert system for the selection of assistive communication devices. In *Proceedings of the 13th Annual RESNA Conference* (pp. 348–349). Arlington, VA: RESNA Press.

Gogia, P.P., Bratz, J.H., Rose, S.J., & Norton, B.J. (1987). Reliability and validity of goniometric measurements of the knee. *Physical Therapy*, *67*(2), 192–195.

Goodenough-Trepagnier, C., Rosen, M., Minneman, C., Chen, K., Felts, T., & Chung, G. (1985). A needs–features spreadsheet for communication device prescription. In *Proceedings of the 8th Annual RESNA Conference* (pp. 332–334). Arlington, VA: RESNA Press.

Hamilton, G.F., & Lachenbruch, P.A. (1969). Reliability of goniometers in assessing finger joint angle. *Physical Therapy*, *49*, 465.

Hughes, C.J., Weimar, W.H., Sheth, P.N., & Brubaker, C.E. (1992). Biomechanics of wheelchair propulsion as a function of seat position and user-to-chair interface. *Archives of Physical Medicine and Rehabilitation*, *73*, 263–269.

Kapandji, I.A. (1982). *The physiology of the joints: Vol. 1. Upper limb*. New York: Churchill Livingstone.

Kauzlarich, J.J., Thacker, J.G., & McLaurin, C.A. (1985). *Wheelchair tire rolling resistance theory and tests* (REC Report 102-85). Charlottesville: University of Virginia.

Kendall, F.P., McCreary, E.K., & Provance, P.G. (1993). *Muscles: Testing and function* (4th ed.). Baltimore: Williams & Wilkins.

Kondraske, G.V. (1988, September). Rehabilitation engineering: Towards a systematic process. *Engineering in Medicine and Biology Magazine*, 11–15.

Kraat, A., & Silver, M. (1987). *Features of commercially available assistive devices*. Poster chart for the Augmentative Communication Program, Speech and Hearing Center, Queens College, Flushing, NY.

Orpwood, R.D. (1990). Design methodology for aids for the disabled. *Journal of Medical Engineering and Technology*, *14*(1), 2–10.

Owen, J., & House, L. (1984). Decision making processes in augmentative communication. *Journal of Speech and Hearing Disorders*, *49*(1), 18–25.

Payton, O.D., Nelson, G.E., & Ozer, M.N. (1990). *Patient participation in program planning: A manual for therapists.* Philadelphia: F.A. Davis.

Ragnarsson, K.T. (1990, March). Prescription considerations and a comparison of conventional and lightweight wheelchairs. *Journal of Rehabilitation Research and Development, Clinical Supplement 2*, 8–16.

Shane, H., & Bashir, A. (1980). Election criteria for the adoption of an augmentative communication system: Preliminary considerations. *Journal of Speech and Hearing Disorders, 45*(3), 408–413.

Smith, L.K., Iddings, D.M., Spencer, W.A., & Harrington, P.R. (1961). Muscle testing: 1. Description of a numerical index for clinical research. *Physical Therapy Review, 41*, 99–105.

Sprigle, S., Morris, B., Nowachek, G., & Karg, P. (1995). Assessment of the evaluation procedures of drivers with disabilities. *Occupational Therapy Journal of Research, 15*(3), 147–164.

Swanson, G. (1993). Functional outcome report: The next generation in physical therapy reporting. In D.L. Stewart & S.H. Albeln (Eds.), *Documenting functional outcomes in physical therapy* (pp. 101–134). St. Louis: Mosby–Year Book.

SECTION IV

INCORPORATING ASSISTIVE TECHNOLOGY INTO CHILD DEVELOPMENT

CHAPTER 15

Locomotor Experience Facilitates Psychological Functioning

Implications for Assistive Mobility for Young Children

Rosanne Kermoian

Providing mobility devices to young children with physical disabilities reflects the cutting edge of pediatric rehabilitation practice (Dietz, 1995; Wright & Egilson, 1996; Wright-Ott, 1995). The assumption underlying this clinical trend is that self-directed mobility, by expanding children's opportunities to interact with their social and physical world, promotes integration into society at an earlier age.

Theoretical support for this assumption comes from philosophers and psychologists who have long hypothesized about the importance of motor activity for the psychological development of young children. In the cognitive domain, Piaget (1960) theorized that motor activity is the basic building block of knowledge, suggesting that learning is entirely dependent on children's actions on the world. In the perceptual domain, Gibson (1979) proposed that

The research described in this chapter was funded in part by grants from the Oregon Medical Research Foundation, the MacArthur Network on Developmental Transitions, and the John D. and Catherine T. MacArthur Foundation.

The author thanks Christine Wright-Ott and the staff at the Stanford Rehabilitation Engineering Center for sharing their extensive clinical experience and astute clinical insights on the role of mobility in the development of children with physical disabilities.

movement enhances the visual information that children receive, thereby permitting extraction of invariants from the environment. In the emotional domain, psychoanalysts (e.g., Mahler, Pine, & Bergman, 1975; Stern, 1985) hypothesized that mobility sets the stage for increases in the expression of positive and negative emotion and subsequent changes in parent–child relationships as a result of new levels of autonomy.

Despite theoretical interest in the functional consequences of motor activity for psychological development and late 1990s trends in clinical practice, there have been remarkably few empirical investigations of this issue (Kermoian, 1997). Consequently, a number of questions fundamental to both theory and practice remain unanswered. Does motor activity facilitate or induce psychological development? Is motor activity of central importance exclusively during the sensorimotor period of life? What domains of psychological development are affected by motor activity, and what are the mechanisms by which motor activity exerts its effects? For children with physical disabilities, does psychological development fail to occur in the absence of specific motor skills, or are there alternative pathways to development? Research addressing such questions has important theoretical implications for better understanding the processes that drive developmental change and clinical implications for the rational design, use, and justification to third-party payers of assistive technology (AT) for young children.

The fundamental premise of the work presented here is that development in early life occurs as a consequence of the dynamic interplay between children and their environments. Each major motor milestone in early life—reaching, creeping, and walking—thus would be expected to have profound consequences for development by virtue of the fact that all interactions with the world are mediated through motor activity. When children begin to reach, for example, the world on which they can act expands to just beyond arm's length (Rochat, 1992); when they begin to locomote, the world on which they can act expands to as far as they can crawl or walk (Kermoian, in press). Each new motor acquisition, therefore, should serve as a nodal skill that generates myriad new experiences and demands that, in turn, result in specific gains in cognitive, perceptual, and socioemotional functioning (Campos, Kermoian, & Witherington, 1995).

EFFECTS OF MOBILITY ONSET
ON PSYCHOLOGICAL FUNCTIONING

In the 1990s, it has become clear that the onset of one motor skill, hands-and-knees creeping, facilitates widespread important changes in infant psychological functioning. Among the changes that have been identified, there is evidence that mobility can bring about heightened sensitivity to objects or events beyond arm's reach and increases in goal-oriented behavior that are mirrored by concomitant increases in parental expectations of their infants and new patterns of communication.

The evidence that locomotor experience facilitates development and is not merely a correlate of change in these domains comes from converging study results provided by two research designs:

1. Findings from studies using an age-held-constant design reveal that *locomotor* infants perform at higher levels than *prelocomotor* infants of the same age.
2. Findings from studies using an enrichment research design, in which prelocomotor infants have the artificially induced experience of moving in a baby walker, reveal that *prelocomotor* infants with walker experience perform more similarly to *locomotor* infants than to *prelocomotor* infants without walker experience of the same age.

Effects in Typically Developing Infants

Heightened Sensitivity to Objects or Events Beyond Arm's Reach
With the onset of locomotion, we propose that the expansion of infants' functional space to locations beyond arm's reach results in more differentiated responding to objects or events in distant space. Support for this hypothesis comes from studies that demonstrate that locomotor infants need less visual stimulation for postural control than do prelocomotor infants (Higgins, Campos, & Kermoian, 1996; Witherington, Campos, & Kermoian, 1995). At 7 months of age, infants can coordinate visual stimulation with vestibular stimulation to control their posture in a seated position. However, the amount of visual stimulation needed must fill the entire visual field: The infants' responses to partial optic flow fields remain undifferentiated (Bertenthal & Bai, 1989; Higgins et al., 1996), despite their ability to perceive motion (Aslin & Shea, 1990; Bertenthal & Bradbury, 1992) and their muscular ability to make postural adjustments (Bertenthal & Bai, 1989). In contrast, by 9 months of age, infants' visual–vestibular coordination becomes less diffuse. Infants establish more specific visual–vestibular relations in which specific patterns of optic flow, such as peripheral optic flow, are associated with specific patterns of vestibular information. These coordinations serve to improve postural control in a seated position, which in turn permits infants to use their arms freely to reach for and explore objects.

Findings from two studies show that locomotor experience facilitates the process of coordinating spatially delimited portions of the visual field with vestibular information for postural control in 8-month-old infants (Higgins et al., 1996; Witherington et al., 1995). Postural control was measured with the infants seated in a "moving room" apparatus, a small enclosure with moveable walls designed to induce the illusion of self-motion. As seen in Figure 1, all infants, regardless of locomotor status, adjusted their posture in a coordinated response with the movement of the walls when the whole room moved around them, creating global optic flow. In contrast, locomotor infants were significantly more likely than prelocomotor infants to adjust their posture in a coordinated response with the movement of the walls when only the side walls of the room moved, creating peripheral optic flow.

In summary, these findings suggested that locomoting on hands and knees or in a walker sensitizes infants to peripheral optic flow information, and this information becomes correlated with vestibular stimulation specifying self-motion that is used for postural control. Locomotor experience may effect this change in infant visual proprioception as a consequence of the infants' increased

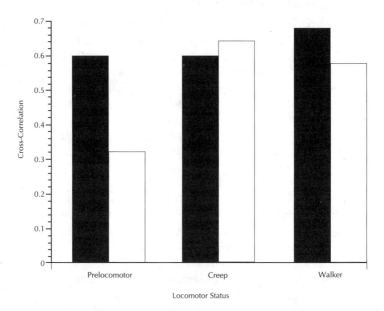

Figure 1. Magnitude of directional and temporal coordination between infants' postural adjustments and wall movement (cross-correlation) under conditions of whole-room movement (global optic flow) and side wall movement (peripheral optic flow), by locomotor status. (■, whole room; □, side walls.)

need to relate specific patterns of optic flow to their own movements in order to maintain their posture while moving and their need to simultaneously monitor their own motion in space as well as the independent movement of objects in the environment to avoid collisions (Bertenthal & Bai, 1989).

Locomotor infants showed a similar heightened sensitivity to locations beyond arm's reach in a laboratory investigation of spontaneous attentional deployment (Freedman & Kermoian, 1993). In this study, attentional deployment was measured in 8-month-old infants who were seated in front of an illuminated display box in a dimly lit room. Infants could explore a novel object within their reach visually, manually, or both, and could visually explore one of three novel objects beyond arm's reach during a brief 60-second trial. Although locomotor and prelocomotor infants did not differ significantly in the duration of time they spent looking to areas beyond arm's reach, the object of attention in distant space differed greatly as a function of locomotor experience. As seen in Figure 2, infants who had experience locomoting, either on hands and knees or in a walker, directed a significantly higher percentage of distal-looking time preferentially to novel objects beyond arm's reach (i.e., look far) than did prelocomotor infants, who, surprisingly, were just as likely to look to the novel objects as to the walls, floor, or ceiling (i.e., look away).

Locomoting independently through space may facilitate infants' understanding of the attention-worthy aspects of distant

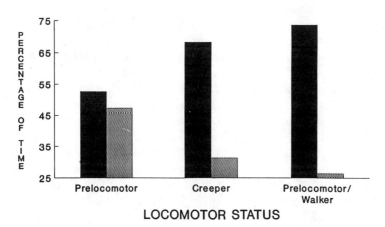

Figure 2.   Percentage of distal-looking time during which infants looked to novel objects beyond arms' reach (i.e., look far) versus the ceiling, walls, or floor (i.e., look away), by locomotor status. (■, look far; ▨, look away.)

space by providing them with experiences that lead them to characterize floors, walls, and ceilings as stable and unchanging. Thus, when placed in an unfamiliar room, infants ignore those features that they have come to expect to be invariant and deploy their attention instead to objects that are novel and potentially manipulable or moveable.

It would seem that, although objects or events in distant space are visually available to prelocomotor infants, the implications of these objects or events for the infants' own activity have yet to be established through action. This explanation is supported by evidence of increased sensitivity of locomotor infants to objects or events beyond arm's reach in the naturalistic setting of the home (Campos, Kermoian, & Zumbahlen, 1992). Parents of 8-month-old locomotor infants were significantly more likely than parents of prelocomotor infants to report that their infants attended to distal events (90% versus 29%), that their infants responded to their departure from the room (71% versus 33%), and that their infants spontaneously checked back with them in situations in which they had previously prohibited their infants or had attempted to get their infants to comply with a request (68% versus 7%).

Taken overall, the more differentiated response of locomotor infants to nonsocial and social events beyond arm's reach is consistent with Gibson's (1979) ecological approach to visual perception. In Gibson's conceptualization, the characteristics of objects or events that are located in distant space afford locomotor infants with information that directly specifies the structures of the environment and the relevance of these structures to their own activities. Although the perceptual correlates of these functional properties of objects or events in distant space are undoubtedly perceived by prelocomotor infants, their implications for the infants' own activity have yet to be established through action.

Increases in Goal-Oriented Behavior   With the onset of locomotion, we propose that changes in goal orientation will arise from the new demands associated with setting and attaining goals that are distant from oneself in time and space (Freedman & Kermoian, 1993). First, locomotor infants are more likely than prelocomotor infants to need to establish goals as a way of organizing the vast number of opportunities that are available to them. Second, locomotor infants are more likely than prelocomotor infants to have experiences in which there is disassociation in time between goal setting and goal attainment. Specifically, when locomoting infants have a goal located in distant space, they must keep the goal in mind and resist distractions for the duration of the time it takes them to locomote to it. Third, locomotor infants are more likely than prelocomotor infants to encounter obstacles to goal attainment and have the need to use multiple means to overcome such obstacles. If these three changes in goal setting and goal attainment follow locomotor onset, then locomotor infants should be more likely than prelocomotor infants to persist in attempts to achieve their goals, even in the face of distraction, and more likely to express frustration when their goals are blocked. In summary, the experiences encountered while locomoting are likely to increase the infants' goal orientation and understanding of self as an intentional being, thereby resulting in major shifts in the infants' expression of negative affect and in their social interaction (Campos, Mumme, Kermoian, & Campos, 1994).

Support for the hypothesis that changes in goal orientation follow the onset of locomotion comes from a study in which locomotor infants were significantly more likely than prelocomotor infants to display negative affect when their goal-directed activity was blocked and to direct their anger to the source of frustration (Lloyd, Kermoian, & Campos, 1994). In this study, an examiner blocked the goal-directed activity of 8-month-old infants by placing an attractive toy that the infants were reaching toward behind a barrier for three 20-second trials. The infants' expressions of positive and negative affect were then indexed by composite scores formed from measures of facial, vocal, and postural responses during the first 5 seconds of each trial.

Locomotor infants displayed significantly more negative affect than prelocomotor infants of the same age when the toy was placed behind a barrier (mean of .84 versus .08) and were significantly more likely to look to the examiner when expressing negative affect (mean of 1.0 versus .27). The two groups did not differ in affective expression during a control condition or in the total number of times that they looked at the examiner when the toy was behind the barrier, indicating that the difference between groups was not due to baseline differences in affective expression or willingness to look at the examiner.

This increase in the expression of negative affect in locomotor infants was also observed in the naturalistic setting of the home. Significantly more parents of locomotor infants reported an increase in the expression of anger by their infants than did parents of prelocomotor infants (89% versus 40%) (Campos et al., 1992). Subsequent discussion with parents confirmed that locomotor infants typically manifested anger when frustrated in an attempt to reach or maintain a goal and that their displays of displeasure were intense. For example, locomotor infants were no longer content to accept another object or activity in place of the one they were unable to reach or partake in and expressed their displeasure by screaming or having tantrums.

Changes in Parental Expectations and Communications   As parents observe their children's increasing goal orientation, they attribute to their infants a new form of purposefulness and expect their infants to begin assuming responsibility for their own actions (Campos et al., 1992). Parents of locomotor infants were significantly more likely to spontaneously report that they expected their infants to comply with their rules than were parents of prelocomotor infants (69% versus 23%). The frequency and manner in which parents of locomotor infants attempted to communicate their expectations to their infants also differed significantly from those of parents of prelocomotor infants: Every parent of a locomotor infant reported using verbal prohibitions, compared with 60% of parents of prelocomotor infants. They also reported an increase in the use of their voice for disciplinary purposes significantly more often than did parents of prelocomotor infants (75% versus 18%).

A striking change reported by parents of locomotor infants involved the use of anger to regulate their infants' behavior (Campos et al., 1992). Significantly more parents of locomotor infants reported expressing verbal anger when prohibiting their infants than did parents of prelocomotor infants (90% versus 50%), with some parents noting that the onset of crawling marked the first time that they had expressed anger toward their infants. Some parents of locomotor infants (39%) reported that their anger extended to physical punishment in response to repeated infant infractions of parental rules, such as when their infants repeatedly touched the oven door or carried off the remote control despite numerous warnings, whereas no parents of prelocomotor infants reported using physical punishment. In summary, significant changes are seen in the affective climate of the family following locomotor onset, with parents beginning to treat their infants as autonomous individuals who are responsible for their actions.

Summary   Locomotor experience is composed of many new experiences that have specific consequences for development. Although gains occur in a number of separate domains of psychological functioning, including sensitivity to objects or events beyond arm's reach and increases in goal orientation, each behavioral development reflects a step-function increase in the child behaving as an agent in the physical and social world that is mirrored by increases in parental expectations. In summary, mobility seems to exert its effect on development by providing infants with new means by which they can actively construct their world as well as by providing new physical and social contexts for these acts (Bidell & Fischer, 1996; Fischer & Hencke, 1996).

Effects in Children with Locomotor Disabilities

If the onset of mobility facilitates development by greatly increasing the probability that specific new infant–environment transactions will occur, then one would predict that young children who are delayed in the onset of mobility would be less likely to have such experiences and that specific developments, therefore, would likely be delayed. This hypothesis is supported by clinical reports of dramatic behavior change associated with the use of mobility aids by preschool and school-age children who have physical disabilities severe enough to preclude the onset of locomotion. Such reports include large increases in engagement in the social and physical world, such as greater curiosity and more exploratory behavior (e.g., Butler, Okamoto, & McKay, 1983), and equally large gains in children's autonomy following locomotor onset with a mobility device. Children are described as more self-confident, more independent, more likely to express opinions and desires, more likely to make choices, and naughtier (e.g., Thiers, 1994; Trefler & Taylor, 1987).

It is particularly intriguing that the reported changes following self-directed mobility in children with motor disabilities are strikingly similar to those identified in infants following locomotor onset: Self-directed mobility seems to bring with it a more mature understanding of the self as an actor in the world with independent wishes and wants that extend across time and space. Although further work is needed to confirm these initial clinical investigations, this pattern of greater engagement in the world is in clear contrast to the marked passivity reported for people who reach adolescence or adulthood without an opportunity for self-directed mobility (Becker, 1975; McDermott & Akina, 1972). Such individuals are described as helpless even in conditions in which their disability per se does not interfere with the activity in which they are engaged— behavior that is not consistent with increasing societal interest in fostering independence and greater integration into the community for individuals with disabilities.

Conclusions

Self-directed mobility brings with it a complex experiential package that seems to greatly facilitate specific and enduring changes in infants both with and without a locomotor disability. Although it is unlikely that self-directed mobility is necessary for change, the experiences associated with self-directed mobility appear to be particularly powerful because they both increase children's exposure to sensory stimulation and provide an environmental press to attend to and organize this new sensory input. As children adapt to these experiences, their behavior changes, and, in turn, they are perceived and responded to by others as more mature and autonomous.

BARRIERS TO MOBILITY DEVICE USE BY YOUNG CHILDREN

If locomotor experience is a powerful facilitator of early psychological development, then the most direct means of preventing delays in psychological development is to provide independent mobility as close to the normative age of locomotor onset as possible. Indeed, in the 1990s, there has been an increased interest in providing mobility aids to young children with locomotor disabilities. This trend is reflected by a sharp increase in the types of manual and powered mobility devices available for use by young children (Taylor & Monahan, 1988; Trefler & Marcrum, 1987; Wright, 1993; Wright & Bigge, 1991), by an increase in the number of schools and therapy units adopting intervention programs that promote assisted mobility (e.g., Project Move [Thiers, 1994]), and by newly developed assessments for young children with disabilities that are designed to evaluate children's mobility in assistive devices (McNeal, 1994; Tefft, Furumasu, & Guerette, 1995; Wolf, Massagli, Jaffe, & Deitz, 1991). An increased interest in assistive mobility devices for children is also reflected at the federal level in law (e.g., Technology-Related Assistance for Individuals with Disabilities Act of 1988 [PL 100-407]) and in the priorities of the National Center for Medical Rehabilitation Research (1993).

Despite an increased interest in providing early mobility, few children are given mobility aids. Even children whose motor involvement is severe enough that the prognosis of ambulation is poor typically do not have an opportunity to use a mobility aid until they receive their first power wheelchair. This does not occur until 10.3 years of age, on average (Wright, 1993), and is frequently preceded by months or even years of therapy devoted to wheelchair driver training.

The most significant barriers to young children attaining mobility devices have been concerns about the cost-effectiveness of devices, the potential motivational changes in children who use assistive devices, and the safety of mobility devices. The lack of empirical data needed to evaluate each of these concerns highlights the importance of research that is designed to inform treatment decisions.

Cost-Effectiveness

Given the rising costs of health care and the likelihood that assistive equipment that is acquired will not be used, it is particularly important that the costs of providing devices to young children, who can rapidly outgrow equipment, be compared to the benefits. Butler (1988), Colangelo (1994), and Thiers (1994), among others, have suggested that early assisted mobility will reduce the personal and societal cost of disability by increasing children's independence and the probability of integration into the community at an earlier age; however, empirical data are needed to test this hypothesis. The encouraging findings from basic research and clinical investigations on the effects of mobility to date suggest that cost-effectiveness studies are worth pursuing.

Motivation

Many clinicians are concerned that the ease with which children can move in assistive devices will reduce their motivation to move independently and thereby interfere with therapeutic goals for motor development (Trefler & Marcrum, 1987). Although it is possible that using a mobility aid may lessen children's motivation to move independently, a study by Paulsson and Christofferson (1984) found that moving in a device seemed to increase children's motivation to move. The author's clinical impression is consistent with the latter hypothesis. The author has observed a number of children who, after moving in a powered mobility device for several hours in a therapy setting, have returned home and moved in their manual mobility aid for the first time, even though moving in the manual aid is much more effortful than moving in the powered device. The parents of these children reported that their children struggled to move in their manual device because they wanted to go places and do things by themselves. These reports suggest that brief exposure to self-directed mobility may increase children's motivation to move by helping them establish the critical link between independent movement and attainment of goals in the same way in which sign language, although much less motorically demanding than vocal communication, can facilitate the onset of speech (Acredolo & Goodwyn, 1996). Clearly, empirical data are needed to address this important issue.

Safety

It is extremely important that mobility devices do not exacerbate children's physical problems or create new physical problems. Although this has been a primary reason that therapists have been reluctant to recommend that young children use mobility devices, these concerns have been diminishing in the 1990s because of the wide range of devices on the market that have been designed for children with specific diagnoses (Wright & Egilson, 1996). Thus, it is increasingly possible to find mobility devices that do not interfere with therapeutic goals.

Although locating an appropriate mobility device is less problematic than it once was, there are still many unanswered questions regarding young children's abilities to navigate safely. Ironically, many skills that are thought to be essential to the successful and safe use of AT overlap with those that are typically learned via early mobility (Berhmann, Jones, & Wilds, 1989; Schiaffino & Laux, 1986). Intentional behavior and the ability to make independent choices, for example, are skills that have been proposed as essential to safe mobility and are facilitated by mobility. If children cannnot drive a power wheelchair safely unless they have acquired these fundamental skills, and if such skills are usually gained via locomotor experience, then young children with physical disabilities and their parents, teachers, and therapists are confronted with a problem for which there is no obvious solution, a Catch-22.[1]

Extrapolating from the experiences infants have when they first begin to locomote on hands and knees or in a walker, it may be possible to help young children with disabilities acquire safe mobility, and the skills gained via mobility, by designing mobility devices that are limited in initial function but that increase in function with gains in psychological competence. A second way that it may be possible to support safe assistive mobility skill acquisition via mobility is to devise training experiences that provide high levels of feedback from the physical and social environment.

DESIGNING MOBILITY DEVICES THAT GROW IN SIZE AND FUNCTION

Increasingly, children's mobility devices are being designed to meet the physical requirements of childhood: They are lightweight, sta-

---

[1]Although locomotor experience is possibly the most common route to gaining specific psychological skills, it seems unlikely that locomotor experience is necessary for development. Indeed, some children learn to drive a power wheelchair safely with minimal training as young as 36 months of age (e.g., Butler, 1986). The majority of children who can benefit from mobility aids, however, have mutiple disabilities (e.g., visual impairments, cognitive limitations) in addition to delays in locomotor onset that make safe mobility and the skills generally gained via mobility potentially more difficult to learn.

ble, and durable and can be adapted to rapid changes in physical growth (Wright & Egilson, 1996). In contrast to the attention that has been given to designing devices that can adapt to the physical requirements of childhood, minimal attention has been given to designing devices that meet the changing psychological needs and competencies of childhood.

One exciting model for the design of mobility devices that "grow" with psychological development comes from rehabilitation engineering approaches to the design of upper-body prostheses for infants and children. The design goal for many of these devices has been to create a prosthesis that is simple enough to be mastered by young children, yet complex enough to permit those interactions with the environment that are essential precursors to more mature patterns of adaptation. Thus, a prosthetic hand that permits just one form of grasp, the pincer grasp, limits the possible degrees of freedom of movement yet maintains the essential psychological function of grasp—object manipulation. With age and experience, as the functional requirements of the child increase, additional grasp capabilities can be added. Hu, Naumann, Cleghorn, and Reid (1996), for example, began the process of designing a prosthetic hand for children by identifying the functional requirements, control ability, and grasping patterns of able-bodied children of different ages. Based on these data, they are now designing a hand that provides pincer grasp capabilities to children under the age of 7. With children's increasing age, three additional grasp capabilities will be added to permit more sophisticated interaction with objects—specifically, better orientation of the object held for use, improved stability of the object being held, and minimized compensatory motions during prehension.

Designing mobility devices for young children presents even greater challenges than those of upper-body prostheses. Mobility not only serves more diverse functions than prehension but also, when uncontrolled, is more dangerous to the child and the immediate physical and social environment. Manual mobility devices and transitional powered devices, such as motorized toy cars or power standing frames, have been a creative solution to providing young children with a means of independent movement without the complexity and cost of a power wheelchair (see Chapters 16 and 17). These devices differ greatly from one another, and, to date, there have been no attempts to evaluate them for the degree to which they permit self-directed movement or the degree to which they maximize psychological development. Developing guidelines for the design of assistive mobility devices for young children and evaluating the effects of these devices on children's physical and psychological development thus remain important issues open for fruitful collaboration between clinicians and basic researchers.

INTRODUCING MOBILITY AIDS
TO INFANTS AND YOUNG CHILDREN

In contrast to the efforts that have been made to identify the prerequisite skills that children must have to be safe wheelchair drivers, little effort has been directed toward identifying features of the environment that are likely to support or to hinder the transition to safe wheelchair driving. Able-bodied infants learn the skill of hands-and-knees creeping or moving in a baby walker in a rich physical and social context. When infants do not simultaneously monitor their own motion in space as well as the independent movement of objects in the environment, for example, they are likely to collide with objects in their path. The experience of inattention and subsequent collision is associated with physical pain, parental anger when furniture is damaged, and fear when the dog growls after being hit. Although newly locomoting infants indeed do collide with people and objects, each of the many experiences associated with collision make the need for visual vigilance more personally relevant and subsequent lapses of attention less likely to occur.

If context is as important for the transition to mobility as suggested by findings to date on the transition to mobility in able-bodied infants, then it may be possible to scaffold the performance of young children who are being introduced to assistive mobility by increasing the salience of critical features of the environment. Given that prelocomotor children are not particularly sensitive to objects or events beyond arm's reach, exaggerating specific perceptual cues in the environment to which they are unlikely to attend may help children become safe wheelchair drivers. In clinical practice, children typically are introduced to mobility devices in a decontextualized environment, such as a play area or large room, so that they will not collide with objects or experience frustration when their attempts to control the device fail. However, providing a highly contextualized environment in the form of a clearly demarcated asphalt path is more likely to result in self-directed forward movement than is an open field setting. Presumably, the dark surface of the path draws the children's visual attention downward, and the optical flow texture provided by the parallel edges of the path provides perceptual cues of self-movement that are sufficient to permit continuous forward progression. In summary, identifying the physical and social features of the environment that can regulate behavior in able-bodied infants and then increasing the salience of these environmental cues may provide useful, albeit sometimes counterintuitive, training strategies for the transition to safe mobility.

FUTURE DIRECTIONS

The years ahead provide a unique window of opportunity for clinical practice to inform research and for research to inform clinical practice. Increasingly, very young children with physical disabilities are receiving mobility aids; however, the potential effects of this practice are somewhat controversial and remain largely unstudied (Butler, 1988; Trefler & Taylor, 1987). This lack of empirical data on which to base treatment decisions suggests an immediate and profound need for systematic research that evaluates the effects of mobility devices on the development of children with different diagnoses. There is an equally compelling need, however, for basic research that goes beyond studies that demonstrate a link between mobility and psychological functioning to research that specifies the mechanisms by which mobility exerts such powerful effects on development. Knowledge gained from clinical practice and from research, jointly considered, can provide a powerful rational base from which to design AT devices and early interventions that assist children in reaching their full neurobehavioral potential.

REFERENCES

Acredolo, L., & Goodwyn, S. (1996). *Baby signs: How to talk with your baby before your baby can talk.* Chicago: Contemporary Books.

Aslin, R.N., & Shea, S.L. (1990). Velocity thresholds in human infants: Implications for the perception of motion. *Developmental Psychology, 26,* 589–598.

Becker, R.D. (1975). Recent developments in child psychiatry: 1. The restrictive emotional and cognitive environment reconsidered: A redefinition of the concept of therapeutic restraint. *Israel Annals of Psychiatry, 13,* 239.

Berhmann, M.M., Jones, J.K., & Wilds, M.L. (1989). Technology intervention for very young children with disabilities. *Infants and Young Children, 1,* 66–77.

Bertenthal, B., & Bai, D. (1989). Infants' sensitivity to optic flow for controlling posture. *Developmental Psychology, 25,* 936–945.

Bertenthal, B., & Bradbury, A. (1992). Infants' detection of shearing motion in random-dot displays. *Developmental Psychology, 28,* 1056–1066.

Bidell, T.R., & Fischer, K.W. (1996). Between nature and nurture: The role of human agency in the epigenesis of intelligence. In R. Sternberg & E. Grigorenko (Eds.), *Intelligence: Heredity and environment* (pp. 193–242). Cambridge, England: Cambridge University Press.

Butler, C. (1986). Effects of powered mobility on self-initiated behaviors of very young children with locomotor disability. *Developmental Medicine and Child Neurology, 28,* 472–474.

Butler, C. (1988). High tech tots: Technology for mobility manipulation, communication, and learning in early childhood. *Infants and Young Children, 2,* 66–73.

Butler, C., Okamoto, G., & McKay, T. (1983). Powered mobility for very young disabled children. *Developmental Medicine and Child Neurology, 25,* 472–474.

Campos, J., Kermoian, R., & Witherington, D. (1995). The epigenesis of emotion in infancy. In R. Kavanaugh, B. Zimmerberg-Glick, & S. Fein (Eds.), *Emotion: Interdisciplinary perspectives* (pp. 119–138). Hillsdale, NJ: Lawrence Erlbaum Associates.

Campos, J., Kermoian, R., & Zumbahlen, M. (1992). Socio-emotional transformations in the family system following infant crawling onset. In N. Eisenberg & R. Fabes (Eds.), *New directions for child development: No. 55. Emotion and its regulation in early development* (pp. 25–40). San Francisco: Jossey-Bass.

Campos, J., Mumme, D., Kermoian, R., & Campos, R. (1994). A functionalist perspective on the development of emotion. *Monographs of the Society for Research in Child Development, 59*(2-3, Serial No. 240), 284–303.

Colangelo, C. (1994). Powered mobility and the child with cerebral palsy. *Advance/Rehabilitation, 3*(7).

Deitz, J. (1995, April). *Mobility devices and play.* Paper presented at the Conference on Behavioral Adaptation to the Use of Assistive Technology: Enhancing Human Movement in the 21st Century for People with Disabilities, Baltimore.

Fischer, K.W., & Hencke, R.W. (1996). Infants' construction of actions in context: Piaget's contribution to research on early development. *Psychological Science, 7*(4), 204–210.

Freedman, D., & Kermoian, R. (1993, March). *Locomotor experience and deployment of attention to near and distant space.* Paper presented at the meeting of the Society for Research in Child Development, New Orleans.

Gibson, J.J. (1979). *The ecological approach to visual perception.* Boston: Houghton Mifflin.

Higgins, C., Campos, J., & Kermoian, R. (1996). Effect of self-produced locomotion on infant postural compensation to optic flow. *Developmental Psychology, 32,* 836–841.

Hu, P., Naumann, S., Cleghorn, W., & Reid, D. (1996). *Development of a multi-degree of freedom prosthetic hand for child user* (Annual Report No. 1995-6, Rehabilitation Engineering Department). Toronto, Ontario, Canada: Bloorview Macmillan Centre.

Kermoian, R. (1997). Locomotor experience and psychological development in infancy. In J. Furamasu (Ed.), *Childhood powered mobility: Developmental, technical, and clinical perspectives* (pp. 7–21). Washington, DC: RESNA Press.

Lloyd, R., Kermoian, R., & Campos, J. (1994, June). *Effects of locomotor experience on emotional display during a manual detour search task.* Paper presented at the Ninth International Conference on Infant Studies, Paris.

Mahler, M., Pine, F., & Bergman, A. (1975). *The psychological birth of the human infant.* New York: Basic Books.

McDermott, J.F., & Akina, E. (1972). Understanding and improving the personality development of children with physical handicaps. *Clinical Pediatrics, 11*, 134.

McNeal, D. (1994). RERC on technology for children with orthopedic disabilities. *Technology and Disability, 3*, 307–339.

National Center for Medical Rehabilitation Research. (1993). *Research plan for the National Center for Medical Rehabilitation Research* (NIH Publication No. 93-3509). Washington, DC: National Institute of Child Health and Human Development.

Paulsson, K., & Christofferson, M. (1984). Psychosocial aspects of technical aids: How does independent mobility affect the psychosocial and intellectual development of children with physical disability? In *Proceedings of the 2nd International Conference on Rehabilitation Engineering* (pp. 282–286). Washington, DC: RESNA Press.

Piaget, J. (1960). *The psychology of intelligence.* Paterson, NJ: Littlefield, Adams & Co.

Rochat, P. (1992). Self-sitting and reaching in 5- to 8-month-old infants: The impact of posture and its development on early eye–hand coordination. *Journal of Motor Behavior, 24*, 210–220.

Schiaffino, S., & Laux, J. (1986, June). Prerequisite skills for psychosocial impact of powered wheelchair mobility on young children with severe handicaps. *Developmental Disabilities, 9*, 1.

Stern, D.N. (1985). *The interpersonal world of the infant.* New York: Basic Books.

Taylor, S., & Monahan, L. (1988). *Considerations in assessing for powered mobility.* Washington, DC: RESNA Press.

Technology-Related Assistance for Individuals with Disabilities Act of 1988, PL 100-407, 29 U.S.C. §§ 2201 *et seq.*

Tefft, D., Furumasu, J., & Guerette, P. (1995, February). *Powered mobility and young children.* Paper presented at the Eleventh International Seating Symposium, Pittsburgh.

Thiers, N. (1994, May). Hope for rehab's forgotten child. *OT Week*, 16–18.

Trefler, E., & Marcrum, J. (1987). Trends in powered mobility for school aged physically handicapped children. In K. Jaffe (Ed.), *Childhood powered mobility: Developmental, technical, and clinical perspectives: Proceedings of the RESNA First Northwest Regional Conference* (pp. 510–511). Washington, DC: RESNA Press.

Trefler, E., & Taylor, S. (1987). Powered mobility for severely disabled children: Evaluation and provision practices. In K. Jaffe (Ed.), *Childhood powered mobility: Developmental, technical, and clinical perspectives: Proceedings of the RESNA First Northwest Regional Conference* (pp. 117–126). Washington, DC: RESNA Press.

Witherington, D., Campos, J., & Kermoian, R. (1995, March). *What makes infants become wary of heights?* Paper presented at the meeting of the Society for Research in Child Development, Indianapolis, IN.

Wolf, L., Massagli, T., Jaffe, K., & Deitz, J. (1991). Functional assessment of the Joncare Hi-Lo Mater power wheelchair for children. *Physical and Occupational Therapy in Pediatrics, 11*, 57–72.

Wright, C. (1993). *Engineering the environment to provide mobility experiences for young children with disabilities.* Paper presented at the RESNA 16th Annual Conference, Las Vegas, NV.

Wright, C., & Bigge, J. (1991). Avenues to physical participation. In J.L. Bigge (Ed.), *Teaching individuals with physical and multiple handicaps* (pp. 132–174). New York: Macmillan.

Wright, C., & Egilson, S. (1996). Mobility. In J. Case-Smith, A. Allen, & P. Pratt (Eds.), *Occupational therapy for children* (3rd ed., pp. 562–580). St. Louis: Mosby–Year Book.

Wright-Ott, C. (1995, April). *Human factors consideration in product design.* Paper presented at the Conference on Behavioral Adaptation to the Use of Assistive Technology: Enhancing Human Movement in the 21st Century for People with Disabilities, Baltimore.

CHAPTER 16

Pediatric Augmented Mobility

Jean Crosetto Deitz

The design and implementation of pediatric mobility devices merit evaluation relative to the development of the infant's or child's attitudes (perception of self as a person who has control); the addressing of the parent's or care provider's attitudes and concerns; the enhancement of the infant's or child's perceptual and cognitive skills; and the adjustment and inclusion of the infant or child with a mobility impairment within the family, the school, and the community. This evaluation requires a developmental perspective specific to the three domains of human occupation: self-care, school, and play and leisure.

MOBILITY AND THE DEVELOPMENT OF ATTITUDES

Children's Attitudes

When we know a child has a severe motor impairment that has an impact on mobility, how young or at what developmental level should we introduce a mobility device? Many children with disabilities, especially those without parents or other adults who aggressively advocate for them, spend their first 5 or more years without a mobility device that they can control independently. Thus, their movement typically is controlled by adults in their environments, especially if the children also have communication impairments. This practice seems contrary to findings in the literature suggesting feasibility and possible benefits of earlier introduction of mobility technology.

By age 7 or 8 months, children who are typically developing begin to crawl and creep, and, through this movement, environmental exploration is potentiated. They learn that they can control their movement and, in many cases, the environment. Butler, studying the effects of power mobility on young children, noted that onset of a passive-dependent pattern "coincided with failure of the normal development of locomotion about 12 months of age, and was increasingly manifested as inhibited locomotion progressively interfered with normal childhood activities" (1986, p. 325).

Systematic observation of young infants with motor impairments may demonstrate that the restricting influences of inhibited locomotion begin even earlier than 12 months of age. In consequence, the development, testing, and use of alternative forms of mobility as an important aspect of therapeutic intervention should be explored. The feasibility of using switch-activated forms of mobility for infants with motor impairments is suggested by the research of Glickman, Deitz, Anson, and Stewart (1996) and Swinth, Anson, and Deitz (1993). The former study suggested that the majority of infants who are typically developing and between ages 6 and 9 months can access a computer by using a hand switch to play a simple cause-and-effect game, whereas in the latter study only one third of the infants ages 9–11 months demonstrated competency in accessing a computer by using a head switch to play a cause-and-effect game. Although the results from this research suggest that use of a head switch is more difficult than use of a hand switch, some infants less than 1 year of age in both conditions were successful in using switch controls. Therefore, it seems feasible for infants with motor impairments to use similar controls to activate specially designed mobility devices, thus allowing for self-initiated movement experiences.

Parents' and Care Providers' Attitudes and Concerns

Often parents of young children with disabilities are still involved in the grieving process. They view power mobility in traditional designs as a sign of disability and additional confirmation that their children will not walk. This attitude is further confirmed by the wheelchair being an international symbol for disability. Health care providers and researchers need to be sensitive to this concern and to consider two strategies: 1) methods for introducing mobility device use in ways that facilitate the family's transition from use of mobility devices powered by family members to use of mobility devices operated by infants and children, and 2) design and evaluation of new mobility devices specifically created to meet the needs of infants and young children with disabilities and their families. For example, relative to the former, Butler (1991) suggested that, following diagnosis, professionals should begin to educate parents that the primary issue is not whether their child will walk, but rather how to provide a variety of mobility options to facilitate the overall development of the child. The potential impact of this refocusing of priorities merits examination relative to parent acceptance, understanding, and implementation of alternative mobility options for their children with mobility impairments.

Relative to the design and evaluation of new mobility devices sensitive to parents' or care providers' attitudes and concerns, the question of whether the use of mobility toys as transitional mobility devices encourages earlier parent or care provider acceptance of the devices should be addressed. Also, the development and use of devices with a more playful appearance could be studied relative to parent or care provider acceptance.

In clinical practice, some parents who resist traditional power mobility devices for their children, especially those with some ambulatory potential, readily embrace the use of power mobility toys such as motorized cars that enable mobility play with peers on school playgrounds and in neighborhoods. One mother of a child with whom I have worked initially resisted power mobility for her child after explaining her concerns that the sight of a person using a wheelchair communicates disability. However, witnessing her child's success and increased abilities when supplied with a mobility toy, the mother pursued power mobility for her daughter. Anecdotally, other therapists describe similar experiences, thus suggesting the need to explore attitudes relating to power wheelchairs and disability and methods for introducing wheeled mobility to children and their families.

In conjunction with this, it is important not only to examine parental attitudes regarding wheeled mobility for their children but also to examine parent and teacher perceptions of children with mobility impairments when the children are using augmented mobility. Kermoian suggests that parents respond differently to their children once they are mobile, and, as a result, hypothesizes that this has implications for the social development of children with motor impairments (see Chapter 15). Also, as children become more able through the use of mobility devices, it seems logical that parents and others are likely to perceive them as more able. This merits investigation in terms of both 1) parents' and other adults' perceptions of infants and children as they make the transition to self-initiated mobility, and 2) children's dependence on care providers and educators as reflected through type and quality of interactions with adults.

MOBILITY AND PERCEPTUAL AND COGNITIVE SKILLS

The literature supports the relationship between self-produced locomotion and the acquisition of some perceptual and cognitive skills (Bertenthal, Campos, & Barrett, 1984; Kermoian & Campos, 1988). According to Campos and Bertenthal, "the emergence of wariness of heights, as assessed on the visual cliff, is not innate, but follows the acquisition of self-produced mobility" (1987, p. 17). Furthermore, the findings from the Kermoian and Campos (1988) study supported the close link between self-produced locomotion and object permanence, whereas the relationship between self-produced locomotion and the shift to an object-referenced search strategy was supported by research by Telzrow, Campos, Shepherd, Bertenthal, and Atwater (1987). Seven children with myelodysplasia were longitudinally followed from a prelocomotor stage at the onset of the study through self-produced locomotion. Results for this sample indicated that, independent of age, there was a relationship between self-produced locomotion and the shift from a predominantly egocentric search strategy to a predominantly object-referenced strategy. Although these studies suggested a relationship between the onset of self-produced locomotion and the subsequent acquisition of certain perceptual and cognitive skills, there is a need for further confirmation and expansion of these findings with infants and children with motor impairments.

Many clinicians recommend that a child have certain prerequisite visual-spatial skills prior to the introduction of a power mobility device. However, in view of the previously cited research suggesting a link between self-produced mobility and some visual-spatial skills and observation of the mobility experiences of children who are typically developing, the current recommendations seem to be contraindicated. Rather, it seems more appropriate to enable self-initiated mobility experiences for children with motor impairments through the supervised use of augmented mobility and to do this prior to the children's development of object permanence and wariness of heights. Before allowing children who are typically developing to creep or crawl, we do not require specific prerequisite skills. Instead, we supervise their movement and "childproof" the environment. This same approach deserves consideration for children with motor impairments, except that, at the appropriate developmental stage, we need to provide devices to enable mobility and then allow supervised self-initiated movement exploration.

MOBILITY AND INCLUSION

Many children with significant mobility impairments spend the majority of their waking hours in mobility devices. Therefore, we need to evaluate each device in terms of function and the extent to which the device facilitates inclusion in the home, school, and community. This can be addressed for children from the perspective of the three domains of occupation mentioned previously: self-care, school, and play and leisure. Relative to all three domains, the child–device–environment match merits examination, and, in many cases, the benefit of using a variety of mobility devices for one child in order to maximize the child's function and inclusion in diverse environments should be explored.

The ability of children with motor impairments to successfully engage in self-care occupations such as dressing, eating, toileting, and hygiene activities is often compromised. Hence, there is a need to develop augmented mobility devices that facilitate participation in these activities. In developing and evaluating these devices, questions such as the following should be addressed:

- Does the device allow for positioning at the kitchen table such that the child is included at an equal level with other family members?
- Does the match between the device and the environment allow for adequate positioning at sinks and access to cupboards and shelves of importance to the child within the home and in public buildings?
- If appropriate, does the device support ease in transfer from bed to device and back again, from device to toilet, and so forth?
- Does the device allow for use of additional adaptive equipment as needed?

Children and adolescents spend many of their waking hours at school or in school-related occupations. Therefore, the impact of power mobility on the children's abilities to function and perceptions of self within the school environment merit study. In addition, the impact of children's use of power mobility on teachers and peers is of importance. In the school environment, some of the relevant questions are

- When children are using the mobility device, can they be appropriately positioned at school desks?

- Do the devices allow children to be positioned at the same level as their peers?
- What does it mean to children if the design of their mobility devices necessitates positioning away from the group?
- What wheelchair designs facilitate ability to independently obtain access to work surfaces and school supplies and play materials positioned on shelves of varying heights (Deitz, Jaffe, Wolf, Massagli, & Anson, 1991)?
- Can the children travel in a timely, efficient, and independent manner within the school (e.g., from the classroom to the lunchroom or library)?
- In the school environment, what are the energy demands for using independent ambulation, assisted ambulation, manual wheelchairs, and power mobility devices for children with various types and degrees of motor impairment?
- What are the distance and speed criteria necessary for success in the preschool, the elementary school, the middle school, and the high school environments?
- What environmental designs and adaptations optimize function and participation?

All of the domains of occupation are important, but play is the domain that is least often addressed. According to Simon and Daub, play is "an activity voluntarily engaged in for pleasure" (1993, p. 118) and is one of the primary occupations of childhood. Also, it has been noted that exploratory play contributes to the acquisition of knowledge and skills necessary for competent performance. In conjunction with this domain of occupation and the use of augmented mobility, questions such as the following are important to address:

- Are children who use specific types of devices able to travel independently on all surfaces of the school playground, or do these children have to wait on the periphery, never joining in a game of chase or unable to reach the baseball field to serve as scorekeepers?
- What impact does use of power mobility devices have on children's abilities to gain access to preschool play areas (e.g., sensory tables, toy shelves, homemaking areas)?
- How do other children respond to various augmented mobility technologies used by children with motor impairments?
- When technologies have a playful appearance, do other children respond more favorably?

- How can mobility devices be adapted (e.g., adding sirens, racing strips, baskets) to increase their play potential?
- Does use of specific mobility devices contribute to or detract from the play environment?
- What impact does use of mobility devices have on the quality of peer interactions, the maturity of the children's behavior, and the roles assumed by the children in the play environment (e.g., roles of parent, firefighter, baby, dog)?
- What types of mobility devices (e.g., adapted bicycles, sit skis) facilitate inclusion in family and peer recreational activities?

The developer of augmented mobility devices should maintain a developmental perspective, recognizing the changing needs of children as they move from infancy through adolescence. There is a need 1) to start with devices allowing for experiencing self-initiated mobility and environmental exploration; 2) to progress to devices allowing for continuous movement and participation in games of seemingly random movement and chase in the preschool environment; and 3) to continue on to devices for the school-age child that allow for traveling to and from neighbors' homes and inclusion in family, school, and peer outings involving activities such as bicycling and skiing. As adolescents, devices are needed that allow for participation in extracurricular activities and increased independence through adapted driving. Relative to the latter, studies focusing on development, refinement, and evaluation of vehicle adaptations and specialized driver education programs are important.

RESEARCH AND DEVELOPMENT NEEDED TO OPTIMIZE PEDIATRIC AUGMENTED MOBILITY

Pediatric Mobility Design Issues

Too often mobility devices for children are just smaller versions of those designed for adults. Although this is appropriate in some instances, in others the designs are not sensitive to the unique needs of children. For example, typically, when a power wheelchair is purchased for a toddler or young preschooler, the size is such that the child is cocooned in the chair and cannot reach beyond it to interact with other children and to gain access to objects in the environment. Innovative designs such as the Chairman Robo (Permobil) and the GoBot (Innovative Products, Inc.) are encouraging efforts to design mobility devices to meet the needs of children. The former resembles a small forklift with the child controlling the vertical position of the seat, facilitating positioning at desks and tables and access to play materials and other objects on the floor and on shelves of varying heights. The primary limitations of the device relate to 1) the turning radius, which may be prohibitively large in many home and preschool environments; and 2) the weight of the device. The GoBot, by contrast, shows promise for toddlers and preschoolers because it is small; it positions the child to facilitate access to the environment and peers; it has an adjustable frame allowing for growth and for positioning in sitting, semistanding, and standing; and it can be disassembled for ease in transport. Furthermore, it has a playful appearance, comparable to riding toys typically seen in preschool environments. Its use is limited primarily to indoors.

These designs are excellent; however, more variety is essential in order to meet the needs of younger children and children with diverse abilities. New designs should be developed and evaluated for the infant at the developmental age when crawling and creeping are emerging and being refined. For example, both manually propelled and motor-powered scooter boards could be considered. Relative to these and other designs, research questions such as the following warrant investigation:

- What impact does positioning in a mobility device (prone versus supported sitting) have on the development of 6- to 12-month-old infants?
- What impact does use of a mobility device by infants with motor impairments have on the infants' interactions with siblings?
- How do parents or other caregivers feel about their infants with motor impairments when their infants are using mobility devices? What impact does use of mobility devices have on the parents' or care providers' interactions with their infants and the infants' responses to the parents or other care providers?
- How can use of mobility devices by infants be safely incorporated into home environments?

Another major design issue related to pediatric mobility devices concerns portability. Modular designs merit development. Consider a power mobility device for use at age 2 or 3 years. Most are heavy and require purchase of a van with a ramp or lift. This additional expense is prohibitive for many families; as a consequence, the use of early mobility devices often is restricted to one environment (e.g., home, school). Even if families can afford an adapted van, this has an impact on inclusion. For example, consider the child in an inclusive preschool program. Often, especially in parent cooperative situations, children take regular field trips to the zoo, the grocery store, and so forth. Typically there are two alternatives for a child with a disability: either the parent can attend all of the field trips so that the child can use his or her mobility device, or the child can be transported in a stroller and thus will lack independent mobility. While other children run, play, and explore the new environment, the child with the disability is left in the care of an adult and is dependent on that adult for all movement.

In order to facilitate transport, pediatric mobility devices must be modular. Assembly and disassembly should be easy and quick, requiring no tools. When disassembled, each piece should be of a weight that can be picked up and moved without stress by an adult female of average strength. Also, all parts should fit together in the trunk of a compact car. This may require exploration of alternative power sources because most batteries are heavy and large. It is hoped that power sources can be developed that are smaller and lighter, while still maintaining durability and containing costs.

Also, relative to design, pediatric mobility devices must interface easily and economically with other assistive devices used by the children (e.g., communication augmentation systems, environmental control systems). Simple, standardized components are needed that allow for ease in changing parts of the systems as the children grow and develop without having to change other parts that are still appropriate.

Further challenges include the need to develop and evaluate mobility devices specific to rural environments with rough terrain and environments involving unusual challenges, such as frequent snow or steep hills. In addition, cultural factors warrant consideration in the design and evaluation of the effectiveness of power mobility devices.

Evaluation of Pediatric Mobility Devices

Both current devices and new devices require evaluation. This evaluation should focus on safety, durability, and portability as well as on the impact of the device on mobility, environmental access, cognition, socialization, and attitudes (i.e., of the user, peers, parents, other care providers, teachers). In addition, evaluation of the device should occur concurrently with the evaluation of training needs and the development of training approaches for infants and children and their parents, other care providers, and teachers.

We need to start by evaluating the devices that are available relative to what pediatric users and their families want to do and need to do. We need to systematically evaluate all pediatric mobility devices in terms of function in the home, school, and community environments so that parents and professionals can make informed decisions (Deitz et al., 1991). Because one device may be more effective relative to one recognized need and another might be better with respect to a second need, the final choice often involves trade-offs. Only with knowledge about the respective strengths and limitations of various devices can consumers make optimal decisions.

For pediatric users, this systematic evaluation of mobility devices should extend to others in the children's lives: parents, teachers, siblings, and peers. We need to ask practical questions such as

- Does the device track in too much dirt from outside?
- What are the consequences when children using the device accidentally bump into other children or adults? Does the design of the device minimize the potential for injury to others in the children's environments?
- To what extent does the device have safety features designed to protect children and the physical environment? Are these features effective?
- Does the mobility device position children so they have maximal access to the environment?
- What features of mobility devices facilitate function (e.g., gaining access to objects on shelves of varying heights, getting in and out of small spaces such as restrooms and elevators)?
- Is the mobility device too heavy for the care providers to manage?
- To what extent does the device interface efficiently and effectively with other devices (e.g., communication augmentation systems, environmental control systems)?
- To what extent does the design of the device allow for modification as children grow and their needs change?
- To what extent can the mobility device be adapted to facilitate play? For example, can red sides, ladders, and a siren be added to turn a wheelchair into a fire engine?
- Do mobility devices that look like toys encourage inclusion on playgrounds and in neighborhoods?
- Is the mobility device attractive to other children of a similar age?
- Does the mobility device allow children to be positioned at eye level with peers?
- To what extent is the device appropriate to different cultures and environments?

A systematic evaluation system, focusing on these and other questions, is needed in order to identify strengths and limitations in existing mobility devices. This is important for two reasons. First, as previously mentioned, it provides information for consumers and health care providers so that they can make informed choices. Second, it provides information necessary for modifying existing devices and designing new devices to better meet the needs of children with disabilities.

On the basis of this initial evaluation, existing devices should be modified and new devices should be designed. Factors to be considered in the design of these devices include, but should not be limited to, the following:

- Safety (e.g., bumper guards or electronic stops to protect other children and adults in the child's environment as well as walls and furniture; anti-tipping mechanisms; sensors to detect stairs and dropoffs)
- Potential for adaptation (e.g., modular designs that allow for growth and the changing needs of the child)
- Potential for easy interface with other technologies
- Cosmesis from the perspectives of pediatric users, family members, and peers, and flexibility in appearance as the child's concept of "cool" changes
- User friendliness from the viewpoints of pediatric users and adults and children in their environments
- Biomechanical efficiency
- Durability
- Cost

Environmental Adaptation to Enhance Self-Initiated Functional Mobility

In addition to focusing on the design of mobility devices, focus is necessary on environmental characteristics and adaptations that optimize function and on the interrelationships between mobility device designs and environmental characteristics. For example, questions such as the following need to be addressed:

- To what extent is functional positioning facilitated by using classroom and cafeteria tables without skirts or by having, in each setting, one or more tables with sections allowing for height adjustments?
- How does positioning of classroom furniture and placement of toys and work materials enable participation?

- What factors, such as sturdy tables and bars on the walls, permit pull to stand and propping for nonambulatory children who can stand with support?
- What playground equipment and features encourage participation by children with mobility impairments?
- How can others in the environment facilitate inclusion?

These and related questions deserve examination in order to optimize participation in self-care, school, and play and leisure activities.

Service Provision Models

Many young children with motor impairments do not have appropriate mobility devices, whereas others have appropriate devices but do not have adequate services (e.g., training, repair) available to them so that they can optimally use the devices. A major underlying concern is cost, especially for young children requiring constant assistance and changing continuously as a result of growth and development. Thus, it is necessary to design and evaluate models of service delivery to reduce costs. For example, regional systems for "trading" used mobility devices or parts should be considered. Trading could be facilitated through the use of modular designs with interchangeable parts; hence, it might be possible to trade in an outgrown seating system but maintain the power base. Current Internet systems facilitating "trading" should be refined and evaluated, and "technology swaps" modeled after annual "ski swaps" organized in regions of the country where winter sports are popular could be tried.

Equally complex is the issue of providing children with mobility impairments and their parents or other care providers with an enjoyable introduction to mobility technology and a continuous system of support. It seems that movement away from the medical model is indicated both to contain costs and to encourage early, successful introduction of mobility technology in the lives of children with motor impairments and their families. Consider the possibility of child/parent mobility clubs with therapists and rehabilitation engineers serving as resource people. Many parents of children without disabilities spend one or more mornings, afternoons, or evenings driving their children to dance classes; watching them engage in soccer, gymnastics, or T-ball; or participating with them in cooperative preschools. Comparable activities could be created for very young children with disabilities, or for late preschool-age or early school-age children with both motor and cognitive impairments. Mobility club families could meet once or twice a week in school gyms or play courts to "drive" mobility vehicles (e.g., toy cars, power wheelchairs). Structured games involving stop signs and paths to follow could be interspersed with free movement in a playful atmosphere encouraging comfort and competence with technology. Children in this supervised environment could explore self-initiated movement, with more experienced children serving as role models. Furthermore, they could learn to drive safely, could develop spatial skills (e.g., amount of space consumed by the mobility device, which direction to turn in order to drive to Dad), and could gain social skills (e.g., turn taking, importance of not running into other people).

Parents, in this supportive environment, could learn from each other about how to select, adapt, and maintain mobility technology and how to integrate the technology into the lives of their children and their families. In many cases, the mobility technologies employed could be commercially available motorized toy vehicles with inexpensive customized controls and seating systems. For example, for very young children, seating systems can be developed using discarded car seats or customized foam inserts fashioned from medium-density foam using an electric carving knife. Likewise, for children requiring more external supervision (e.g., children with severe motor impairments and blindness, very young children with motor impairments), remote controls can provide added safety while still allowing the children to experience self-initiated movement at a distance from the supervising parents.

It is hoped that use of mobility technology in the "club" environment would carry over into the home environment, starting with driving in the recreation room or joining siblings or neighbor children riding tricycles in the cul-de-sac or driveway. In summary, the primary overall goals of such groups would be fun for children and parents; potentialities for self-initiated movement for the children; possibilities for the children to learn mobility, spatial, and social skills important for participation in home, school, and community environments; and opportunities for the parents or other care providers to become "technology smart."

Related to service provision models, we need to examine our current systems for funding mobility technologies for infants and children with motor impairments. The current systems are complex and tedious, with delays in obtaining request approvals common. Infants and children lacking strong advocates who aggressively pursue technology funding and related services often go without appropriate assistive devices for extended periods of time during critical stages in their development. The current systems should be evaluated 1) by examining the perspectives of parents and professionals working with children who have disabilities regarding what is and is not working within these systems, 2) by determining how many children at each level (birth to 3 years, preschool, elementary school, middle school, and high school) do not have the mobility devices they need, 3) by systematically documenting the amount of time that elapses between when a need is identified and when a child receives the appropriate mobility device, and 4) by identifying the barriers to obtaining multiple mobility aids for an individual child. Based on this information, the current system should be refined or new models developed to ensure prompt and appropriate funding of mobility devices for all children with mobility impairments.

CONCLUSIONS

In the area of pediatric augmented mobility, there are endless questions to answer and directions to explore. This requires a multifaceted approach involving the evaluation of existing technology and the design and evaluation of new assistive devices; the identification, use, and evaluation of environmental adaptations that enhance self-initiated functional mobility for children with disabilities; and the creation and evaluation of service provision models intended to maximize access. In addition, the interrelationships of all of these factors should be examined. In all stages of this process, consumers should be involved in the identification and defining of research and development priorities. This could be accomplished by using a focus group process similar to the one described by Bricnza, Angelo, and Henry (1995). In addition to including the pediatric users of mobility devices, parents, teachers, peers, and siblings of children using mobility devices should be included in the focus groups. All of these individuals are affected by the child's use of a mobility device, and, if their concerns are not considered, the effectiveness of the device for the child will be affected.

REFERENCES

Bertenthal, B., Campos, J., & Barrett, K. (1984). Self-produced locomotion as an organizer of perceptual, cognitive and emotional development in infancy. In R. Emde & R. Harmon (Eds.), *Cognitive and emotional development in infancy* (pp. 175–210). New York: Plenum.

Brienza, D., Angelo, J., & Henry, K. (1995). Consumer participation in identifying research and development priorities for power wheelchair input devices and controllers. *Assistive Technology, 7*, 55–62.

Butler, C. (1986). Effects of powered mobility on self-initiated behaviors of very young children with locomotor disability. *Developmental Medicine and Child Neurology, 28*, 325–332.

Butler, C. (1991). Augmented mobility: Why do it? *Physical Medicine and Rehabilitation Clinics of North America, 2*, 801–815.

Campos, J., & Bertenthal, B. (1987). Locomotion and psychological development in infancy. In K.M. Jaffe (Ed.), *Childhood powered mobility: Developmental, technical, and clinical perspectives: Proceedings of the First Northwest Regional Conference* (pp. 11–42). Washington, DC: RESNA Press.

Deitz, J., Jaffe, K., Wolf, L., Massagli, T., & Anson, D. (1991). Pediatric power wheelchairs: Evaluation of function in the home and school environments. *Assistive Technology, 3*, 24–31.

Glickman, L., Deitz, J., Anson, D., & Stewart, K. (1996). The effect of switch control site on computer skills of infants and toddlers. *American Journal of Occupational Therapy, 50*, 545–553.

Kermoian, R., & Campos, J. (1988). Locomotor experience: A facilitator of spatial cognition. *Child Development, 58*, 908–917.

Simon, C.J., & Daub, M.M. (1993). Knowledge bases in occupational therapy, Section 2A: Human development across the life span. In H.L. Hopkins & H.D. Smith (Eds.), *Occupational therapy* (pp. 95–130). Philadelphia: J.B. Lippincott.

Swinth, Y., Anson, D., & Deitz, J. (1993). Single-switch computer access for infants and toddlers. *American Journal of Occupational Therapy, 47*, 1031–1038.

Telzrow, R., Campos, J., Shepherd, A., Bertenthal, B., & Atwater, S. (1987). Spatial understanding in infants with motor handicaps. In K.M. Jaffe (Ed.), *Childhood powered mobility: Developmental, technical, and clinical perspectives: Proceedings of the RESNA First Northwest Regional Conference* (pp. 62–69). Washington, DC: RESNA Press.

CHAPTER 17

Designing a Transitional Powered Mobility Aid for Young Children with Physical Disabilities

Christine Wright-Ott

Assistive technology (AT) devices intended for children, including wheelchairs, orthopedic seat systems, walkers, and commodes, typically are designed as smaller versions of devices originally designed for adult users. An important unmet need, particularly with mobility aids, is to design these products to better meet the specific needs of children with disabilities and their families. In this chapter, the experiences and knowledge gained during the 3-year Transitional Powered Mobility Aid (TPMA) Project are discussed to provide insights into factors that should be considered before designing AT for children with physical disabilities.

TPMA is a device designed specifically for children with physical disabilities younger than age 5 years (see Figure 1). The TPMA consists of an adjustable positioning frame attached to a battery-powered base. The frame is designed to be adjustable for growth and to accommodate various positioning needs of children with weak or low muscle tone and children with spasticity or reflexive posturing. The positioning frame can be adjusted to enable a child to move

The Transitional Powered Mobility Aid (TPMA) Project, on which this chapter is based, was funded by Grant H180P00018-91 from the U.S. Department of Education, Office of Special Education Programs.

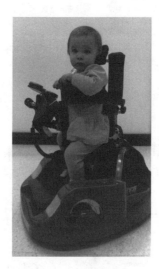

Figure 1.   A 14-month-old child is positioned in the original prototype of the Transitional Powered Mobility Aid. Switches for moving the device are mounted on an adjustable tray placed under the right hand.

while in a sitting, semistanding, or standing position. The positioning frame is removable for transport in a vehicle. The control system includes a joystick or four switches that, when activated, move the TPMA either forward, in reverse, to the left, or to the right. The switches are mounted on an adjustable tray that can in turn be mounted in any location, allowing the child to maneuver the TPMA using movements of the hands, head, or feet. The TPMA is designed for indoor use or on level outdoor surfaccs.

The purpose of the TPMA is to provide a child who has a physical disability with an opportunity to explore the environment using upright, self-initiated mobility. It is designed to enable the child to get close to objects for reaching and touching. The TPMA may provide a course of development for children with physical disabilities that parallels that of their peers without disabilities by encouraging early exploratory or transitional mobility opportunities. This period of transitional mobility may be the precursor to functional mobility (see Chapter 15). The transitional mobility period is the time when children first begin to experience the consequences of self-initiated mobility. Being able to manipulate their environment provides greater opportunities for development in the areas of communication, visual-perceptual skills, socialization, upper-extremity function, and self-esteem.

DESIGNING FOR NEED

Generally, the initial process of designing and developing a product begins with an idea or solution for a particular need or problem. Next, one determines if products already exist that would meet the needs of the user or if similar products were tried, did not solve the problem and were discarded. The functions that the product will enhance or supplement are then described. Finally, physical characteristics of people who might benefit from the product are analyzed. Once these phases are completed, a design concept is developed and data are gathered to identify specific features that should be considered in the design of the prototype. In developing the TPMA, the project team covered these design steps by including individuals with skills and past experiences that provided a link between clinical knowledge of children's physical and functional needs and technical knowledge of engineering possibilities. The design team included a mechanical engineer, an electrical engineer with a rehabilitation engineering background, and an occupational therapist experienced in AT and pediatrics. The role of the occupational therapist was to match the functional needs of the users with the features of the product.

Observation of Need

During the development of a project, it is important to maintain a continuous dialogue with the consumers for whom the AT device is intended. If the product is intended for the pediatric population, the primary consumers will be the child and their caregivers. Because many children with disabilities cannot communicate effectively, consumer feedback depends on the design team's skills in observing the children and communicating with their caregivers. In addition, the design team must interact with others who influence the children's selection and use of AT, including their caregivers, community teachers, aides, speech-language pathologists, physical therapists, and occupational therapists. These individuals appear to have the greatest influence on whether a device should even be considered for a particular child. Although physicians are the primary referral for an assistive device, they often depend on the experience of the therapists to make the recommendations. Third-party payers also depend on these professionals for justifying purchase of a device. If any of these individuals believe that the features of a device do not appropriately meet the needs of the child, in all likelihood the device will not be recommended for purchase.

The TPMA team dedicated significant amounts of time throughout the project gathering feedback and ideas from a wide variety of sources. Members of the team visited schools, therapy sites, and children's homes. In these settings, they interviewed key informants who influence product acquisition and use. These included teachers, aides, therapists, caregivers, and extended family members. This process continued until the project was completed. Communication of this nature required a significant amount of time to schedule appointments, to travel to the sites, and to interview key informants. However, the TPMA team found it to be the best method for acquiring an understanding of what features should and should not be considered for a device to be functional for children in their settings.

Survey of Need

Interviews and surveys are often used as a means for identifying specific features that should be considered during the product design process. Because children are dependent on adults to make recommendations for a device, it is of equal importance to identify attitudes and opinions of professionals regarding their thoughts on the need for such a device and what impact they believe it will have on the user. This was accomplished by including questions in the initial needs assessment survey that gathered information from professionals on their attitudes and opinions regarding the use of powered mobility devices for children less than 5 years of age. Data were collected using a needs assessment survey that was sent to professionals throughout the nation.

The 150 responses to this survey indicated that the majority of those professionals surveyed agreed with the premise that the development of a child with a physical disability could be adversely affected if that child had no means for self-initiated mobility in the early years. The survey respondents did not consider the devices available on the market as adequate for meeting children's developmental and mobility needs. Several reasons were identified that explain why children are not using powered mobility devices: lack of portability, concern over safety issues (e.g., driving around other young children), and cost. Additional concerns inhibiting recommendation for the use of powered mobility devices were the difficulty of maneuvering these devices indoors, the problems associated with positioning children with severe disabilities in power wheelchairs, and the inability to provide training in use of a powered mobility device before recommending it for purchase. This valuable information led to design specifications that provided for portability, maneuverability indoors, an easily adjustable position-ing frame, extensions for growth adjustments, options for position-ing in sitting or standing to augment development, and a projected lower cost as compared with powered wheelchairs. The survey indi-cated that the average age of a child with a disability for whom a powered wheelchair is purchased is 10 years.

Another very interesting finding from the survey was that pro-fessionals were concerned that parents and caregivers were not ready to see their child use a powered wheelchair. The use of a wheelchair was seen as a sign to the caregivers that they should give up hope that eventually their child will walk. The most consis-tent feedback obtained from caregivers was the desire to have the device look so attractive that other children would want to use it as well. The appearance of the device had to be "kid-friendly." Parents frequently commented during the project that durable medical equipment for children looks too disabling and not inviting to other children. The parents reported that some AT tends to isolate a child with physical disabilities from his or her peers. This information led the project team to design the TPMA with an aesthetic appear-ance that would motivate children and not intimidate caregivers. The TPMA was intentionally designed to look different from a powered wheelchair. The project team set a goal that the TPMA should look like it came off the shelf of a toy shop rather than from a durable medical equipment shop.

Consumer-Centered Design

The TPMA project team found it challenging to use a consumer-centered approach to design because each feature of the product had to be prioritized according to cost, benefit, and consumer prefer-ence. The ultimate solution was to use a modular design that al-lowed inclusion of optional features for addition at different points in the child's development. For the TPMA, these options included a remotely operated joystick that would override the child's ability to use the controls on the device, laptrays, foot placement guides, and knee pads. Although other features were considered, manufacturers consulted by the project team cautioned that too many features in the TPMA would complicate the manufacturing process, increase the cost, and make it difficult to find a manufacturer.

Successful product designs incorporate individual preferences and needs. This is particularly necessary for pediatric products be-cause children may be at various stages of physical development and abilities. The greatest challenge for the project team was to de-sign the TPMA's positioning frame to accommodate a variety of physical characteristics ranging from low muscle tone (i.e., children with muscle diseases and spina bifida) to extremely high muscle tone and strength (i.e., children with severe spasticity from cerebral palsy). The frame had to secure the child in an upright and desirable position with a minimum of restraints to avoid interfering with the child's ability to explore the environment. The same positioning frame had to adjust easily and quickly in a clinical setting to fit children of various sizes from as young as 12 months to as old as 5 years. Another critical design feature was to provide children using the TPMA with a body position that would accomplish their therapeutic goals and also allow them to move their bodies when leaning to reach for and touch objects, moving their legs to kick balls, and playing with other children. The project team was able to build the features related to therapeutic goals into the design of the TPMA by carefully considering the ideas expressed by physical therapists and occupational therapists during the design process. Equally important in designing the TPMA was the caregivers' feedback. Caregivers focused more on ease of use and whether one person could safely put the child in and out of the TPMA.

Multiple-Use Devices

The trend in designing infant products for use by the general public is to incorporate several functions into one unit. For example, new infant carrying seats are designed to be used as car seats in a vehicle. When the infant seat is removed from the car, it may be converted to a stroller by attaching it to a base with wheels. This concept of incorporating the function of several different devices into one unit is beneficial not only for the general public but also for AT products. Children with disabilities tend to use numerous pieces of equipment at school and in their homes for therapeutic and functional purposes. If one device can appropriately replace the function of two devices, there is greater likelihood it will be viewed favorably by consumers and third-party payers. The TPMA was designed to serve multiple functions, including a therapeutic standing frame (typically prescribed for children with mobility impairments) and an early mobility exploration device. The TPMA can also be modified to incorporate a child's existing standing frame.

Previous Attempts

The project team found it useful to research the history of other powered mobility products that were or were not successfully brought to the marketplace. A powered mobility caster cart, designed for children with mobility impairments, had been introduced 10 years earlier by a wheelchair manufacturer. The project team solicited feedback obtained from industry professionals who had been involved in previous projects. Their insights into design considerations provided valuable information for designing the TPMA. For example, the caster cart appeared to look too much like a toy for consideration as an assistive device for reimbursement from third-party payers. In addition, the caster cart was so low to the ground that children could not interact appropriately with peers. Finally, children with moderate to severe disabilities could not be positioned appropriately or use the joystick.

TIMING AND DEVELOPMENT OF ASSISTIVE TECHNOLOGY

Developing a new idea into a successful product depends on doing it at the right time. If an idea is too innovative, people will have a difficult time accepting it. Potential consumers should be educated during the product design and testing phases, and after the product is developed, to assist them in understanding the innovative concept behind the technology. The TPMA is an innovative product designed to facilitate exploration and learning for toddlers and preschool children who have mobility impairments or delays. Studies of child development have found that children need to interact with their environments through self-initiated exploration (see Chapters 15 and 16). Acceptance of this concept rested, in part, on convincing potential users that the TPMA is specifically designed to allow these explorations to occur and is not just another type of powered wheelchair. This required professionals to shift from the traditional paradigm that the child must demonstrate excellent driving skills using a powered wheelchair in order to have self-initiated mobility experiences. Thus, driving skills were the standard criteria for acquiring a powered wheelchair. The new paradigm relies on therapists accepting the premise that development is enhanced by early intervention and opportunities to interact with the environment. Furthermore, they must be convinced that the TPMA provides children who have mobility impairments with the opportunity to self-initiate exploration of their environments and to learn by doing. To be successful, the TPMA needed to be considered as a device that provides the essential functions of exploratory and transitional mobility rather than the type of functional mobility provided by a powered wheelchair.

The right time for an idea also depends on the attitudes of society. If the TPMA had been designed 10 years earlier, it would have been difficult or even impossible for it to become a successful product. Two pieces of legislation passed in the late 1980s and early 1990s have contributed to the development of AT, access to information on existing devices, and services for maintaining AT. The Technology-Related Assistance for Individuals with Disabilities Act of 1988 (PL 100-407) established an information network that promotes increased consumer awareness of existing and newly developed products. This information network provided an avenue for dissemination of TPMA availability. A second essential legislative initiative was contained in Part H of the Individuals with Disabilities Education Act (IDEA) of 1990 (PL 101-476) (now redesignated Part C under the IDEA Amendments of 1997 [PL 105-17]). This act mandated appropriate education and intervention for very young children, birth to 3 years of age. The educational and therapeutic uses of the TPMA can be seen to address the very intent of the legislation. Both of these acts helped to bring the TPMA to the attention of professionals and third-party payers who are essential in making purchasing decisions for AT.

EVALUATION OF ASSISTIVE TECHNOLOGY

For the TPMA to gain acceptance as a therapeutic tool that could meet the intent of improving educational interventions for young children with physical disabilities, two methods were used to evaluate its function and features. The first was a structured environment model that was incorporated in a mobility camp. The structured environment was necessary to allow the design team to concentrate on evaluating the features of the device through first-hand experiences of using the TPMA prototype with children and to compare performance with other mobility aids. This was accomplished by establishing a series of mobility experience day camps in which children with mobility impairments from various communities were invited to participate. Response to invitations to attend the mobility camp was extremely favorable. Families came from great distances and made considerable efforts to attend. For example, one family had no means of transportation other than riding a bus for 2 hours each way, which they did even during winter storms. Their child had cerebral palsy with severe spastic quadriplegia. The family carried her on the bus.

Children with a variety of diagnoses, ages (from ages 15 months to 6 years), and socioeconomic backgrounds attended the mobility camp. Children participated in a 90-minute daily session for 2 weeks. During these sessions, they experienced self-initiated mobility using the TPMA and other devices. A total of 37 children (18 girls and 19 boys) attended the mobility camp over a 3-year period. The average age was 2 years, 10 months. Thirty-two children had a diagnosis of cerebral palsy. Other diagnoses included muscular dystrophy, arthrogryposis, Down syndrome, atelosteogenesis syndrome type III, and chromosome 13X syndrome; one child had an unknown diagnosis. Caregivers were required to attend the sessions and siblings were encouraged to participate. Two children "campers" attended each session. The mobility camp allowed the project team to evaluate features of the TPMA on one day, make needed adjustments, and reevaluate the device with the same users the following day. The structured environment also provided uninterrupted time and few distractions, which are common when testing a device in the child's natural environment.

An additional benefit of using the mobility camp model for evaluation was the collection of observational data of the children using the device over a period of time. If parents or caregivers commented on their children's behavior, the comments were noted. These included an increase in the child's language and verbalization, more frequent eye contact, longer periods of sleep at nap time, and an increase in smiling and laughing. The mobility camp experience also provided insight into variations of behavior of the children in their interactions while using the TPMA. The staff noted differences in ability to operate the TPMA by children with cerebral palsy, spastic quadriplegia, and athetoid quadriplegia. This was an unexpected finding that was possible to discern only by observing the children in the device over time. Several children had owned a mobility device that they had not been able to use effectively. These experiences clearly illustrate the need for more research to study the best methods for matching the needs of the child with the capabilities of the AT. These studies should include cost–benefit analyses of using mobility aids that consider the effects of using such devices on a child's emotional, social, and physical development. With these findings in hand, criteria can be developed for selecting a mobility device that enhances the multitude of functions essential for a child to fully develop.

A second evaluation technique was used to assess the effects of the TPMA in the natural environments of the child's school, home, and therapy settings. Both the engineer and the occupational therapist were always present during these trials. The project team found it important for a design team to obtain feedback directly, for its members to be present at the same time, and for the team to experience firsthand the variations between environments and users. Observing users in their natural environments is critical for evaluating the effectiveness of the prototype and how it functions. Home trials were conducted by bringing the device to the child's home and observing the child use the TPMA. These sessions were videotaped to record feedback from the caregivers. The design team found that most of the homes were small and inaccessible for the children. In addition, several TPMA prototypes were placed in local preschool special education classrooms, therapy clinics, and a community preschool. These settings enabled the design team to observe children using the TPMA with adults who were not family members. This evaluation method had the advantage of obtaining immediate and direct feedback on TPMA use. The disadvantages in using these environments were the limited amount of time for TPMA use and the schedules and disruptive nature of the many concurrent activities taking place in these settings.

The TPMA project team found using both the structured and natural environment methods valuable because each offered unique advantages. The structured environment (the mobility camp model) provided uninterrupted time, reduced costs for traveling, allowed evaluation of users over a period of time, and provided more information about the behavioral aspects of using the device. The natural environment settings (i.e., the child's home, classroom, therapy settings) provided more feedback on the ability of the device to function effectively under various conditions. Both methods allowed adults to provide feedback on the use of the TPMA. Family members and caregivers tended to be very positive and excited about the TPMA. They provided little feedback that was critical of the device. Teachers and aides spoke positively about the need for such a device, which they viewed as a learning opportunity. However, they did not offer ideas for how the TPMA might improve the child's function. Therapists focused their feedback on the physical aspects of the child and the device's ability to provide an appropriate position for the child while augmenting function. They were most likely to look at specific features of the TPMA and to make recommendations for additional features that might meet their clients' individual needs.

CONCLUSIONS

Several factors have been identified that can contribute to successful product designs of AT devices for children. A multidisciplinary, experienced project team should be assembled that includes engineers with technical knowledge of device capabilities and pediatric therapists who have clinical knowledge of client needs. An essential task for the project team is to maintain a continuous dialogue with the consumers during the entire design process. Consumers should include caregivers, professionals who recommend the technology, and third-party payers. Needs assessment surveys should seek information regarding attitudes and opinions of professionals who will be making recommendations for the purchase and use of AT. Designs that use modular components and incorporate functions of several devices into one should be considered. The TPMA project team discovered that feedback from prototype testing and evaluation is dependent on who is being interviewed and where the test is made (a structured or natural environment setting). Further research is needed to establish design criteria for AT for children, study the effects and outcomes of using AT on children's development, design and develop more user-friendly devices, improve the aesthetic appearance of devices, and develop selection criteria for AT that match user needs.

REFERENCES

Individuals with Disabilities Education Act (IDEA) of 1990, PL 101-476, 20 U.S.C. §§ 1400 *et seq.*

Individuals with Disabilities Education Act Amendments of 1997, PL 105-17, 20 U.S.C. §§ 1400 *et seq.*

Technology-Related Assistance for Individuals with Disabilities Act of 1988, PL 100-407, 29 U.S.C. §§ 2201 *et seq.*

SUMMARY

CHAPTER 18

Conclusions

Moving to the Next Stage of Assistive Technology Development

David B. Gray,
Louis A. Quatrano,
and Morton L. Lieberman

The National Center for Medical Rehabilitation Research (NCMRR; 1993; Pope & Tarlov, 1991) developed a model for classifying domains of research (see Figure 1). This model provides a heuristic tool for understanding the importance of assistive technology (AT) to people with disabilities and to those who might best address issues involved in designing, developing, testing, selecting, training, using, and paying for AT. The five domains set forth in this model are societal limitation, disability, functional limitation, impairment, and pathophysiology. With regard to AT, societal limitations include restrictions in AT purchase by government entitlement and eligibility programs, inadequate funding of design and development of AT, poor funding of training programs for professionals and consumers, and liability laws that virtually prohibit development of high-technology AT. Making changes within the societal limitations domain will require information gleaned from studies of the composite costs and benefits to society of providing improved AT to citizens with disabilities. Matching AT to activities that a person with a disability chooses to do is a function of complex interactions of many factors.

The disability domain of the NCMRR model captures the importance of evaluating the whole person (strengths and weaknesses)

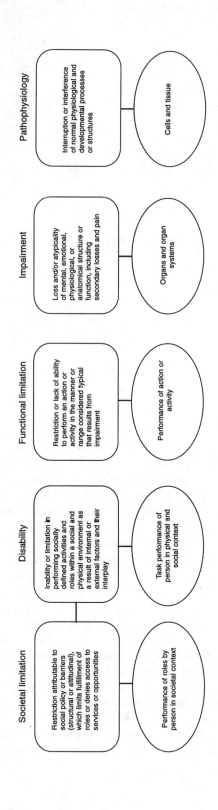

Pathophysiology

Interruption or interference of normal physiological and developmental processes or structures

Cells and tissue

Impairment

Loss and/or atypicality of mental, emotional, physiological, or anatomical structure or function, including secondary losses and pain

Organs and organ systems

Functional limitation

Restriction or lack of ability to perform an action or activity in the manner or range considered typical that results from impairment

Performance of action or activity

Disability

Inability or limitation in performing socially defined activities and roles within a social and physical environment as a result of internal or external factors and their interplay

Task performance of person in physical and social context

Societal limitation

Restriction attributable to social policy or barriers (structural or attitudinal), which limits fulfillment of roles or denies access to services or opportunities

Performance of roles by person in societal context

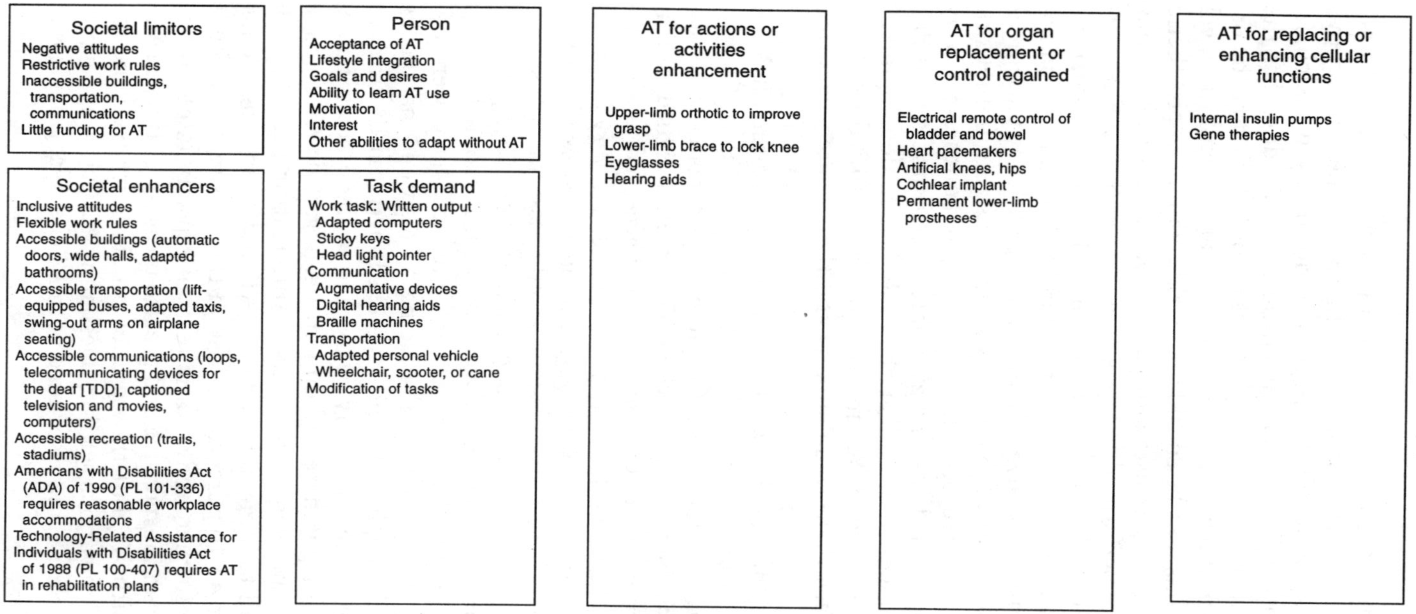

Societal limitors

Negative attitudes
Restrictive work rules
Inaccessible buildings, transportation, communications,
Little funding for AT

Societal enhancers

Inclusive attitudes
Flexible work rules
Accessible buildings (automatic doors, wide halls, adapted bathrooms)
Accessible transportation (lift-equipped buses, adapted taxis, swing-out arms on airplane seating)
Accessible communications (loops, telecommunicating devices for the deaf [TDD], captioned television and movies, computers)
Accessible recreation (trails, stadiums)
Americans with Disabilities Act (ADA) of 1990 (PL 101-336) requires reasonable workplace accommodations
Technology-Related Assistance for Individuals with Disabilities Act of 1988 (PL 100-407) requires AT in rehabilitation plans

Person

Acceptance of AT
Lifestyle integration
Goals and desires
Ability to learn AT use
Motivation
Interest
Other abilities to adapt without AT

Task demand

Work task: Written output
Adapted computers
Sticky keys
Head light pointer
Communication
Augmentative devices
Digital hearing aids
Braille machines
Transportation
Adapted personal vehicle
Wheelchair, scooter, or cane
Modification of tasks

AT for actions or activities enhancement

Upper-limb orthotic to improve grasp
Lower-limb brace to lock knee
Eyeglasses
Hearing aids

AT for organ replacement or control regained

Electrical remote control of bladder and bowel
Heart pacemakers
Artificial knees, hips
Cochlear implant
Permanent lower-limb prostheses

AT for replacing or enhancing cellular functions

Internal insulin pumps
Gene therapies

Figure 1. Assistive technology (AT) in the context of terminology used in the National Center for Medical Rehabilitation Research model. (Adapted from Pope and Tarlov [1991]; National Center for Medical Rehabilitation Research [1993].)

in the evaluation of the best fit of person to technology. The functional limitations domain includes AT that is designed to improve performance of specific actions (e.g., locomotion by wheelchair, writing by orthotic splints). The impairment domain describes the loss or atypicality of an anatomical structure or function at the organ level. AT that allows the user to regain control over lost bowel or bladder functions may be considered in this domain. A prosthetic lower limb that gives the user similar or even enhanced functions that are typically performed by a leg might fit within the impairment domain. Indwelling pumps that replace lost or abnormal tissue or cellular products (e.g., insulin) would fall within the pathophysiology domain. Although one might argue with the placement of specific AT within the five NCMRR domains, the framework does allow for some categorization and discussion of the vast array of AT discussed in this book and available to consumers with disabilities. The model makes clear that the design, development, selection, and purchase of AT, and the training required to use it, present challenges that cross domains and their related scientific disciplines.

A variety of themes that apply to AT in each of the NCMRR domains emerge from the chapters contained in this book. Clearly, AT does not and will not answer all problems associated with disabling conditions. Nevertheless, when AT is well designed, taught in appropriate contexts, made affordable, and accepted by the consumer, the lives of individuals with disabilities are very often enhanced. Essential to the positive outcome of AT use is the notion that the selection of assistive devices should take into consideration the whole person and his or her chosen level of participation in major life activities. Although AT abandonment is too high, only a few studies of how AT abandonment can be reduced have been conducted. One area of consensus for reducing AT disuse is that during the design of AT, people with the targeted functional limitations need to be incorporated in nearly every step of the process. Financial support for AT purchase and difficulties in getting AT repaired are serious limiting factors in AT use. Anticipating the effects of clinical or school training in how to use AT in determining the nature and type of AT to purchase for use in the consumer's home is an area needing further study. Static tests of capacity in controlled settings provide an inexpensive and precise measure of the person's performance with AT, but they do not predict very well the dynamic use of AT in various settings. Designing AT that is age appropriate, reducing the stigma associated with AT use, recognizing that

AT has a "shelf life," and understanding that body shapes and sizes as well as life goals change over time are but a few of the factors likely to contribute to understanding how AT can best meet the needs of people with disabilities. Multidisciplinary efforts are required to address AT needs that change over time (e.g., pediatrics through old age). The lack of multisite clinical trial networks hampers the ability of scientists to collect large samples for statistical comparisons of the differential effectiveness of various assistive technologies.

The nature of AT ranges from mass-produced, universally designed products to individually designed, function-specific devices that require high technology. For the latter types of AT, the presumption that AT is cost-effective needs scientific study at several levels. The individuals using these high-cost orphan technologies need to be a part of the decision-making process. The expected outcomes of AT use need to be made clear. Some macroeconomic studies need to be made if increased provision of AT is to become incorporated into national government, private employment, managed care, and private insurance benefit programs. If high-tech AT is to be considered a small market (e.g., orphan drugs), then the standards for provision of AT need to be clear, public, and malleable. A necessary step in gaining support for increased availability of AT is to improve the quality control used in producing AT. The feedback on AT product performance from consumers, therapists, and third-party payers is nearly nonexistent. By applying scientific methods in the development of AT, increasing the quality of AT, and establishing reasonable safety standards for AT, the cost of liability insurance and thus the cost of AT development may be significantly reduced.

Technology development has provided the cornerstone for many of the advances that have been made in AT. Indeed, technology continues to offer the potential of providing further advances in AT and thereby improved functional outcomes for people with disabilities. However, input from clinicians and people with disabilities is essential to avoid technological successes that fail to improve the lives of people with disabilities. Such disappointments are not technological failures, but rather failures to adequately define the problems that the technologists must address. There are vast technological resources available in federal laboratories, universities, and private industry. Utilization of these resources is dependent on funding earmarked for specific applications. Tapping into these resources requires funding defined for AT. Established funding channels are one avenue for seeking support. Another potential source is conversion of technology originally developed for national defense purposes. The transfer of technology from the defense research laboratories to use in developing commercial products follows no single, well-defined paradigm and is strongly affected by third-party payers. Thus, the evaluation of AT must capture the user's perspective, third-party payer's concerns, and the scientist's expectation for the devices to improve function in order to be cost-effective and meet technical performance standards. Advances in technology designed specifically for people with disabilities may have an impact on individuals without disabilities. This has the effect of broadening the market, reducing price, diminishing stigma, easing acquisition of skills needed for device use, and gaining rapid acceptance by consumers.

The chapters in this book raise a number of questions that need to be answered to improve the quality, quantity, function, and cost of AT used by people with disabilities. The issues cited provide the reader with an idea of the enormity of the tasks that need to be considered in developing, producing, selecting, teaching, and using AT. The next several paragraphs contain a number of research projects recommended for consideration for further investigation. This list is neither exhaustive nor comprehensive but is suggestive of areas ripe for exploration.

CONCEPTUALIZING, CLASSIFYING, AND COUNTING AT

A national classification system for assistive technology devices and services is being developed by the Research Triangle Institute (Curtin, 1997). However, few conceptual or classification models provide a clear notion of how to connect the classification of AT with the differing models of disability (e.g., medical, economic) used to justify AT purchase. Without a classification system that includes AT specifications, costs, durability, consumer satisfaction, and outcomes of AT use as a therapeutic intervention, no clear justification can be built for the purchase of AT by governments, insurers, and employers. In turn, this lack of information discourages industry from investing in the development of AT. Linking AT use to increased independence in personal self-care, improved job performance, higher employment, more control over communications, and better transportation may provide empirical evidence for recognizing AT as the preferred therapeutic intervention both for individual cases and for making the built environment more accessible for all Americans. Recommendations for conceptualizing, classifying, and counting AT are to construct a model that encompasses AT in the rehabilitation process, develop a classification scheme that allows AT to be counted, study environments that encourage maximal use of AT, and encourage national databases to include AT in their surveys.

SELECTION OF AT DEVICE

Several chapters of this book make the point that if the consumer is not involved in the choice of AT device, then the chances of the AT device being discarded are high. The process for matching AT with consumer needs is not well developed. Some chapters advocate developing expert systems that take into account personal characteristics and needs as major factors in selecting an AT device. Others suggest providing detailed descriptions of AT capabilities and working with the consumer to select the device that fits their lifestyles. Most often, however, a salesperson or therapist makes a decision to recommend AT based on clinical experience. The controversy over AT selection—by whom and on what basis—suggests several research projects. Recommendations for selection of AT are to establish effectiveness of different types of AT selection processes, determine professional and consumer responsibilities in the selection processes, develop methods for matching people with disabilities and AT, and study critical periods in development and aging when AT is needed and accepted.

DESIGN OF ASSISTIVE TECHNOLOGY

The great diversity in what is considered to be assistive technology requires several approaches to the design process. In many cases, involving the consumer from initiation through completion of the project seems wise. For other products, consumers are asked to evaluate the finished AT device. Some devices are individualized for personal use to improve a single function (e.g., bladder control); other products are designed for use by a broad market (e.g., level door handles). Recommendations for design of AT are to study the steps from design to market at which people with disabilities can have positive effects; examine new and existing products for reliability, redundancy, and safety; determine design features that promote universal use; develop mobility devices that improve social interactions, especially for children; and encourage designs that promote health and prevent secondary conditions.

ACQUISITION OF SKILLS FOR AT USE

Learning to use assistive technology is a challenge for the consumer. Adapting to a new mode of interacting with his or her environment (e.g., use of a wheelchair for mobility) after injury means developing a whole new set of skills to perform old, familiar tasks. Teaching people with disabilities these new skills is a complex activity involving understanding the person's self-concept, prior interests, physical capacities, device characteristics, and task requirements. Several chapters in this book make the point that teaching the use of AT in settings (e.g., hospital, rehabilitation facility, workshop) other than those where the AT will eventually be used (e.g., home, work) often results in AT abandonment. Recommendations with regard to acquisition of skills for AT use are to study adaptation to and use of AT for different types of AT in different settings, examine critical periods for introducing AT to infants and children, determine the design features of AT that are most easily learned and retained, and develop virtual reality training devices for environmental simulation of AT use.

EVALUATION OF ASSISTIVE TECHNOLOGY

In order for a device to be considered AT, the device must improve the function of the user. As discussed by several chapter authors, evaluation of changes in function attributable to AT use is not a trivial task. Measuring the person's capacity to perform without using AT devices may not reveal much if the task is impossible without the AT. Tests of AT use by individuals without the target impairment may miss important operating requirements that people with disabilities cannot perform. Standardization of tests of AT capacities based on static conditions will not evaluate AT performance under dynamic conditions on such important factors as speed, endurance, reliability, and safety. Recommendations for evaluation of AT are to develop standards of AT performance based on successful use by consumers with similar impairments; conduct comparative studies of AT devices that are designed to improve similar functions for acquisition and ease of use as well as change in performance; design studies to determine optimal balance of AT device control by the consumer and the device itself; measure the effects of provision of wheeled mobility devices to infants on their development; examine different AT designs for cosmetic effects and social acceptance by users and their friends, families, colleagues, and strangers; and analyze national databases for the effects of increased use of AT on employment, health care use, transportation system demands, and duration of returning and remaining in the home after injury or disease.

MOVING TO THE NEXT STAGE OF AT DEVELOPMENT

Americans with disabilities are a large and growing minority with an increasing need for assistive technology. More individuals survive traumatic injuries, fewer infants with impairments die, people with cancer and other diseases live longer, and the number of older adults with disabilities is increasing. The direct and indirect economic costs of this growing minority is several hundred billion dollars annually. Yet, funding for medical research to restore the biological and psychological functions of these survivors is less than $200 million annually; few advances in reversing chronic conditions have been made; and the funding of AT development by federal agencies is less than $100 million annually (Institute of Medicine, 1997). However, the pace of discovery of new technologies has opened many new possibilities for individually designed, component-manufactured AT that maximizes improved functioning in multiple activities for individuals with disabilities. AT has reduced the need for personal assistance, decreased caregiver burden, increased employment opportunities, lowered total costs, and even provided easier access to activities for people with disabilities.

The result has been a broadening of the concept of assistive technology to include any device that improves the function of people with or without disabilities. Several pieces of legislation have recognized the importance of AT to people with disabilities. The Technology-Related Assistance for Individuals with Disabilities Act of 1988 (PL 100-407) and the Rehabilitation Act Amendments of 1992 (PL 102-569) improved access to information on existing AT (West, 1991). The Americans with Disabilities Act (ADA) of 1990 (PL 101-336) requires that accessible housing, transportation, and communication be provided to people with disabilities. In addition, ADA, a historic civil rights law for people with disabilities that has provided an impetus for increasing the availability and effectiveness of AT, requires that reasonable accommodation be provided for employees with disabilities.

Justification for AT purchase is beginning to change from narrow medical necessity to broader human needs, and the market for AT spans the age range from infants to older adults. Changing the federal and state tax codes to allow for the purchase of AT to be claimed as a tax credit instead of a medical deduction would go a long way toward improving the demand side of the AT market. If entitlement programs (e.g., Social Security Disability Insurance, Supplemental Security Income) were to provide AT to people with disabilities as incentives for returning to work, the AT market would expand. Yet, even if AT-friendly social policy changes were made to improve access to and funding of AT, considerable difficulty would remain in matching AT to personal needs, desires, and capabilities. The chapters in this book have described the importance of using an inclusive conceptual model for assessing AT need. Providing a classification system that can track the provision of AT and the change in outcomes that are related to the use of AT is essential if governments and third-party payers are to be convinced of the long-term benefits of AT. Equally important is the AT provider's skill in knowing which AT to recommend, at what time during rehabilitation or development to introduce AT, and how best to train AT users to avoid injury, disuse, and abandonment. Designing, developing, manufacturing, and marketing AT requires the involvement of the consumer to ensure that the product fits the need, is accepted, and is used.

This book has delineated the importance of assistive technology for the lives of people with disabilities. AT makes it possible for people with disabilities to perform vital life functions (e.g., breathe, urinate), participate in activities of daily living (e.g., grasp, parent, work, play), and age with dignity. In short, AT plays a key role in empowering people with disabilities to live as contributing members of society. Providing support for developing new AT needs must be a national priority.

REFERENCES

Americans with Disabilities Act (ADA) of 1990, PL 101-336, 42 U.S.C. §§ 12101 *et seq.*

Curtin, T. (1997). *National Classification System for Assistive Technology Devices and Services.* Research Triangle Park, NC: Research Triangle Institute.

Institute of Medicine. (1997). *Enabling America: Assessing rehabilitation science and engineering.* Washington, DC: National Academy Press.

National Center for Medical Rehabilitation Research (NCMRR). (1993). *Research plan for the National Center for Medical Rehabilitation Research* (Publication No. 93-3509). Washington, DC: U.S. Department of Health and Human Services.

Pope, A.M., & Tarlov, A.R. (Eds.). (1991). *Disability in America: Toward a national agenda for prevention.* Washington, DC: National Academy Press.

Rehabilitation Act Amendments of 1992, PL 102-569, 29 U.S.C. §§ 701 *et seq.*

Technology-Related Assistance for Individuals with Disabilities Act of 1988, PL 100-407, 29 U.S.C. §§ 2201 *et seq.*

West, J. (1991). The social and policy context of the Act. In J. West (Ed.), *The Americans with Disabilities Act: From policy to practice* (pp. 15–18). New York: Milbank Memorial Fund.

Index

Page numbers followed by "f" and "t"
indicate figures and tables, respectively.